Primer on Transplantation

Companion website

Purchasing this book entitles you to access to the companion website:

www.astprimer.com

The website includes:
- Interactive Multiple Choice Questions for each chapter
- Figures from the book as Powerpoints for downloading
- All chapters online

How to access the website:
1. Carefully scratch away the top coating on the label on the inside front cover of the book to reveal PIN code.
2. Go to www.astprimer.com to register your PIN and access the site.

Primer on Transplantation

Edited by

Donald Hricik MD

Third edition

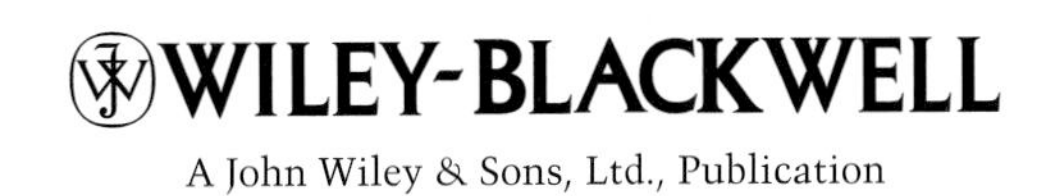

Blackwell Publishing was acquired by John Wiley & Sons in February 2007. Blackwell's publishing program has been merged with Wiley's global Scientific, Technical and Medical business to form Wiley-Blackwell.

Registered office: John Wiley & Sons Ltd, The Atrium, Southern Gate, Chichester, West Sussex, PO19 8SQ, UK

Editorial offices: 9600 Garsington Road, Oxford, OX4 2DQ, UK
The Atrium, Southern Gate, Chichester, West Sussex, PO19 8SQ, UK
111 River Street, Hoboken, NJ 07030-5774, USA

For details of our global editorial offices, for customer services and for information about how to apply for permission to reuse the copyright material in this book please see our website at www.wiley.com/wiley-blackwell

Library of Congress Cataloging-in-Publication Data

Primer on transplantation / edited by Donald Hricik.
p. cm.
Includes bibliographical references and index.
ISBN 978-1-4051-4267-0 (hardback)
1. Transplantation of organs, tissues, etc. I. Hricik, Donald E.
RD120.7.P735 2011
617.9′5–dc22

2010043300

ISBN: 9-781-4051-4267-0

A catalogue record for this book is available from the British Library.

This book is published in the following electronic formats: ePDF 9781444329780; Wiley Online Library 9781444329773; ePub 9781444329797

Set in 9 on 11.5 pt Sabon by Toppan Best-set Premedia Limited
Printed and bound in Singapore by Markono Print Media Pte Ltd

01 2011

Contents

Companion website

Purchasing this book entitles you to access to the companion website:

www.astprimer.com

The website includes:
- Interactive Multiple Choice Questions for each chapter
- Figures from the book as Powerpoints for downloading
- All chapters online

Preface

The transplantation community has witnessed a number of important anniversaries since the last edition of the Primer on Transplantation was published by the American Society of Transplantation (AST) in 2001. These have included the 50th anniversary of the first successful kidney transplant, the 25th anniversary of the AST (initially known as the American Society of Transplant Physicians), and most recently, the 10th anniversary of the American Transplant Congress. Celebrations of these anniversaries have provided opportunities to reflect upon the rapid growth of solid organ transplantation over the past five decades and the accompanying need for training transplant professionals. These professionals not only care for the growing number of solid organ transplant recipients, but also perform the research necessary to advance the field, ultimately improving patient outcomes. The AST's commitment to research and training is captured in the Society's mission statement:

> "The American Society of Transplantation is an international organization of professionals dedicated to advancing the field of transplantation and improving patient care by promoting research, education, and organ donation."

This edition of the Primer represents just one of the AST's many educational initiatives targeted to the next generation of transplant professionals. Like other endeavors of the AST, creation of this edition of the Primer was challenging because of the diverse information necessary to cover each organ-specific transplant specialty. In addition to organ-specific chapters (kidney, pancreas, heart, lung and liver), we have included generic chapters that should be of interest to all readers, irrespective of their organ-specific specialty. These include chapters on immunobiology, pharmacology, donor management, infectious complications, pediatric transplantation, and general principles of patient management. New features of this edition include clinical vignettes, "key point" boxes to emphasize major teaching points, and self-assessment multiple choice questions for each chapter. We hope that this third edition of the AST Primer on Transplantation will serve as an important reference for students, postgraduate trainees, and other transplant professionals with an interest in advancing the field of transplantation.

Donald Hricik, M.D.,
on behalf of the contributing authors

Contributors

Joshua J Augustine, MD
University Hospitals Case Medical Center and Case Western Reserve University, Cleveland, Ohio, USA

Robin K Avery, MD
Department of Infectious Disease, The Cleveland Clinic and Cleveland Clinic Lerner College of Medicine of Case Western Reserve University, USA

Joseph L Bobadilla, MD
University of Wisconsin School of Medicine and Public Health, Madison, Wisconsin, USA

Kenneth A Bodziak, MD
University Hospitals Case Medical Center and Case Western Reserve University, Cleveland, Ohio, USA

Kimberly Brown, MD
Division of Gastroenterology and Hepatology, Henry Ford Hospital, Detroit, Michigan, USA

Connie L Davis, MD
Kidney Care Line, Kidney and Pancreas Transplantation University of Washington School of Medicine, Seattle, Washington, USA

Niloo M Edwards, MD
University of Wisconsin School of Medicine and Public Health, Madison, Wisconsin, USA

Jay A Fishman, MD
Transplant Infectious Disease and Compromised Host Program, Massachusetts General Hospital and MGH Transplantation Center, Harvard Medical School, Boston, Massachusetts, USA

Gregg A Hadley, PhD
Division of Transplantation Comprehensive Transplant Center, The Ohio State University Medical Center, Columbus, Ohio, USA

William Harmon, MD
Pediatric Nephrology Department, Children's Hospital Boston and Harvard Medical School, Boston, Massachusetts, USA

Donald E Hricik, MD
University Hospitals Case Medical Center and Case Western Reserve University, Cleveland, Ohio, USA

Mary Ann Huang, MD
Division of Gastroenterology and Hepatology, Henry Ford Hospital, Detroit, Michigan, USA

Maryl R Johnson, MD
University of Wisconsin School of Medicine and Public Health, Madison, Wisconsin, USA

Walter G Kao, MD
University of Wisconsin School of Medicine and Public Health, Madison, Wisconsin, USA

Marwan Kazimi, MD
Intestinal Transplant Program, Division of Transplant Surgery, Henry Ford Hospital, Detroit, Michigan, USA

Elizabeth A Kendrick, MD
University of Washington School of Medicine, Seattle, Washington, USA

Takushi Kohmoto, MD
University of Wisconsin School of Medicine and Public Health, Madison, Wisconsin, USA

John McCartney, MD
Department of Medicine, University of Wisconsin School of Medicine and Public Health, Madison, Wisconsin, USA

Keith C Meyer, MD, MS, FACP, FCCP
Adult Cystic Fibrosis Clinic Section of Allergy, Pulmonary and Critical Care Medicine, Department of Medicine, University of Wisconsin School of Medicine and Public Health, Madison, Wisconsin, USA

Dilip Moonka, MD
Liver Transplantation, Division of Gastroenterology and Hepatology, Henry Ford Hospital, Detroit, Michigan, USA

James M Neuberger, MD
Liver Unit, Queen Elizabeth Hospital, Birmingham, UK

Aparna Padiyar, MD
University Hospitals Case Medical Center and Case Western Reserve University, Cleveland, Ohio, USA

Ian AC Rowe, MRCP
Hepatitis C Virus Research Group, University of Birmingham, and Queen Elizabeth Hospital, Birmingham, UK

James A Schulak, MD
University Hospitals Case Medical Center and Case Western Reserve University, Cleveland, Ohio, USA

Jonathan E Spahr, MD
Children's Hospital of Pittsburgh and the University of Pittsburgh School of Medicine, Pittsburgh, Pennsylvania, USA

Qiquan Sun, MD
Comprehensive Transplant Center, The Ohio State University Medical Center, Columbus, Ohio, USA

Elaine M Winkel, MD
University of Wisconsin School of Medicine and Public Health, Madison, Wisconsin, USA

Kenneth E Wood, DO
Gessinger Medical Centre, Danville, Pennsylvania, Department of Medicine, University of Wisconsin School of Medicine and Public Health, Wisconsin, and Department of Medicine, Temple University School of Medicine, Philadelphia, Pennsylvannia, USA

Jason M Zimmerer, PhD
Comprehensive Transplant Center, The Ohio State University Medical Center, Columbus, Ohio, USA

Acknowledgments

I would like to thank the present and past officers and councilors of Board of the American Society of Transplantation, for their dedication to and support for publication of this edition of the Society's Primer.

I am grateful to Susan Nelson, Elizabeth McDannell and other members of the Staff of the American Society of Transplantation, for their administrative assistance and oversight.

Donald Hricik

1 Immunology of transplantation

Qiquan Sun, Jason M Zimmerer, and Gregg A Hadley
The Ohio State University Medical Center, Columbus, Ohio, USA

The transplantation of internal organs has been feasible since the turn of the nineteenth/twentieth centuries when surgical techniques for construction of vascular anastomoses were first developed. However, the early results of organ transplantation were abysmal. In 1908, Alexis Carrel reported the results of kidney transplantation in a series of nine cats. Despite normal early graft function, all grafts ultimately failed after 1 month. The first human kidney transplantations were performed in the 1950s with similarly disappointing results. There is no technical reason why organ transplants from other individuals should not be compatible with the host's own tissues; indeed, organ transplants exchanged between genetically identical individuals are uniformly successful. Rather, it is now recognized that rejection of a graft is a manifestation of a complex immune mechanism that serves to recognize and eliminate foreign (non-self) antigens, and which evolved to protect the host against pathogens. With the availability of immunosuppressive drugs that efficiently blunt the recipient's immune system, clinical organ transplantation is now routine, and indeed is the preferred treatment for end-stage failure of the kidneys, heart, liver, and lungs. In the USA, over 25 000 such transplantations are now performed each year. However, currently available immunosuppressive drugs do not completely prevent immune injury to a graft. For all organ types, graft loss rates approach 50% after 10 years. The purpose of this chapter is to detail the immunologic basis of this important clinical problem.

All authors contributed equally to the preparation of this chapter.

Primer on Transplantation, 3rd edition.
Edited by Donald Hricik.

Terminology

Here is a list of key terms used to communicate ideas in the field of transplantation immunology:

- *Allografts:* grafts transplanted between individuals of the same species
- *Isografts:* grafts transplanted between genetically identical (*syngeneic*) individuals
- *Autografts:* grafts transplanted in the same individual, i.e., the donor is the recipient
- *Xenografts:* grafts transplanted between individuals of different species
- *Graft rejection:* immunologic destruction of transplanted tissues
- *Histocompatibility (H) antigens:* antigens that evoke graft rejection; a graft is histocompatible if all of its H antigens are expressed by the recipient (i.e., none is foreign), histoincompatible if they are not
- *First-set graft:* a first graft from a given individual or inbred strain
- *Second set graft:* a second graft of the same type from the donor of the first, or from a donor genetically identical to the first; the second set is also used to describe the accelerated rejection of a graft by a specifically sensitized recipient
- *Orthotopic:* graft placed at the normal anatomical site
- *Heterotopic:* graft placed at site distinct from the normal anatomical site.

Immunologic nature of allograft rejection

The immune system is composed of two components referred to as innate and adoptive immunity. The innate system involves cells such as macrophages and natural killer (NK) cells that constitutively express a limited set of receptors recognizing common elements of a broad range of pathogens. The innate system is capable of a rapid response. The adaptive system involves T and B cells that express a very broad range of receptors, each cell's receptor having very a narrow specificity. As the frequency of cells expressing any one receptor is low, the cells recognizing a particular antigen must replicate before they can mount an effective response. Once this expansion has occurred, however, the adaptive system is capable of a rapid memory response if the antigen is encountered a second time. Although both components of the immune system contribute to graft rejection, the adaptive system is more important in transplant-related immune responses, and therefore is the primary target of most immunosuppressive therapy.

That allograft rejection has an immunologic basis was established initially through the studies of Sir Peter Medawar. As a physician treating burn patients during World War II, Medawar noted that skin allografts were rejected in an accelerated fashion if the recipient had previously received an allograft from the same donor. He followed these observations with an elegant series of skin grafting experiments in mice and rabbits. Through these studies, Medawar conclusively demonstrated that allograft rejection encompasses both memory and specificity, the classic features of adaptive immunity.

Memory

This feature is well illustrated by the behavior of skin allografts (Table 1.1). First-set skin allografts exchanged between different mouse strains survive for approximately 10 days. During the first few days after transplantation, first set skin allografts are indistinguishable from isografts or autografts by either gross inspection or histological criteria. However, second set skin allografts transplanted onto specifically immunized hosts are rejected in approximately 3 days, and there is little or no latent period because immunity is acquired. This memory response is analogous to the primary versus secondary response to conventional antigens (e.g., measles virus), and is likely mediated by memory T cells. There is now compelling evidence that memory T cells play an important role in immune responses to transplanted organs.

Table 1.1 Behavior of skin allografts

Donor strain	Recipient strain	Treatment	Rejection
A	B	None	Slow (10 days)
A	B	Sensitized with strain A graft	Rapid (3 days); exhibits *memory*
C	B	Sensitized with strain A graft	Slow (10 days) exhibits *specificity*

Specificity

Allograft rejection is exquisitely specific. For example, accelerated rejection occurs only when the second-set graft shares mismatched H antigens with the first set graft. Moreover, the immune system easily distinguishes between histocompatible and histoincompatible grafts even when they are contiguous, e.g., a skin autograft placed on the same bed or even interspersed with an allograft is accepted despite vigorous rejection of the adjacent allograft.

Histocompatibility antigens

Historical perspective

Studies of tumor and skin grafts exchanged between inbred strains of mice led to formulation of the "laws of transplantation." These observational studies led to the recognition that H antigens are encoded by polymorphic loci (i.e., loci that differ between individuals of the same species). In addition, the expression of H antigens is co-dominant (i.e., both alleles are expressed). Subsequent studies estimate the total number of independently segregating H antigen loci at >100, although, as discussed below, some H-antigen loci are more immunogenic than others.

Key points 1.1 Laws of transplantation

Transplantations within inbred strains will succeed

Transplantations between different inbred strains will fail

Transplantations from an inbred parental strain to an F1 offspring will succeed, but those in the reverse direction will fail

Three sets of antigens play dominant roles in stimulating graft rejection: major histocompatibility complex (MHC) antigens, minor histocompatibility antigens (mHAs), and blood group antigens.

Major histocompatibility complex molecules

MHC molecules, as their name implies, are the most important antigens responsible for graft rejection. Every vertebrate species has MHC molecules. In humans, they are called HLA (human leukocyte antigens). There are two basic forms of MHC molecules: class I and class II. Class I MHC molecules are expressed on almost every type of cell whereas MHC class II molecules are expressed primarily on a subset set of cells that have "antigen-presenting" capacity, including dendritic cells, B cells, and macrophages. Class I HLA molecules are encoded by three separate genetic loci referred to as A, B, and C in humans. There are also three separate loci (called DR, DQ, and DP) that encode class II molecules. Both of the alleles inherited at all six of these loci are expressed on the cell surface, a phenomenon referred to as co-dominant expression. One of the striking features of MHC molecules is their extraordinary polymorphism. There are dozens of different alleles in the human population that can be expressed in each of the MHC loci, making MHC-encoded genes the most polymorphic loci known to humans.

The gene products of six different MHC loci can be expressed on the surface of a given cell, and two alleles are expressed per locus. Thus, an individual's MHC genotype technically should be described by a list of 12 alleles. However, the A, B, and DR loci exert a more powerful effect in transplantation than the C, DP, and DQ loci. Therefore, only HLA antigens encoded by the A, B, and DR loci are typically identified before transplantation. For example, one individual might be A2, A4, B3, B7, DR3, DR4 and another might be A18, A24, B7, B21, DR6, DR9. As there are so many different alleles in humans for each locus, the chances of two unrelated people expressing the same six HLA antigens is very small – of the order of one in a million. However, within families, the mother's and father's MHC alleles tend to be inherited as a group, called haplotypes. As a result, among siblings, a quarter are likely to share no haplotypes (no HLA antigens), a half are likely to share one of the two haplotypes (half of the HLA antigens or "haploidentical"), and a quarter are likely to share both haplotypes, in which case they will be "HLA identical" (Figure 1.1).

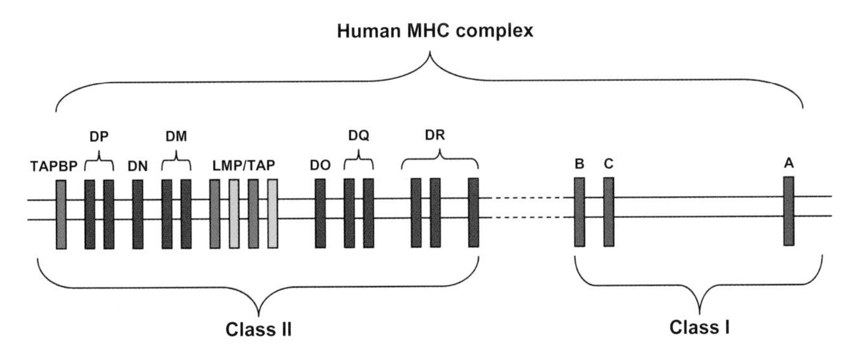

Figure 1.1 Schematic map of human MHC (major histocompatibility complex) loci. Located on chromosome 6, several polymorphic gene loci are clustered together. Note that this genetic region includes a variety of loci encoding proteins involved in antigen processing and presentation (LMP, TAP, DM) in addition to class I (A, B, C) and class II (DR, DP, DQ) MHC molecules. Sizes of genes and intermediate DNA segments are not shown to scale.

Although MHC molecules are important in causing graft rejection, and were originally discovered as a result of transplantation experiments, their intended function in the immune system has nothing to do with transplantation! The molecular structure of MHC molecules is critical to their physiologic function. All MHC alleles share in common the expression of four extracellular domains, the outer two of which are configured to form a groove or "cleft." This cleft has the capacity to carry within it short peptides of 8–22 amino acids in length. The many different MHC alleles in the human population each have clefts that are configured slightly differently, making each of them capable of carrying a different set of peptides. After HLA molecules are first constructed inside a cell they are then transported to the cell surface where they will be expressed. During this transport, the HLA molecules encounter elaborate intracellular machinery that samples all the proteins within the cell, breaking them down into peptide fragments, and loading those peptides into the clefts of the new HLA molecules if they have a suitable size and structure. Thus, when MHC molecules are expressed on the surface of a cell, they carry with them a sampling of all the proteins that exist within that cell. Most of those proteins are normal components of a healthy cell, but in some cases they may be foreign proteins picked up from the environment, produced endogenously by viruses, or resulting from malignant transformation. Thus, one of the primary functions of MHC molecules is to provide an external display of the internal cellular elements both in health and during disease (Figure 1.2). Generally, class I MHC molecules present peptides derived from cytoplasmic

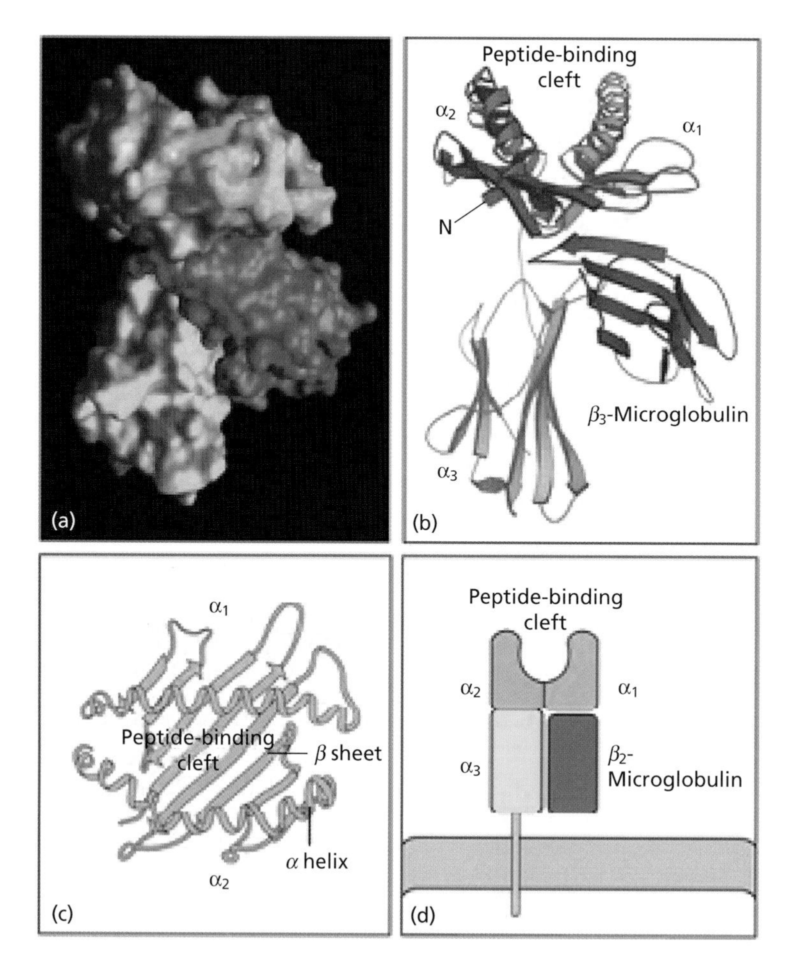

Figure 1.2 Structure of a class I MHC (major histocompatibility complex) molecule. Class I molecules are composed of a polymorphic alpha chain noncovalently bound to the nonpolymorphic β_2-microglobulin. The amino-terminal α_1- and α_2-segments of the α chain interact To to form a cleft large enough to bind peptides that are 8 to 11 amino acids in size. (Reproduced from *Immunology*, 6th edn. New York: Garland Science, 2005.)

proteins whereas all II MHC molecules present peptides derived from extracellular proteins.

Minor histocompatibility antigens
Even in situations where the transplant donor and recipient share all their MHC alleles (i.e., a perfect HLA match), other antigens, referred to as minor histocompatibility antigens (mHAs) can provoke rejection. In contrast to MHC-mismatched allografts, which are generally rejected in a matter of days, allografts exchanged between MHC-identical mouse strains that differ at a single minor H antigen may survive for weeks or months before they are rejected. These antigens are generated by allelic differences for some of the non-MHC proteins within a cell. Slight amino acid differences in a cytoplasmic protein generate peptides when that protein is broken down for display by the MHC molecules of the donor that are distinct from the set of peptides previously encountered by the recipient. These MHC/peptide complexes can therefore be recognized by host T cells that mediate rejection of the transplanted organ.

This is analogous to recognition of viral or tumor antigens, i.e., foreign peptides derived from endogenous proteins enter the class I presentation pathway. Note that recognition of minor H antigens occurs only in situations where donor and recipient are at least partially MHC matched for MHC-encoded antigens. It has been estimated that there are more than 100 loci for mHAs.

Blood group antigens
Red blood cells and vascular endothelial cells express surface glycoproteins, called blood group antigens, that can also cause transplant rejection by serving as targets of anti-donor antibodies. In humans, there are three important forms of these antigens, called blood groups O, A, and B. The blood group O glycoprotein represents a common backbone expressed by all humans. This backbone can be modified by enzymes to produce the A, B, or both (AB) determinants. As the A and B determinants are very similar to glycoprotein determinants expressed by intestinal microbes, humans who do not themselves express either A or B begin producing anti-A or anti-B antibodies relatively soon after birth. If there is a blood group incompatibility, these naturally occurring antibodies can bind to the A and B determinants on the vascular endothelium of a donor organ and cause hyperacute rejection (see below).

Key points 1.2 General course of transplantation

Recognition of mismatched histocompatibility antigens

T-cell activation and the production of cytokines; B-cell activation and production of anti-donor antibodies

Effector mechanisms: delayed-type hypersensitivity (DTH) mediated by host CD4+ T cells, cytotoxicity mediated by host CD8+ T cells, antibody-mediated injury

B cells and humoral rejection

B-cell biology

Although allograft rejection was traditionally held to be a T-cell-mediated process, it is now widely recognized that B cells play a key role in promoting destruction of transplanted tissues and organs by the production of anti-donor antibodies that bind to allografts. The antibody response to transplanted tissues and other foreign antigens is referred to as the humoral immune response. Antibodies are polypeptides with the ability to bind foreign antigens, thus tagging them for removal by the immune system. However, before B cells can secrete antibodies, they generally require interaction with other cell populations including CD4+ T cells. The antigen receptor of the B cells is membrane-bound IgM and IgD, which recognizes the native conformation of foreign antigen. When these receptors engage a foreign antigen, with the assistance of CD4+ T cells, the B lymphocyte is stimulated to differentiate into an antibody-secreting plasma cell. Plasma cells represent the final phase of B-cell differentiation and secrete antibodies with the same specificity as the original B lymphocyte. Each B-cell clone expresses a unique receptor and is present in the body at very low frequency. Consequently, B-cell clones recognizing a particular antigen must replicate before they can mount an effective response.

Antibodies

Antibodies comprise four polypeptide chains, two light chains and two heavy chains. According to differences in the heavy chains, there are five different types of antibodies, referred to as isotypes: IgM, IgG, IgA, IgD, and IgE. Once B cells are stimulated by a specific antigen, the secreted antibodies initially are of the IgM isotype, but eventually IgG antibodies are secreted, a process referred to isotype switching, which requires interaction of B cells with helper T cells. After the initial response, memory B cells are preserved and can maintain production of specific antibody for many years. IgG and IgM antibodies both can play important roles in the pathogenesis of transplant rejection.

The most important antibodies that stimulate allograft rejection are those directed to donor MHC (or, in humans, HLA) molecules. Anti-HLA antibodies can be induced by a previous transplant, pregnancy, or blood transfusion. There is increasing evidence that autoantibodies and antibodies to non-MHC proteins also take part in the humoral alloimmune response to transplanted tissues. As discussed above, antibodies to ABO incompatibilities also can trigger hyperacute rejection of organ allografts.

Mechanisms of antibody-mediated graft damage

After antibodies (IgM or IgG) bind to antigens on the allograft endothelium, they can initiate the complement cascade via the classic pathway, leading to production of the membrane attack complex (MAC) from its terminal components. The MAC can directly cause endothelial cell lysis and subsequent graft injury. In addition, chemoattractants such as C3a and C5a liberated by the complement cascade can attract inflammatory cells to the graft and mediate graft injury (Figure 1.3). C4d, a fragment of C4 produced during the classic complement activation pathway, is highly stable and persists at the cell surface well after the time at which antibody is no longer detectable. As C4d is readily detected, and correlates with the existence of donor specific anti-HLA antibodies, it is widely utilized as an *in situ* marker of antibody-mediated rejection. However, it is important to note that C4d deposition in the graft is merely a marker of rejection and that other, more labile, complement components are likely responsible for actual graft injury.

Another important effect of antibody and complement fixation to the graft vasculature is activation of graft endothelial cells. Complement components increase adhesion molecule expression by graft endothelial cells, can trigger proliferation of endothelial cells via release of growth factors and chemokines, and can induce synthesis of tissue factors that regulate the extrinsic clotting system. Thrombotic injury can dominate in severe cases, such as hyperacute rejection mediated by pre-existing anti-donor antibodies. Such injury is characterized by thrombotic microangiopathy with diffuse vascular damage and thrombosis. There is also evidence that antibodies can mediate graft damage through a complement-independent mechanism, which is thought to cause chronic graft injury. Anti-donor antibodies may also lead to destruction of target cells by a process of antibody-dependent cell-mediated cytotoxicity (ADCC).

Pathogenesis of antibody-mediated rejection

Antibody-mediated rejection (AMR) can occur in any time period after transplantation and is manifest of one of several distinct syndromes (Table 1.2), depending on the titer or the pattern of antibody. High-titer, pre-existing, donor-specific antibodies can cause hyperacute rejection, which can destroy a transplanted kidney within minutes. In hyperacute rejection, pre-existing circulating antibodies to donor MHC or blood group antigens lead to rapid binding of large quantities of antibodies to the graft vasculature, resulting in activation of the classic complement cascade and production of the MAC as described above. The MAC, in turn, stimulates endothelial activation that can become manifest within minutes to hours. This type of endothelial activation (type I) causes the cells to retract from each other, and to express procoagulant factors. As a result, leakage of blood into the interstitium produces a swollen blue organ with subsequent intravascular thrombosis. Hyperacute rejection is the most severe type of rejection after organ transplantation. There is no therapy that can reverse this process once it has started. In some cases infarction of the organ occurs before the completion of surgery.

A second form of rejection caused by antibodies is referred to as acute antibody-mediated rejection (AAMR). This clinical entity is thought to represent an important cause of early kidney transplant failure.

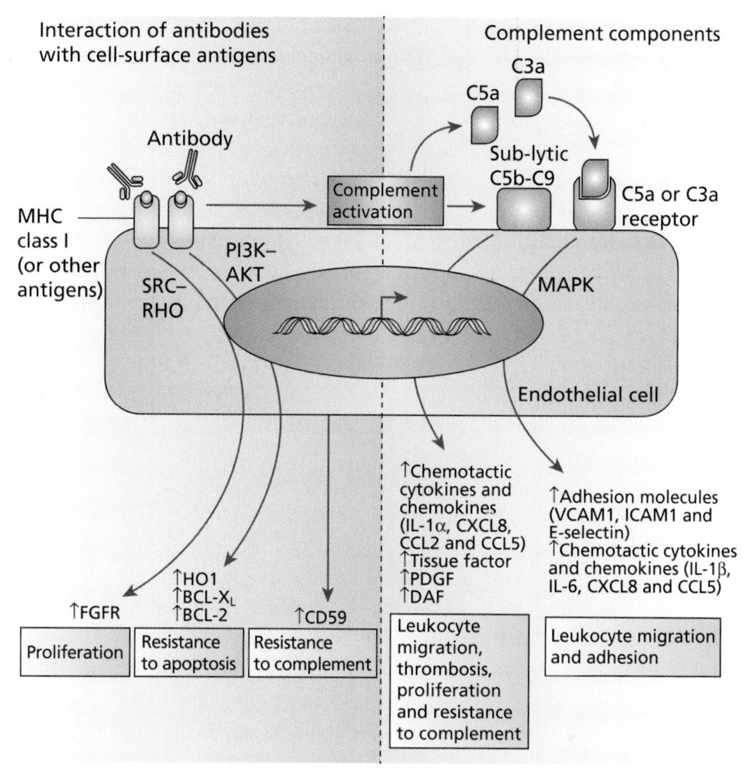

Figure 1.3 Effects of antibody and complement components on human endothelial cells. Effects mediated by the interaction of antibody with antigen at the surface of endothelial cells are shown on the left and the effects caused by complement components on the right. Target antigens may be MHC (major histocompatibility complex) class I and II molecules, ABO blood-group antigens, or other non-MHC antigens. BCL, B-cell lymphoma; CCL, CC-chemokine ligand; CXCL8, CXC-chemokine ligand 8; DAF, decay-accelerating factor; E-selectin, endothelial-cell selectin; FGFR, fibroblast growth-factor receptor; ICAM-1, intercellular adhesion molecule 1; IL, interleukin; MAPK, mitogen-activated protein kinase; PDGF, platelet-derived growth factor; PI_3K, phosphatidylinositol 3-kinase; RHO, RAS homolog; VCAM-1, vascular cell-adhesion molecule 1. (Reproduced from Colvin RB, Smith RN. Antibody mediated organ allograft rejection. *Nature Rev Immunol* 2005;5:807–17.)

Table 1.2 Clinical syndromes of antibody-mediated rejection (AMR)

Syndromes	Antibody involved	Time course	Clinical manifestations
Hyperacute rejection	Pre-existing antibodies	Immediately after reperfusion, takes minutes to hours	Immediate graft loss, cannot be treated
Acute AMR	Pre-existing or new antibodies	Any time after transplantation, takes days to weeks,	Rapid graft dysfunction, can be reversed
Chronic/late AMR	Mostly new antibodies	Months to years	Slow but progressive loss of graft function, difficult to be controlled

AAMR can occur when antibodies appear in the circulation very early after the transplantation, usually within a few days. The antibodies involved may be pre-existing antibodies present initially at very low concentrations, or antibodies produced anew after transplantation. The binding of these anti-donor antibodies over time causes a second type of endothelial activation (type II), which occurs more slowly than the type I activation responsible for hyperacute rejection. In this case, the two major consequences of the activation are generation of procoagulant factors and the appearance of fibrinoid necrosis of the vessels. The hallmark of this type of rejection is diffuse C4d staining, especially in peritubular capillaries (Figure 1.4). AAMR can sometimes be reversed by some combination of treatment with plasmapheresis, anti-CD20 monoclonal antibody (rituximab), intravenous immune globulin (IVIG) and increased pharmacologic immunosuppression.

A third syndrome induced by antibodies is chronic antibody-mediated rejection (CAMR). In this situation, antibodies develop very slowly, usually over the course of years. The pathologic picture includes myointimal hyperplasia in the vessels and progressive interstitial fibrosis, with additional features that are organ specific (Figure 1.5). In some cases of chronic rejection, anti-donor antibodies can be detected in the transplanted organ or in the circulation, suggesting a pathogenic role. However, there appear to be multiple potential etiologies for chronic rejection and determining the contribution of any one is not practical currently.

Key points 1.3 Antibody-mediated rejection

Can be mediated by antibodies to MHC molecules, ABO blood group antigens, and a variety of non-MHC molecules

Can occur at any time after transplantation

Risk factors include prior transplantation, multiple pregnancies, and a history of blood transfusions

C4d deposition in the graft peritubular capillaries correlates with the presence of circulating anti-donor antibodies and is thus a widely accepted marker of antibody-mediated rejection, but there is no evidence that C4d deposition is causally related to graft injury

Detection of antibodies

Several methods are currently employed to identify and/or monitor the development of anti-donor antibodies in clinical transplant recipients. The cross-match assay is widely used to select recipients for renal transplantation. In the cytotoxic cross-match assay, cells from the potential donor are mixed with serum from the recipient along with an exogenous source of complement. If the recipient serum contains anti-

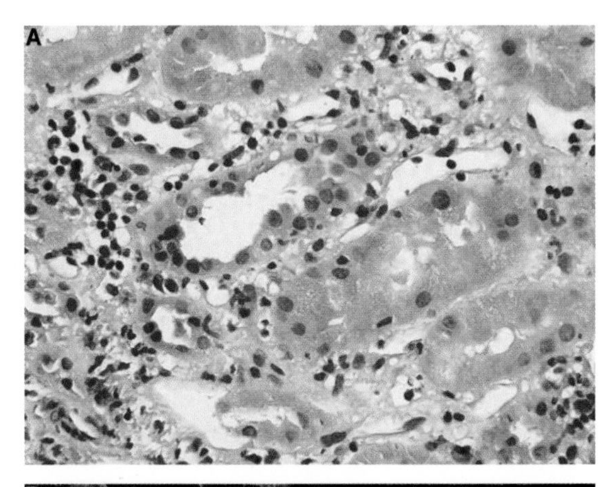

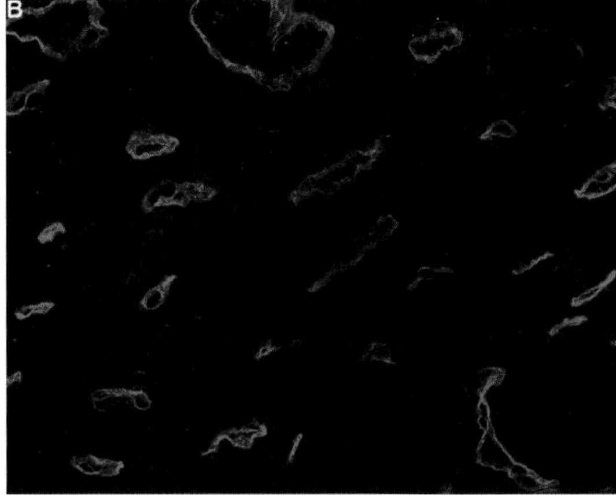

Figure 1.4 Histological features of acute humoral rejection. (a) Light microscopy shows interstitial edema, tubular injury, and infiltration of neutrophils and mononuclear cells into the peritubular capillaries (PTCs). (b) Immunofluorescence (IF) microscopy demonstrates widespread, bright, linear staining of PTCs for C4d. (From Colvin RB. Antibody-mediated renal allograft rejection: diagnosis and pathogenesis. *J Am Soc Nephrol* 2007;**18**:1046–56.)

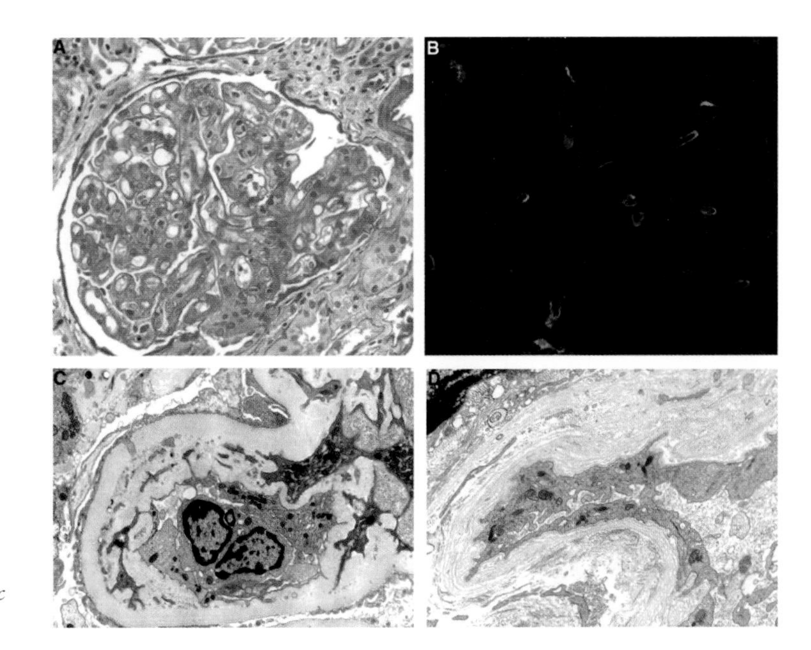

Figure 1.5 Chronic humoral rejection: (a) transplant glomerulopathy with duplication of the glomerular basement membrane (GBM) and accumulation of mononuclear cells in glomeruli (periodic acid–Schiff stain). (b) Immunofluorescence staining shows patchy distribution of C4d positivity in peritubular capillaries (PTCs). (c) Electron microscopy shows duplication of the GBM and reactive endothelial cells. (d) The PTCs have prominent multilamination of the GBM. (From Colvin RB. Antibody-mediated renal allograft rejection: diagnosis and pathogenesis. *J Am Soc Nephrol* 2007;**18**:1046–56.)

donor antibodies, these will fix the complement and lyse the donor cells. Death of the donor cells signifies a "positive cross-match," in which case organ transplantation is generally not performed because of the high risk of hyperacute rejection. The cross-match assay can also be employed to monitor development of anti-donor antibodies post-transplantation, which is important in diagnosing AMR. Increasingly, more advanced and sensitive techniques are being employed to perform the cross-match assay, such as flow cytometry using either donor cells or antigen-coated beads.

In an effort to predict the likelihood of a positive cross-match, it is common to test recipient sera against a panel of HLA antigens derived from donors expressing a broad range of the human MHC antigens. This method is called panel reactive antibody (PRA) detection. High PRA values are associated with an increased risk of acute rejection after transplantation.

Table 1.3 T-cell subsets and their role in allograft rejection

T-cell subset	Function	Role in allograft rejection
CD8+ (CD4–)	Cytotoxic T cells	Mediate direct killing activity
CD4+ (CD8–)	Orchestrate the overall immune response by facilitating the activation and differentiation of other immune cells	Mediate DTH and provide help for B cell and CD8+ T-cell responses
FoxP3+ (CD4+ or CD8–)	Inhibitor of T-cell activation/function	Instrumental in T-reg induction

T cells and T-cell-mediated rejection

Basic elements of T-cell biology

T cells are a subset of lymphocytes that play a central role in allograft rejection. The abbreviation "T," in T cell, stands for the thymus gland because it is the principal organ responsible for the development of these lymphocytes. In contrast to B cells, which accomplish their function by secreting antibodies into the circulation, T cells accomplish their function by direct cell-to-cell contact or by the secretion of soluble factors (i.e., cytokines) that regulate other cells in the local environment. T cells can be divided into subpopulations, defined primarily by their surface phenotype (Table 1.3). The most characterized subpopulations are CD4+ and CD8+ T cells.

T cells can be distinguished from other lymphocyte types, such as B cells and macrophages, by the presence of a unique receptor on their cell surface, called the T-cell receptor (TCR). Unlike B-cell receptors, which are essentially membrane-bound antibody, TCRs recognize foreign peptides only in the context of self-MHC molecules. CD4+ T cells respond to foreign peptides associated with class II MHC molecules whereas CD8+ T cells respond to foreign peptides presented by class I MHC molecules. Foreign peptides not expressed in association with MHC molecules do not induce a T-cell response.

This mechanism, in which TCRs recognize only foreign proteins when their peptides are presented by self-MHC antigens, is referred to as MHC restriction. T cells can be activated only by contact with other cells, because MHC molecules are expressed primarily on surface of cells. As a result, T cells can function only in relation to other cells, whereas B cells – through production of antibody – can respond to any foreign protein, bound or unbound to another cell.

T cells are educated to recognize foreign peptides in the context of host (self) MHC molecules in the host thymus. When pre-T cells enter the thymus, they randomly recombine TCR gene segments to generate a diverse TCR repertoire. Consequently, the vast majority of the newly generated T cells (referred to as thymocytes) are not restricted by self-MHC molecules. The first step of thymic maturation requires that the T cells express TCRs that effectively bind to self-MHC antigens expressed on the surface of that individual's thymic endothelium. A binding of adequate affinity allows for the T cell to receive survival signals. Developing thymocytes that do not have sufficient affinity for self-MHC cannot serve useful functions in the body and therefore die by apoptosis (programmed cell death) as a result of the lack of the aforementioned survival signals. This process is called positive selection. Whether a thymocyte becomes a CD4+ cell or a CD8+ cell is also determined during positive selection. Double-positive cells (CD4+/CD8+) that are positively selected on MHC class II molecules will become CD4+(CD8–) cells, and cells positively selected on MHC class I molecules will become CD8+(CD4–) cells. Thymocytes that survive positive selection are again presented with self-antigen in complex with MHC molecules on antigen-presenting cells (APCs), such as dendritic cells. Thymocytes that interact too strongly with the self-antigen receive an apoptotic signal that causes cellular death. This process is called negative selection, an important mechanism that prevents the formation of self-reactive T cells capable of generating autoimmune disease. The remaining T cells then exit the thymus as mature naïve T cells.

Key points 1.4 Important properties of T cells

- T cells have specific T-cell receptors that recognize foreign proteins
- T cells recognize foreign protein only on other cells as a MHC–peptide complex
- T cells cross-react at high frequency with MHC alloantigens

T-cell activation through APC interaction

After thymic maturation, naïve T cells migrate into the peripheral lymphoid organs where they are potentially activated in response to foreign antigens. Although the specific mechanisms of activation vary slightly between different types of T cells, the three-signal model in T cells holds true for most. The first signal is provided by binding of the TCR to a short peptide presented by the MHC on another cell. This ensures that only T cells expressing a TCR specific to that specific peptide are activated. The partner cell is usually a professional APC, generally a dendritic cell, although B cells and macrophages also can be important APCs (Table 1.4). As discussed above, CD8+ T cells recognize peptides in the context of MHC class I molecules whereas CD4+ T cells respond to peptides associated with MHC class II molecules.

The second signal comes from co-stimulation, in which surface receptors on the APC are induced and bind to co-stimulatory receptors expressed by naïve T cells. Co-stimulation involves reciprocal and sequential signals between cells. Low constitutive levels of B7.1 and/or B7.2 on the APC activate CD28 on the T cell, inducing upregulation of CD40L on the T cell. CD40L in turn binds to CD40 on the APC, enhancing B7.1/B7.2 expression and reinforcing the CD28/CD40-positive feedback loop. Other co-stimulatory and inhibitory molecules regulated by the initial co-stimulatory signals can further shape the specific outcome of the interaction. The second signal

Table 1.4 Types of antigen-presenting cells

Type	Unique characteristic
Dendritic cell	Constitutively express MHC class I and class II molecules as well as co-stimulatory ligands for optimal activation of host CD4+ and CD8+ T cells
B cell	Can concentrate and present antigen, to which the clonotypic B-cell receptor (surface antibody) is directed, to host CD4+ T cells
Macrophage	Phagocytose cellular debris and present resulting peptides in association with self-MHC class II molecules to host CD4+ T cells

MHC, major histocompatibility complex.

licenses the T cell to respond to an antigen. Without it, the T cell becomes anergic and reactivation in the future becomes more difficult. This mechanism prevents inappropriate responses to self, because self-peptides will not usually be presented with suitable co-stimulation.

The third signal follows the interactions of the T cell with MHC/peptide and co-stimulatory molecules, and involves a cascade of biochemical events in the T cell that subsequently results in the expansion and differentiation of the specific T cell clone. This occurs primarily through an increase in interleukin IL-2 secretion by the T cell and an increase in the density of IL-2 receptors on the T-cell surface. IL-2 is a potent T-cell growth cytokine that acts in an autocrine fashion to promote the growth, proliferation, and differentiation of the T cell recently stimulated by antigen (Figure 1.6).

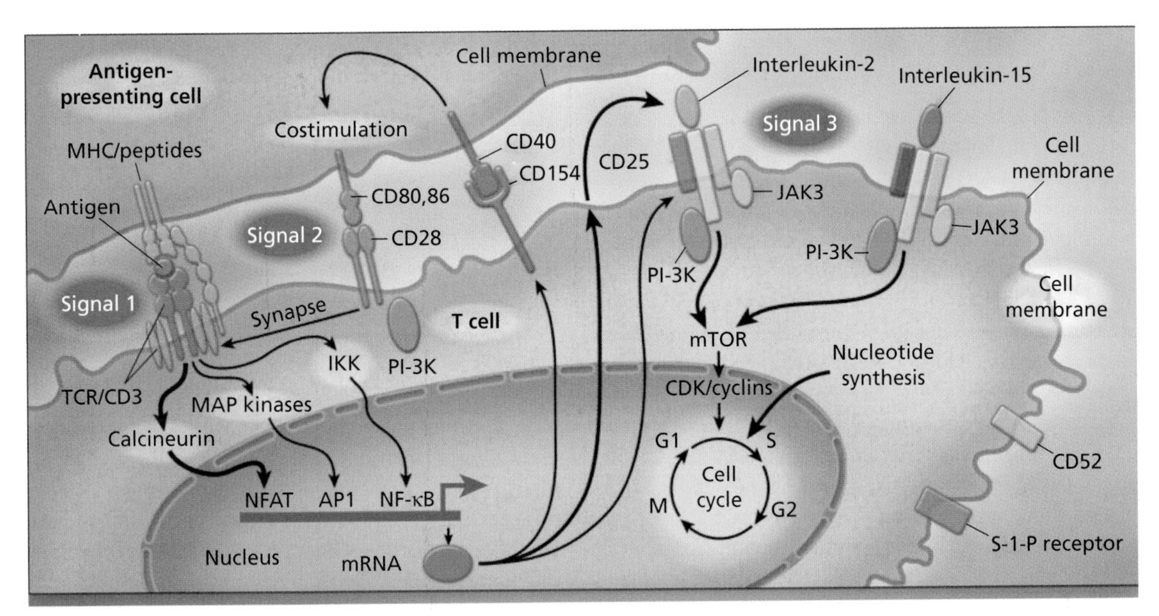

Figure 1.6 Three-signal model of T-cell activation: antigen-presenting cells (APCs) of host or donor origin migrate to T-cell areas of secondary lymphoid organs. These T cells ordinarily circulate between lymphoid tissues where APCs present donor antigen to naive T cells. Antigen triggers T-cell receptor (TCR) signaling (signal 1) and synapse formation. (See https://content.nejm.org/cgi/content/full/351/26/2715–R5#R5.) CD80 (B7–1) and CD86 (B7–2) on the APCs engage CD28 on the T cells to provide signal 2. These signals activate various signal-transduction pathways that activate transcription factors. The result is expression of CD154 (which further activates APCs), interleukin-2 receptor α chain (CD25), and interleukin-2 (IL-2). IL-2 and IL-15 deliver growth signals (signal 3) that initiate the cell cycle. T cells, then, are fully activated and undergo clonal expansion and differentiation to mature T effector cells. (From Halloran PF. Immunosuppressive drugs for kidney transplantation. *N Engl J Med* 2004;351:2715–29.)

Key points 1.5 T cells require multiple signals to mature into effector T cells

Signal 1 is recognition of the APC's MHC–peptide complex by the T-cell receptor

Signal 2 is binding of the T cell to co-stimulatory ligands expressed on APCs

Signal 3 is cytokine signaling that promotes T-cell expansion and differentiation

Direct and indirect allogeneic antigen presentation in transplantation

T-cell recognition of mismatched MHC alleles is a key event in the pathogenesis of allograft rejection. Allogeneic MHC molecules are presented for recognition by host T cells in two fundamentally different ways. The first, called *direct* presentation, involves the recognition of an intact MHC molecule displayed by the donor and is a consequence of the similarity in structure of an intact foreign MHC molecule and self-MHC molecules. As many as 2% of an individual's T cells are capable of directly recognizing and responding to a single foreign MHC molecule, and this high frequency of T cells reactive with allogeneic MHC molecules is one reason that allografts elicit strong immune responses.

The second pathway of T-cell allorecognition, called *indirect* presentation, involves processing of donor MHC molecules by recipient APCs and presentation of peptides derived from allogeneic MHC molecules in association with self-MHC molecules. CD8+ T cells that are generated by the indirect pathway are self-MHC restricted and therefore cannot directly kill the foreign cells in the graft, so when alloreactive T cells are stimulated by the indirect pathway, the principal mechanism of rejection is thought to be mediated by CD4+ T cells recognizing donor alloantigens, thus stimulating other immune cells (Figure 1.7).

Effector mechanisms of T-cell-mediated graft injury

After activation and proliferation, T cells exit the draining lymphoid compartments and circulate through the body to eliminate cells expressing the specific antigen. Once activated T cells come in contact with the mismatched H antigen, the mechanisms of graft destruction depend on the type of T cell responding. CD4+ T cells initiate an indirect response by helping other immune cells, especially B cells and CD8+ T cells, to respond more efficiently to the graft. One important function of CD4+ T cells is to promote the maturation of B cells, which produce anti-donor antibodies. Such responses require the activation of B cells by helper T cells that respond to the same molecule. This is called linked recognition. This means that, before B cells can be induced to

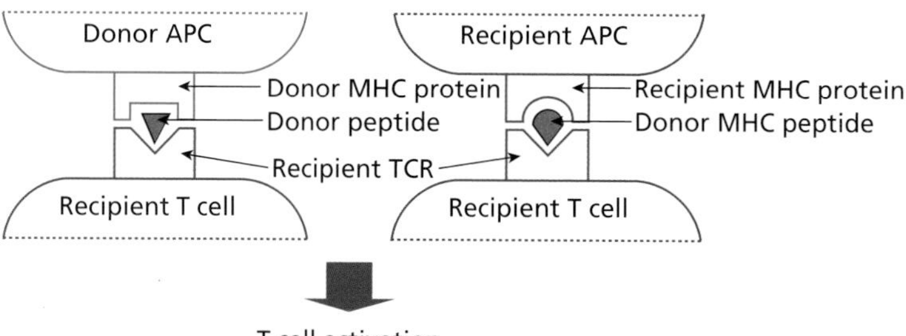

Figure 1.7 Direct and indirect pathways of T-cell allorecognition: direct and indirect pathways of T-cell allorecognition are mediated by different antigen-presenting cells (APCs). Direct antigen presentation involves recognition of intact donor MHC (major histocompatibility complex) molecules by host T cells. Indirect antigen presentation involves recognition of processed donor MHC antigen presented in association with self-MHC molecules by host APCs. Both pathways are important mechanisms of allograft rejection. It is thought that the direct pathway is responsible for T-cell-mediated rejection and that the indirect pathway is responsible for humoral rejection. TCR, T-cell receptor.

Table 1.5 Cytokines in transplantation

Cytokine	Function in transplantation
IL-2	Clonal expansion of activated T cells
IL-4	Induces B cells to produce antibody
IL-12	Enhances cytotoxic activity of activated CD8+ T cells
IFN-γ	Upregulates MHC expression on target cells, activates APCs

IFN, interferon; IL, interleukin; MHC, major histocompatibility complex.

make antibody to a foreign protein, a CD4+ T cell specific for peptides from this pathogen must first be activated to produce the appropriate activated helper T cells. Although the epitope recognized by the activated helper T cell must therefore be linked to the same molecule recognized by the B cell, the two cells need not recognize identical epitopes. CD4+ T cells also provide help to promote CD8+ T-cell responses, and can induce delayed-type hypersensitivity (DTH) responses that can damage the graft. DTH is caused via stimulation of lymphocytes and macrophages, resulting in chronic inflammation and cytokine release (Table 1.5). T cells play an important role in this hypersensitivity, because they activate against the stimulus itself and promote the activation of other cells at the graft site, particularly macrophages.

In contrast, CD8+ T cells can respond directly to cells expressing mismatched H antigens, albeit with help provided by CD4+ T cells. When exposed to a foreign antigen-expressing cells, cytotoxic CD8+ T cells (CTLs) release cytotoxins such as perforin and granzymes that induce target cell apoptosis. Perforin serves to form pores in the target cell's plasma membrane either by directly inducing target cell necrosis or by allowing granzymes to enter the cell, thereby inducing apoptosis by activation of cellular enzymes called caspases. A second way that CD8+ T cells induce apoptosis of donor cells is via cell-surface interactions between the CTL and the antigen-expressing cell. For example, activated CD8+ T cells express the surface protein Fas ligand (FasL), which can bind to Fas molecules expressed on the target cell and thereby induce target cell apoptosis.

In clinical organ transplantation, pharmacologic immunosuppression is imperative to protect the graft from the anti-donor immune response. Indeed, a daily and life-long regimen of immunosuppressive drugs is required to prevent clinical organ allograft rejection. A variety of immunosuppressive drugs is regularly used to inhibit T-cell responses including corticosteroids, antimetabolites, antibodies, drugs acting on immunophilins, among other therapies (Table 1.6). Corticosteroids act by inhibiting transcription factors such as nuclear factor-κB (NF-κB), thus markedly inhibiting genes that code for the cytokines ranging from IL-1 through IL-8 and tumor necrosis factor (TNF)-α, some of which are indispensable for T-cell expansion. Antimetabolites such as azathioprine and mycophenolate mofetil function to inhibit lymphocyte proliferation. Azathioprine was formerly a mainstay of transplant immunosuppression but is increasingly being supplanted by mycophenolate mofetil. Corticosteroids and antimetabolites inhibit downstream T-cell responses by preventing the clonal expansion of lymphocytes in the induction phase of the immune response. In addition, polyclonal antibody treatments such as antithymocyte globulin are widely used to further suppress anti-donor immunity.

Alternatively, monoclonal antibodies (mAbs) can be used to block specific pathways, such as an mAb to the IL-2 receptor which is thought to inhibit T-cell expansion. Finally, drugs such as cyclosporine and tacrolimus act to inhibit calcineurin. Calcineurin inhibitors specifically inhibit IL-2 transcription by host T cells, again leading to reduced T-cell function. It is important to note, however, that all such immunosuppressive drugs have serious side effects, and leave the patient vulnerable to opportunistic infection and malignancy. Consequently, the development of more specific strategies to inhibit the anti-graft immune response remains the Holy Grail in the field of transplantation immunology.

Mechanisms of self-tolerance

Since the pioneering studies of Medawar demonstrating that specific tolerance to allogeneic skin grafts could be produced in mice by *in utero* injection of donor hemopoietic cells, the induction of donor-specific unresponsiveness in transplant recipients has been a major goal of modern transplantation immunology. Immunologic tolerance is defined as

Table 1.6 Commonly used immunosuppressant drug classes used in clinical transplantation and their mechanisms

Immunosuppressant	Mechanisms
Corticosteroids	This general class of immunosuppressants inhibits transcription factors such as nuclear factor-κB (NF-κB) activation, thus markedly decreasing cytokine secretion, and thereby inhibiting immune responses in general
Azathioprine	Antimetabolite; inhibits purine synthesis by converting 6-mercaptopurine to tissue inhibitor of metalloproteinase and thereby prevents proliferation of lymphocytes
Mycophenolate mofetil	Antimetabolite; blocks purine synthesis by inhibiting synthesis of guanosine monophosphate nucleotides, and thereby prevents proliferation of lymphocytes
Cyclosporine	Calcineurin inhibitor; binds to cyclophilin, and thereby inhibits calcineurin phosphatase and T-cell activation
Tacrolimus	Calcineurin inhibitor; binds to FKBP12, and thereby inhibits calcineurin phosphatase and T-cell activation
Sirolimus	Binds to FKBP12; inhibits target of rapamycin, and thereby inhibits IL-2-driven T-cell proliferation
Basiliximab	Anti-CD25 monoclonal antibody; binds to CD25 antigen (IL-2R) expressed on activated T cells, leading to T-cell depletion and inhibition of IL-2-induced T-cell activation
Rituximab	Anti-CD20 monoclonal antibody; binds to CD20 expressed on B cells and thereby mediates B-cell depletion
Muromonab-CD3	Anti-CD3 monoclonal antibody; binds to CD3 expressed on T cells, and thereby blocks T-cell function and/or induces T-cell depletion

IL, interleukin; IL-SR, interleukin-2 receptor.

unresponsiveness to an antigen that is induced by a previous exposure to that antigen. When specific lymphocytes encounter antigens, the lymphocytes may be activated, leading to an immune response, or the cells may be inactivated or eliminated leading to tolerance. There are several mechanisms of tolerance (Table 1.7).

One mode of tolerance induction is *central* tolerance, also known as negative selection. As described above, immature T cells that recognize antigens with high avidity within the thymus are deleted. The two main factors that determine whether a particular self-antigen will induce negative selection of self-reactive thymocytes are the concentration of that antigen and the affinity of the TCRs that recognize the antigen. T-cell recognition of an antigen that is abundantly expressed in the thymus and has a strong association with TCRs will result in apoptosis of the attached T cell. Studies in mouse models indicate that adoptive transfer of donor bone marrow to recipients condi-

Table 1.7 Strategies for tolerance induction

Type of tolerance	Current strategies
Central tolerance	Introduction of donor APCs into the recipient thymus; induction of mixed hemopoietic chimerism
Peripheral tolerance	Administration of drugs that block T-cell co-stimulatory pathways; donor-specific blood transfusions to trigger antigen-induced cell death of alloreactive T cells; induction of regulatory T cells to counter the anti-donor immune response

APC, antigen-presenting cell.

tioned by irradiation or immunotherapy harnesses the phenomenon of negative selection to eliminate donor-reactive T cells by central deletion, after interaction with donor APCs that have accessed the recipient's thymus.

Another mode of tolerance is *peripheral* tolerance. Peripheral tolerance is the mechanism by which mature T cells that recognize self-antigens in peripheral tissues become incapable of subsequent response to the antigen. This mechanism is responsible for T-cell tolerance to self-antigens that are not abundant in the thymus. The same mechanisms may induce unresponsiveness to foreign antigens. Peripheral tolerance is due to anergy, deletion, or suppression of T cells. If T cells recognize peptide antigens presented by APCs in the absence of co-stimulatory molecules, the T cells survive but are rendered anergic, or incapable of responding to the antigen even if it is later presented by competent APCs. Repeated stimulation of T lymphocytes, by persistent antigen, results in the death of activated cells by apoptosis. This form of regulation is called activation-induced cell death. Many current immunotherapies are thought to promote peripheral tolerance to the donor either by blocking the transduction of co-stimulatory signals at the cell surface molecules or via the downstream intracellular signaling events.

Peripheral tolerance can also be mediated through regulatory T cells. Regulatory T cells are a specialized subpopulation of T cells that act to suppress activation of the immune system and thereby maintain immune homeostasis and tolerance to self-antigens. Regulatory T cells actively suppress activation of the immune system and prevent self-reactivity. Interest in regulatory T cells has been heightened by evidence from experimental mouse models demonstrating that the immunosuppressive potential of these cells can be harnessed therapeutically to treat autoimmune disease and facilitate transplantation tolerance.

It is increasingly clear that the immune response that distinguishes self from non-self is regulated at multiple levels. Although it is clear that all individuals have the genetic potential to mount anti-self immune responses at both the T- and B-cell levels, regulatory mechanisms usually prevent such autoreactivity, leading to self-tolerance. It is therefore logical that most methods for inducing tolerance to allogeneic transplants in some way make use of mechanisms that are utilized normally to prevent autoreactivity. A better understanding of the regulation of normal immune responses is thus crucial to understanding the mechanisms for induction of non-responsiveness to transplanted tissues and organs.

Xenotransplantation

An urgent problem in clinical organ transplantation is the shortage of donor organs. This shortage is only expected to worsen in the future, despite improvements in immunosuppressive therapies and/or advances in inducing donor-specific tolerance. A potential solution to this problem is the use of animals as the source of donor organs. Unfortunately, the current barriers to xenotransplantation are formidable. The main barriers to clinical xenotransplantation are summarized in Table 1.8. For one, humans produce natural antibodies to most species that cause hyperacute rejection of xenografts in minutes to hours. The dominant antibodies mediating hyperacute xenograft rejection are directed against a single carbohydrate epitope, Galα1–3-Galβ1–4GlcNAc-R epitope (αGal). The dominant antibody response to

Table 1.8 Main barriers to clinical xenotransplantation

Barrier	Pathogenesis/reasons
Hyperacute rejection	Caused by natural antibodies directed to the αGal carbohydrate moiety; antibody binding to the αGal expressed on the xenograft endothelium results in type I endothelial activation and hyperacute rejection of the xenograft
Acute humoral xenograft rejection	Caused by αGal via type II endothelial activation, may occur within 24 hours after the transplantation, and can lead to xenograft failure within days or weeks
Cellular mechanisms of xenograft rejection	CD4+ T-cell response via the indirect pathway, innate immune responses
Ethical concerns	Mainly focused on the risk of transmission of severe infectious agents from animal to humans

αGal occurs because humans and other Old World primates lack the enzyme (α1–3-galactosyltransferase) that produces the αGal moiety whereas all other vertebrates possess this enzyme. Once αGal-specific antibodies bind to the endothelium of the xenografts they trigger activation and/or necrosis of the graft endothelium, leading to hyperacute rejection of the xenograft. In humans, up to 75% of natural IgM present in normal human serum binds to αGal, with approximately1% of all B cells spontaneously producing anti-αGal antibodies. Thus, anti-αGal antibodies are a major barrier to clinical xenotransplantation. Strategies that remove anti-αGal antibodies and reduce complement activity effectively prevent hyperacute xenograft rejection in experimental models, so there is hope that these problems can be overcome in the future.

The indirect pathway for activation of host CD4+ T cells directed to processed xenoantigens is also very strong. The extent to which direct recognition of xenogeneic MHC antigens occurs is poorly defined. Xenografts also stimulate the innate immune response of the recipient; natural killer (NK) cells, macrophages, and neutrophils can be activated, leading to lysis and/or phagocytosis of xenogeneic cells and eventual graft loss.

One of the great promises of xenotransplantation is the potential to alter the animal donors genetically so that the tissues elicit weaker immune responses and/or are resistant to immune attack. There is hope in the transplant community that transgenic herds of pigs can be developed for use as organ transplant donors, though the feasibility of this goal remains to be determined, e.g., scientists have developed genetically engineered pigs with targeted disruption of the αGal gene. Survival of xenografts from such donors is significantly prolonged in non-human primates. Although such grafts are still subject to rejection, it is expected that these problems may be solved by further gene modification.

Tolerance induction is another potential strategy to overcome the barriers to xenotransplantation: several such strategies are in development in animal models, such as blocking of co-stimulatory signals, donor-specific transfusions, co-transplantation of the donor thymus, and induction of mixed chimerism. However, the utility of such approaches in the human system remains to be established. An additional factor that may limit xenotransplantation is public concern (both real and imagined) that new infectious agents, especially endogenous viruses, may be transmitted from the source animal into the human population.

Bone marrow transplantation

This chapter focused on the immunology of organ transplantation. However, it is important to note that bone marrow transplantations (BMTs) are essentially stem cell transplants that differ from organ transplants in several key respects. For one, BMTs require complete ablation of the recipient's immune system to create "space" and to prevent graft rejection because marrow grafts are much more susceptible to rejection than organ grafts, with the innate arm of the immune system playing a critical role in rejection of bone marrow grafts. For another, graft-versus-host disease (GVHD) directed to minor H antigens – and not graft rejection – is currently the major limitation to broader application of BMTs to treat malignancy and genetic disorders. GVHD occurs when an immunologically competent graft is transplanted into an immunologically compromised host; mature donor T cells present within the marrow inoculum respond to the mismatched histocompatibility antigens (usually mHAs) and subsequently attack the host. The primary sites of attack are the skin, liver, and gut, leading to symptoms such as skin lesions, diarrhea, and wasting, respectively, with the potential for death. Thus, GVHD following BMT is essentially the reverse of organ allograft rejection; consequently, the treatment options are fundamentally similar to those used in organ transplantation.

Further reading

Abbas AK, Lichtman AH. *Cellular and Molecular Immunology*, 5th edn. Philadelphia, PA: Saunders, 2003.

Collins AB, Schneeberger EE, Pascual MA, et al. Complement activation in acute humoral renal allograft rejection: Diagnostic significance of C4d deposits in peritubular capillaries. *J Am Soc Nephrol* 1999;**10**:2208–14.

Colvin RB, Smith RN. Antibody mediated organ allograft rejection. *Nature Rev Immunol* 2005;5:807–17.

Cooper DK, Dorling A, Pierson RN, et al. α1,3-Galactosyltransferase gene-knockout pigs for xenotransplantation: Where do we go from here? *Transplantation* 2007;**84**:1–7.

Davila E, Byrne GW, Labreche PT, et al. T cell responses during pig-to-primate xenotransplantation. *Xenotransplantation* 2006;**13**:31–40.

Davis MC, Distelhorst CW. Live free or die: an immature T cell decision encoded in distinct. Bcl-2. sensitive and insensitive Ca^{2+} signals. *Cell Cycle* 2006;**5**:1171–4.

Hadley GA. Role of the integrin, CD103, in destruction of renal allografts by CD8+ T cells. *Am J Transpl* 2004; **4**:1026–32.

Halloran PF. Immunosuppressive drugs for kidney transplantation. *N Engl J Med* 2004;**351**:2715–29.

Janeway CA, Travers P, Walport M, Shlomchik M. *Immunobiology*, 5th edn. New York: Garland Publishing, 2001.

Jiang H, Chess L. An integrated view of suppressor T cell subsets in immunoregulation. *J Clin Invest* 2004;**114**: 1198–208.

Krensky AM, Weiss A, Crabtree G, at al. Mechanisms of disease: T lymphocyte-antigen interactions in transplant rejection. *N Engl J Med* 1990;**322**:510–7.

Kuwaki K, Tseng YL, Dor FJ, et al. Heart transplantation in baboons using α1,3-galactosyltransferase gene-knockout pigs as donors: Initial experience. *Nat Med* 2005;**11**:29.

Mauiyyedi S, Pelle PD, Saidman S, et al. Chronic humoral rejection: identification of antibody-mediated chronic renal allograft rejection by C4d deposits in peritubular capillaries. *J Am Soc Nephrol* 2001;**12**:574–82.

Najafian N, Albin MJ, Newell KA. How can we measure immunologic tolerance in humans? *J Am Soc Nephrol* 2006;**17**:2652–63.

Racusen LC, Colvin RB, Solez K, et al. Antibody-mediated rejection criteria: An addition to the Banff 97 classification of renal allograft rejection. *Am J Transplant* 2003;**3**: 708–14.

Romagnani S. Regulation of the T cell response. *Clin Exp Allergy* 2006;**36**:1357–66.

Sayegh MH, Carpenter CB. Transplantation 50 years later – progress, challenges, and promises. *N Engl J Med* 2004;**351**:2761–6.

Schwarz BA, Bhandoola A. Trafficking from the bone marrow to the thymus: a prerequisite for thymopoiesis. *Immunol Rev* 2006;**209**:47–57.

Takemoto SK, Zeevi A, Feng S, et al. National conference to assess antibody-mediated rejection in solid organ transplantation. *Am J Transplant* 2004;**4**:1033–41.

Terasaki P, Humoral theory of transplantation. *Am J Transpl* 2003;**3**:665–73.

Tinckam KJ, Chandraker A. Mechanisms and role of HLA and non-HLA alloantibodies. *Clin J Am Soc Nephrol* 2006;**1**:404–14.

Yang YG, Sykes M. Xenotransplantation: current status and a perspective on the future. *Nature Rev Immunol* 2007; **7**:519–31.

2 Pharmacology of transplantation

Ian AC Rowe[1,2] *and James M Neuberger*[2]
[1]University of Birmingham, Birmingham, UK
[2]Queen Elizabeth Hospital, Birmingham, UK

Over the last three decades, there have been major developments in the drugs available for optimal management of the allograft recipient. Regimens for immunosuppression will vary for different organs and within different transplant units. Suggested regimens are described in the organ-specific chapters. Here, the pharmacology of the currently available immunosuppressive agents, and some agents in various stages of development, are discussed. Transplant recipients are often treated with many other drugs, including antiviral, antifungal, and antibacterial drugs used as prophylaxis or as treatment for various infections. Other drug classes commonly administered to transplant recipients include antihypertensives, lipid-lowering drugs, and a variety of medications used to prevent or treat post-transplant osteopenia. These latter drug categories fall out of the scope of this chapter and are covered in other chapters.

It is axiomatic that all drugs are potentially toxic but some have a beneficial effect and those benefits must be balanced against side effects. Most of the therapeutic agents used for immunosuppression are relatively non-specific in their action on the immune system. Side effects of these agents can be considered either as drug or as class specific (such as calcineurin inhibitor [CNI]-related nephrotoxicity) or integral to immunosuppression (such as increased susceptibility to infection and some cancers).

Primer on Transplantation, 3rd edition.
Edited by Donald Hricik.

Drug metabolism in organ failure

Disease of some organs, notably the liver and kidney, may affect both the pharmacokinetics (the relationship between the dose of a drug and changes in concentration over time) and the pharmacodynamics (the relationship between the drug concentration in the blood and the clinical response). The term 'pharmacokinetics' encompasses a number of pharmacologic phenomena including bioavailability, absorption, volume of distribution, clearance, and drug elimination. Each of these parameters may be abnormal in the presence of liver or kidney disease. It is therefore important for the clinician to have some understanding of the potential problems that may arise when prescribing drugs for patients with organ dysfunction. In this chapter, it is not possible to give any more than a superficial account of some of the factors that are of potential importance so the clinician will need to seek specific information in individual cases.

Liver disease

Although the standard liver tests are often referred to as 'liver function tests,' this is a misnomer because the analytes do not accurately reflect liver function nor are they always specific to the liver. Several tests of liver function have been developed and validated (such as the aminopyrine or caffeine clearance tests) but these are rarely used in clinical practice, will reflect only some aspects of liver function, and may not give any useful information about appropriate prescription of drugs in patients with liver impairment. The best, but still not robust, guide to drug handling is probably the serum albumin.

The presence of liver disease may alter the response to drugs by one or more of several different mechanisms.

Absorption
Absorption of some drugs, especially those that are fat soluble, may be affected by the relative lack of excreted bile, or by the co-administration of agents (e.g., cholestyramine) that reduce absorption.

First-pass effect
Cirrhosis itself and intrahepatic stents (e.g., transjugular intrahepatic portosystemic shunts) may be associated with intrahepatic shunting of blood flow. In the presence of such shunts, drugs that are subject to significant first-pass metabolism will exhibit a significantly different profile which may make the patient more susceptible to the drug's effects.

Clearance
Hepatic drug clearance is related to both blood flow and extraction. Blood flow to the liver from the portal vein and hepatic artery may be abnormal in some liver diseases and post-transplantation situations, thus affecting drug clearance

Metabolism
Drug metabolism is potentially affected by liver disease. Distinction must be made between hepatocellular disease (e.g., alcoholic liver disease, viral hepatitis, or acute allograft rejection) and biliary disease (e.g., primary biliary cirrhosis, primary sclerosing cholangitis, or chronic allograft rejection). Most drugs undergo metabolism within the hepatocyte and so will be affected by a variety of factors, including the patient's age, total hepatic mass, and the constituent drug-metabolizing enzymes. The activity of these enzymes may be affected by many factors including concomitant administration of other drugs that may act either as enzyme inducers or inhibitors, or that may compete for metabolic pathways. Drugs may be metabolized to the active agent and/or may be detoxified. Activities of the cytochromes (the major drug metabolizing enzymes) tend to vary during the first 6 months after liver transplantation

Distribution
The presence of ascites and peripheral edema may alter the volume of distribution of a drug. The concentrations of proteins that bind drugs and changes in acid–base balance are affected in liver disease. All of these factors may affect the drug pharmacokinetics and pharmacodynamics, e.g., drugs that are highly protein bound (such as prednisolone and phenytoin) may be more active in patients with low protein concentrations. Understanding the extent of protein binding is important because, for any total plasma concentration of drug, the amount of free (and therefore therapeutically effective) drug will vary with the protein concentration.

Excretion
For drugs that are excreted in the bile, biliary outflow obstruction (whether at the level of the cholangiocyte or the bile duct) may affect elimination, leading to retention of the parent drug and/or its metabolites. Some metabolites may themselves have a therapeutic effect and may or may not be measured in standard assays. For drugs that undergo enterohepatic recirculation, alterations in bile excretion may influence the drug's effects.

End-organ sensitivity
Liver disease may affect end-organ sensitivity, e.g., patients with advanced liver disease may be more likely to develop renal failure when given non-steroidal anti-inflammatory drugs. Those with advanced liver disease are more prone to cerebral depression and encephalopathy when given opiates for analgesia. In some cases, the presence of liver disease itself may be a risk factor for drug toxicity, e.g., methotrexate tends to be more hepatotoxic in the presence of steatosis and steatohepatitis. Of interest, viral infection may affect drug metabolism. It is now clear that tacrolimus levels will be affected when there is evidence of hepatitis C viral replication. The mechanism is not clear but the dose of CNI may need to be altered when the virus reactivates.

Drug hepatotoxicity

Drug hepatotoxicity can be categorized as either type I or II. Type I is predictable and dose related and the classic example is acetaminophen toxicity. When the normal detoxification mechanisms are overwhelmed by the amount of drug to be metabolized, there is retention of a toxic intermediate that binds to cellular macromolecules and causes liver cell necrosis. The level at which toxicity occurs depends on many factors such as the amount of glutathione present (reduced in those with significant liver disease or malnutrition) and the rate at which the toxic metabolites are generated. The latter rate is increased in patients receiving concomitant enzyme inducers (e.g., phenobarbital or alcohol) and decreased when there is concomitant enzyme inhibition (e.g., by cimetidine).

Type II drug toxicity is unpredictable and may be due to idiosyncrasies in drug metabolism (type IIa) or the involvement of immune mechanisms (type IIb). In some transplant recipients, the patient may acquire the idiosyncratic drug responses of the donor, as has been well documented for peanut allergy. It must be stressed that there are no specific tests for adverse drug reactions and the diagnosis is one of exclusion.

Virtually every pattern of hepatic disease can be mimicked by drugs and some drugs may be associated with more than one type of liver damage, e.g., estrogens can be associated with cholestasis, peliosis, vascular thrombosis, adenoma, and even hepatocellular cancer. Azathioprine can be associated with focal nodular hyperplasia and/or hepatitis. If an adverse drug reaction is suspected, the drug should be withdrawn.

Kidney disease

As with liver disease, the presence and extent of kidney damage or reduced kidney function may affect the pharmacology of drugs by a number of mechanisms.

Metabolism

The kidney can metabolize some drugs, but this is rarely of clinical importance. In patients with impaired kidney function, alterations in drug pharmacokinetics and pharmacodynamics may occur as the result of altered acid–base homeostasis and/or with changes in the volume of distribution and concentrations of some drug-binding proteins (e.g., albumin).

Excretion

Impaired kidney function may be associated with reduced excretion of either active or inactive drug or metabolites. These may be pharmacologically significant or give misleading values in some therapeutic drug assays.

Sensitivity

The effects of some drugs may be increased in patients with impaired kidney function, even if metabolism is not affected.

Thus, the significance of impaired kidney function on the pharmacology of drugs will vary according to the extent and type of renal damage, the extent to which the drug is excreted by the kidney, and the therapeutic index (a marker of the ratio of safety to toxicity). The dose or the frequency of dosing for many drugs must be modified in patients with impaired kidney function.

The degree of renal impairment is best assessed by some estimate of glomerular filtration rate (GFR) because serum urea and creatinine concentrations are affected by non-renal factors such as the bulk of muscle mass or the presence of blood in the bowel. Most drug-dosing guidelines are based on the use of timed creatinine clearances to estimate the GFR. However, timed collections are notoriously inaccurate or incomplete. For this reason, many clinicians prefer surrogate estimations using calculations such as the Cockcroft–Gault or MDRD (modification of diet in renal disease) formulae. Neither is ideal nor a very accurate measure of renal function, but they are usually adequate for clinical use. Mild renal impairment is defined as a GFR between 20 and 50 mL/min, moderate impairment as between 10 and 20 mL/min, and severe impairment as <10 mL/min.

Pregnancy

As transplantation has become an established and successful treatment, pregnancy has become an option for more and more female transplant recipients. Many of the commonly used immunosuppressive agents may have adverse effects on the fetus and these effects are summarized for each drug class discussed below. In general, an assessment of drug safety during pregnancy can be made using data from animal models of teratogenicity and mutogenicity before experience is gained in humans.

The US Food and Drug Administration (FDA) introduced a classification of fetal risks due to drugs in 1979 (Table 2.1) based on a similar system introduced in Sweden a year earlier. This classification schema

Table 2.1 The USFDA pregnancy categories of medication-associated risk to the fetus

Pregnancy category	Description
A	Adequate and well-controlled studies have failed to demonstrate a risk to the fetus in the first trimester (or subsequent trimesters) of pregnancy
B	Animal reproduction studies have failed to demonstrate a risk to the fetus and there are no adequate and well-controlled studies in pregnant women, or animal studies, that have shown an adverse effect, but adequate and well-controlled studies in pregnant women have failed to demonstrate a risk to the fetus in any trimester
C	Animal reproduction studies have shown an adverse effect on the fetus and there are no adequate and well-controlled studies in humans, but potential benefits may warrant use of the drug in pregnant women despite potential risks
D	There is positive evidence of human fetal risk based on adverse reaction data from investigational or marketing experience or studies in humans, but potential benefits may warrant use of the drug in pregnant women despite potential risks
X	Studies in animals or humans have demonstrated fetal abnormalities and/or there is positive evidence of human fetal risk based on adverse reaction data from investigational or marketing experience, and the risks involved in use of the drug in pregnant women clearly outweigh potential benefits

does not include any risks conferred by drugs entering breast milk, a phenomenon that is relevant to some of the commonly used immunosuppressants (e.g., cyclosporine, tacrolimus, and mycophenolate mofetil).

Individual immunosuppressive agents

Available immunosuppressants can be classified according to their pharmacologic mechanism of action. It should be noted that the licensed indications will vary over time and between different countries. There is often good evidence for use of drugs 'off-label' or outside their licensed indications.

Key points 2.1 Pharmacological methods of immunosuppression

Depletion of lymphocytes
- Polyclonal antibodies: ALG, thymoglobulin
- Monoclonal antibodies: OKT3

Inhibition of lymphocyte activation
- Antibodies:
  - IL2R antibodies: basiliximab, daclizumab
  - Anti CD80/86 antibodies: belatacept
- Corticosteroids
- Immunophilin–binding drugs
  - Calcineurin inhibitors: cyclosporine and tacrolimus
  - TOR Inhibitors: sirolimus

Inhibition of new nucleotide synthesis
- Purine synthesis inhibitors (IMPDH): mycophenolate
- Pyrimidine synthesis inhibitors (DHODH): leflunomide

Antimetabolites: azathioprine, cyclophosphamide

Inhibitors of lymphocyte trafficking and interaction
- Inhibitor of trafficking: FTY720
- Inhibitors of interactions:
- Antibodies to ICAM–1

ALG, anti-lymphocyte globulin; TOR, target of rapamycin; IMPDH, inosine monophosphate dehydrogenase; DHODH, IL-2R: interleukin-2 receptor; ICAM, intercellular adhesion molecule.

Drugs that cause lymphocyte depletion

These agents are used primarily in induction regimens or in desensitization protocols. Use of these agents for induction therapy varies worldwide, but generally there has been increasing use in the USA for the past decade.

Polyclonal antibodies

Rabbit antithymocyte globulin (Thymoglobulin)

Licensed indication Treatment of acute renal allograft rejection in conjunction with concomitant immunosuppression. The drug is frequently used off-label for induction therapy.

Pharmacodynamics Thymoglobulin is a purified, pasteurized, rabbit IgG antibody preparation, obtained by repeated immunization of rabbits with human thymocytes. The exact mechanism of action is unknown but possible in vivo actions include clearance of activated T lymphocytes and modulation of T-lymphocyte homing, activation, and cytotoxic properties. The preparation includes antibodies against many T-cell antigens including the T-cell receptor, CD2, CD3, CD5, and CD8. In vitro concentrations of >0.1 µg/mL inhibit lymphocyte proliferation. Thymoglobulin has not been shown to be effective in the treatment of humoral (antibody-mediated) rejection.

Pharmacodynamics Thymoglobulin should be administered at a dose of 1.5 mg/kg body weight over a period of 4 hours (6 h for the first dose). The half-life is 2–3 days. Approximately 70% of patients will develop anti-rabbit antibodies though the effect of these is uncertain. In patients who are re-treated with Thymoglobulin measurement of lymphocyte subsets is sometimes recommended to ensure that T-lymphocyte depletion is achieved.

Adverse effects Anaphylactic reactions have been reported rarely. A substantial minority of patients will experience mild infusion reactions (fever, chills), although these may be reduced by premedication with acetaminophen, antihistamine, and/or glucocorticoid. Prolonged use may be associated with profound immunosuppression and an increased risk of opportunistic infections and/or post-transplant lymphoproliferative disease (PTLD)

Pregnancy and lactation Animal reproductive studies have not been performed with thymoglobulin and this drug should be used only if clearly needed.

Monoclonal antibodies

Rituximab

Indications Rituximab is licensed for treatment of patients with follicular lymphoma and PTLD. However, it is also being used off-label to reduce anti-donor antibody titers in highly sensitized renal transplant candidates and occasionally in combination with other modalities (e.g., plasmapheresis) for the treatment of humoral rejection mediated by anti-HLA antibodies or by ABO incompatibility.

Pharmacodynamics Rituximab is a chimeric mouse/human IgG (human IgG1 constant regions and murine light chain and heavy chain variable regions) monoclonal antibody (mAb) directed against CD20. It binds specifically to the transmembrane antigen CD20 located on pre-B and mature B lymphocytes. The antigen does not internalize upon antibody binding and does not circulate in plasma. The Fab domain of the rituximab binds to the CD20 antigen, allowing the Fc domain to recruit immune-mediated effector functions, including complement-dependent cytotoxicity (CDC) and antibody-dependent cellular cytotoxicity (ADCC), resulting in lysis of the cell. Binding of rituximab to CD20 has also been shown to cause apoptosis.

Pharmacokinetics Rituximab is given as an intravenous infusion and should be given in 5% glucose or 0.9% sodium chloride, diluted to 1–4 mg/mL. Serum levels and the half-life are proportional to the dose administered. There are no data on the effects of renal or hepatic dysfunction on the drug's metabolism.

Adverse effects Infusion reactions are common, with up to 10% of patients experiencing systemic symptoms on the first infusion in patients with rheumatoid arthritis, and higher rates in patients being treated for lymphoma. Rituximab may provoke a severe cytokine release syndrome characterized by severe dyspnea, often accompanied by bronchospasm and hypoxia, chills, rigors, urticaria, and angioedema. In patients who develop this syndrome the infusion should be stopped immediately and appropriate treatment instituted. The syndrome is usually reversible although fatalities have been rarely reported. Patients receiving treatment should be closely monitored and antihypertensive medication withheld for 12 h before treatment. These reactions may be significantly reduced by predose administration of intravenous glucocorticoids. Caution is advised when used in patients with a history of cardiovascular disease because of the increased risk of dysrhythmia, angina, and heart failure.

Pregnancy and lactation No data are available in pregnant or lactating women treated with rituximab. However, the immunoglobulin IgG is known to cross the placenta and also enter breast milk, such that systemic effects in the fetus and newborn are to be anticipated.

OKT3

Licensed indications Treatment of acute renal, cardiac, or hepatic allograft rejection refractory to conventional therapy (or where conventional therapy is contraindicated).

Pharmacodynamics OKT3 is a murine monoclonal IgG2 antibody to CD3. CD3 is present on the surface of all human T lymphocytes and is involved in T-lymphocyte activation through its association with the T-cell receptor (together forming the T-cell receptor complex). OKT3 reverses allograft rejection by blocking the function of all T cells and in vitro studies have shown that generation and function of effector T cells are blocked.

Pharmacokinetics No detailed pharmacokinetic information is available. The recommended dose is 5 mg/day as a single intravenous bolus dose for 10–14 days. The drug-containing solution should be drawn up through a sterile, low-protein-binding, 0.2–0.22 μm filter before rapid intravenous bolus injection.

Adverse effects The major side effects are a consequence of cytokine release. The cytokine release syndrome described above for rituximab occurs in most patients treated with OKT3 and may be severe. Pulmonary edema occasionally occurs in euvolemic patients but is more common in those with pre-existing volume overload. All patients should be assessed clinically for signs of volume overload and, if necessary, treated with diuretics or hemofiltration to assure euvolemia before treatment with this drug. The cytokine release syndrome may be prevented or palliated by pre-treatment with glucocorticoids (e.g. hydrocortisone sodium succinate). Hypersensitivity reactions including anaphylaxis have also been described, albeit less frequently than cytokine release syndrome. The two syndromes may be difficult to tell apart.

Neuropsychiatric events including headache (most commonly), seizures, encephalopathy, cerebral edema and herniation, and aseptic meningitis have been reported. Patients with pre-existing neurological disease appear to be at greatest risk. Although headache, seizures, and mild encephalopathy may resolve with continued treatment, fatalities have been reported in those developing cerebral edema, with or without herniation. All patients should be monitored for a period of 24 h after each injection for neurological signs and, if signs of cerebral edema are seen, treatment should be discontinued. Patients treated with OKT3, particularly at high cumulative doses, are at increased risk of infectious complications especially with the human herpes viruses (herpes simplex virus [HSV], cytomegalovirus [CMV], and Epstein–Barr virus [EBV]) and also EBV-mediated post-transplant lymphoproliferative disorders.

Pregnancy and lactation OKT3 is contraindicated in pregnant women, and those who are breastfeeding.

Key points 2.2 Cytokine release syndrome

Characterized by:
- Severe dyspnea, bronchospasm, and hypoxia
- Chills and rigors
- Urticaria and angioedema

Initial treatment:
- Stop treatment
- Oxygen
- Volume expansion
- Intravenous glucocorticoid

Prevention:
- Withhold antihypertensive medication for 12 h before treatment
- Ensure euvolemia
- Premedication with intravenous glucocorticoid

Alemtuzumab (Campath-1H)

Indications Alemtuzumab is licensed for the treatment of chronic lymphocytic leukemia (CLL) in patients who have had a poor response to conventional therapy. It has been used off-label as part of induction therapy, especially in protocols that putatively promote tolerance or immune hyporesponsiveness.

Initial studies, in a variety of organ grafts, show that its use is safe and effective and may allow for reduced exposure to maintenance immunosuppressive drugs. It should not be used in those with chronic hepatitis C viral infection.

Pharmacodynamics This is a genetically engineered humanized IgG1 κ monoclonal antibody directed against CD52. CD52 is a highly expressed, non-modulating antigen which is present on the surface of essentially all B and T lymphocytes, monocytes, thymocytes. and macrophages. The antibody mediates cell lysis through CDC and ADCC. CD52 is found on only a minority of granulocytes (<5%) but not on erythrocytes, platelets, hemopoietic stem cells. or progenitor cells, thus sparing these cell lines from depletion. Administration results in profound depletion of lymphocytes and monocytes. The composition of the reconstituted pool may not resemble that of the original pool of cells.

Pharmacokinetics The available data are from patients receiving treatment for CLL who have been treated with repetitive doses for a much longer period (12 weeks) than is used in transplantation. In transplant recipients, the usual dose is 0.3 mg/kg per day for the first 3–4 postoperative days, but some centers use a single perioperative dose The antibody should be infused in 100 mL 5% glucose or 0.9% sodium chloride over 2 h through a low-protein-binding 5 μm filter. Alemtuzumab is largely distributed in the extracellular fluid and plasma compartments and, because CD52-positive cells are depleted, there is decreased receptor associated clearance and a fall in systemic clearance over time.

Adverse effects The cytokine release syndrome may occur with alemtuzumab and it is recommended that all patients receive pre-treatment with glucocorticoids. Transient hypotension may also occur and antihypertensive medication should be withheld for at least 12 h before administration. Profound lymphocyte depletion inevitably occurs and may be prolonged. During this time patients are at risk for opportunistic infections and all patients should receive appropriate prophylaxis for *Pneumocystis jiroveci* pneumonia and herpes viruses. Hematological monitoring is essential because myelosuppression is common, but monitoring of CD52 is not required.

Pregnancy and lactation Alemtuzumab is contraindicated in pregnant and breast-feeding women due to the potential for the antibody to cross the placenta or into breast milk. The manufacturer advises men and women to use effective contraception during treatment and for 6 months thereafter.

Drugs that inhibit lymphocyte activation

These agents prevent immunological activation through blockade of key signals involved in lymphocyte activation. They include anti-CD25 (the interleukin-2 [IL-2] receptor) antibodies, corticosteroids, the calcineurin inhibitors, and agents that inhibit essential co-stimulatory molecules including CD80/86 and CTLA4.

Basiliximab and daclizumab

Indication Both basiliximab and daclizumab are licensed for the prophylaxis of acute rejection in renal allograft recipients who are also to be treated with cyclosporine and corticosteroids. Their use may allow reduced doses or delayed introduction of CNIs and so may be beneficial in those with delayed graft function and may reduce the risk of late CNI-associated renal failure. Although discussed below, it should be noted that daclizumab was recently removed from the market.

Pharmacodynamics Basiliximab is a murine/human chimeric monoclonal IgG1 antibody directed against the α chain of the IL-2 receptor (CD25) which is expressed on the surface of activated T lymphocytes. The antibody binds with high specificity and affinity to the IL-2 receptor (IL-2R) thus preventing IL-2 binding and cellular proliferation. Complete blocking of the IL-2R is maintained until serum basiliximab levels fall below 0.2 μg/mL (in practice between 4 and 6 weeks). CD25 expression returns and reaches pre-treatment values after an additional 1–2 weeks. Daclizumab is a recombinant humanized IgG1 anti-tac antibody that also acts as an IL-2R antagonist. It also binds to the α or tac subunits of the IL-2R. Daclizumab saturates the IL-2R for approximately 90 days. Antibodies against daclizumab have been detected in 9% of those treated but have no clinical significance.

Pharmacokinetics Basiliximab reaches peak concentrations of 7.1 ± 5.2 μg/mL after intravenous infusion. The terminal half-life is 7.2 ± 3.2 days. Distribution of the drug is not significantly affected by body weight or gender. Basiliximab should be given as a slow intravenous injection or by slow intravenous infusion over 2 h. For adults, the dose is 20 mg before and at 4 days after transplantation. Patients weighing less than 35 kg should receive 10 mg.

Daclizumab given at a dose of 1 mg/kg and the peak concentration after the first dose is 21 μg/mL. A concentration of 0.5–0.9 μg/mL is required to saturate the IL-2R and a dose of 5–10 μg/mL is required to inhibit its biological activity. The recommended dosing regimen of five 1 mg/kg doses, with the first dose given in the 24 h before surgery, is sufficient to saturate the IL-2R for more than 90 days. The terminal elimination half-life is approximately 480 h and is equivalent to that reported for human IgG. Elimination is increased with increasing body weight, hence the need for dosing based on body weight.

Adverse effects In trials of both basiliximab and daclizumab used in combination with cyclosporine and corticosteroids there were no additional adverse effects reported.

Pregnancy and lactation There are some animal data that suggest increased prenatal loss with daclizumab treatment but there are no other data and use of basiliximab and daclizumab is not recommended in pregnancy. The manufacturers advise that women of child-bearing age should use effective contraception during treatment and for 4 months thereafter.

Belatacept

Previously known under the investigational term LEA29YI, belatacept blocks co-stimulation by binding to CD80 and CD86 on the surface of antigen-presenting cells (APCs). This interaction inhibits T-cell activation and promotes anergy and apoptosis (Figure 2.1). The agent is a human fusion protein combining the extracellular portion of CTLA4 (cytotoxic lymphocyte associated antigen-4) with the Fc portion of human IgG1. It has been shown to be of benefit in the treatment of some autoimmune diseases including rheumatoid arthritis and psoriasis. Studies in renal allograft recipients suggest a possible benefit when used in combination with other immunosuppressive agents. The doses used are not fully established: during the early weeks after transplantation, higher doses are given (10 mg/kg) than later in the post-transplant course (5 mg/kg) as a 30-min infusion every 4–8 weeks. Side effects are few.

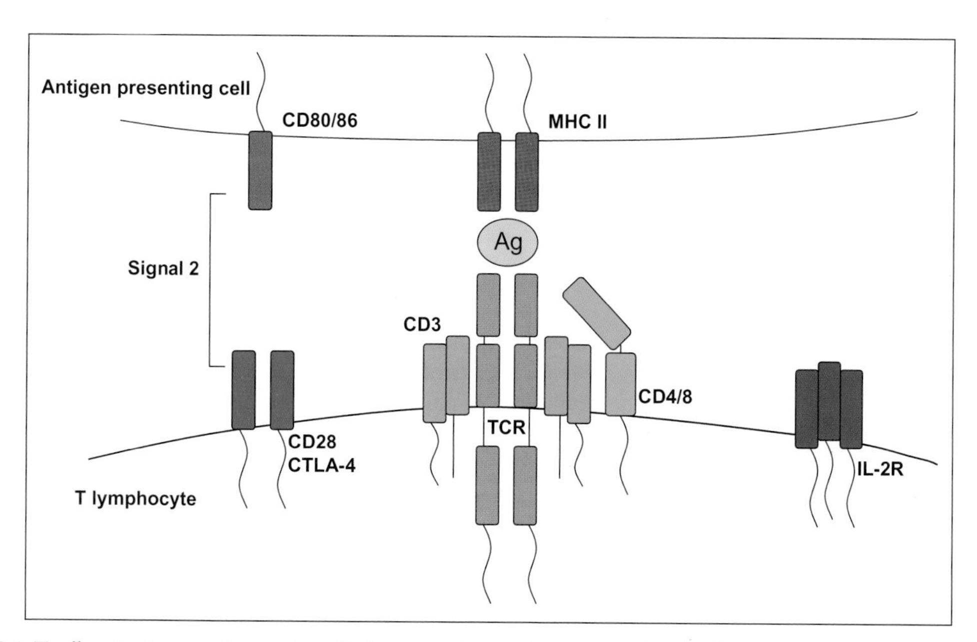

Figure 2.1 T-cell activation requires antigen (Ag) presentation in the context of major histocompatibility complex (MHC) of antigen-presenting cells (APCs) to CD3 T-cell receptor (TCR) complex. A second co-stimulatory signal (signal 2) is also required.

Glucocorticoids

Indication Prophylaxis and treatment of acute rejection following solid organ transplantation.

Pharmacodynamics Glucocorticoids are potent anti-inflammatory and immunosuppressive agents. They enter the cell by diffusion and then bind to high-affinity cytoplasmic glucocorticoid receptors. The glucocorticoid receptor steroid complex enters the nucleus where it binds to the glucocorticoid response element. The glucocorticoid receptor steroid complex may also bind to other regulatory elements, inhibiting their binding to DNA. Both actions lead to alterations in the transcription of genes involved in the immune and inflammatory responses. The most important effects on lymphocytes are mediated through a decrease in expression of the transcription factors nuclear factor (NF)-κB and activator protein-1. Functionally this leads to a decrease in the production of T-cell cytokines that are required to augment the responses of macrophages and lymphocytes. The anti-inflammatory effects are mediated largely through inhibition of phospholipase A_2 by lipocortin, thereby reducing synthesis of prostaglandins and other related compounds. Finally, glucocorticoids cause a decrease in the numbers of circulating lymphocytes by stimulating the migration of T cells from the intravascular compartment to lymphoid tissue.

Table 2.2 Adverse effects of corticosteroids

System	Adverse effect
Cardiovascular	Sodium retention Fluid retention Potassium depletion Hypertension
Endocrine	Carbohydrate intolerance and diabetes mellitus Cushingoid facies Growth retardation Menstrual irregularities
Ophthalmic	Cataract Glaucoma
Musculoskeletal	Osteoporosis and increased fracture risk Aseptic necrosis of femoral head Myopathy Muscle weakness
Dermatologic	Increased bruising Skin thinning Acne
Neurologic	Altered mood Headaches
Gastrointestinal	Peptic ulceration Pancreatitis

Pharmacokinetics Hydrocortisone or methylprednisolone is frequently given intravenously in the first few days after transplantation. Prednisolone, given orally, is well absorbed from the gastrointestinal tract. It is widely used for maintenance immunosuppression in European centers. In the USA, prednisone (the metabolic precursor of prednisolone) is the more popular maintenance agent. Peak plasma concentrations of prednisolone are seen within 1–2 h. Absorption (but not overall bioavailability) is affected by food. The effective half-life of prednisolone is 2–4 h and elimination is in the urine after metabolism in the liver. In general, all corticosteroids are extensively bound to plasma proteins, although prednisolone is bound to a lesser extent than hydrocortisone.

Adverse effects The adverse effects of steroids are well recognized (Table 2.2) and often the physical effects are troubling for the patient. The risk of osteoporosis is great and bone density in all patients receiving long-term steroids should be measured and treatment with calcium supplementation or bisphosphonates considered in those patients at greatest risk.

Pregnancy and lactation There is no evidence that treatment with glucocorticoids increases the risk of congenital malformations. However, prolonged treatment may increase the risk of intrauterine growth retardation. Although most glucocorticoids are inactivated on crossing the placenta, hypoadrenalism in the neonate is theoretically a risk, though rarely clinically important. Mothers with pre-eclampsia should be closely monitored. Only a small proportion of glucocorticoids is excreted in small amounts into breast milk. Doses up to 40 mg of prednisolone are unlikely to cause significant systemic effects in the infant and the benefits of breastfeeding are likely to

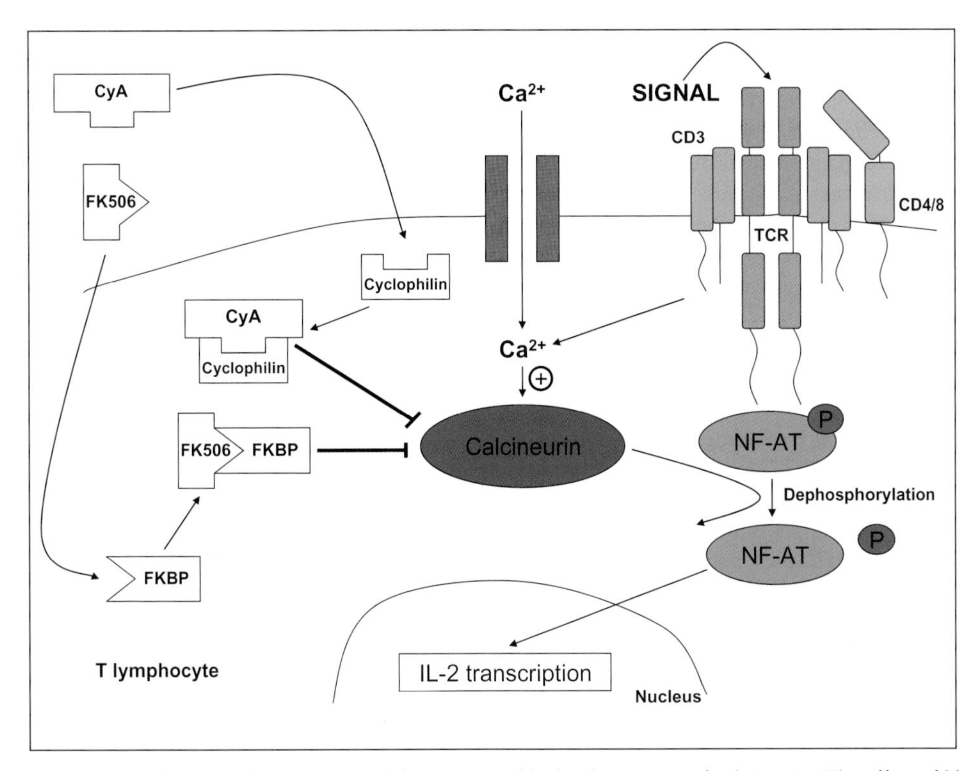

Figure 2.2 Mechanism of action of calcineurin inhibitors. Cyclosporine (CyA) binds to its immunophilin, cyclophilin, forming a complex that blocks the phosphatase activity of calcineurin. Tacrolimus (FK506) binds to the FK506-binding protein (FKBP) and this complex binds to and blocks the activity of calcineurin. The effect of blocking calcineurin is to prevent passage of nuclear factor of activated T cells (NF-AT) into the nucleus, thus preventing transcription of the interleukin-2 (IL-2) gene.

outweigh the theoretical risk to the infant at higher doses.

Immunophilin-binding drugs

Calcineurin inhibitors (Figure 2.2)

The two CNIs used in transplantation are cyclosporine and tacrolimus. Their mode of action is similar but not identical and is described in detail below. Drug interactions may affect levels or toxicity. Metabolism of both CNIs is mediated through the cytochrome P450 system (CYP3A4) and so levels may be affected by enzyme inducers and inhibitors (Table 2.3). With both drugs, therapeutic drug monitoring is required but the correlation between levels and efficacy and toxicity is relatively weak. The side effects of the two CNIs are broadly similar (Table 2.4) but do differ, e.g., hirsutism and gum hypertrophy are seen more frequently with cyclosporine whereas neurological disturbance and diabetes mellitus are more common in patients receiving tacrolimus.

Cyclosporine

Licensed indications Prophylaxis of transplant rejection in liver, renal, heart, combined heart–lung, lung, and pancreas allograft recipients.

Pharmacodynamics Cyclosporine is a small fungal cyclic polypeptide consisting of 11 amino acids and binding to cyclophilin in the cytosol. The cyclosporine–cyclophilin complex binds to calcineurin together with calmodulin and calcium, inhibiting the phosphatase activity of calcineurin. This results in the inhibition of dephosphorylation and translocation of

Table 2.3 Calcineurin inhibitor drug interactions

Effect of interaction	Drug
Increased CNI level (CYP 3A4 inhibitors)	Azole antifungals (ketoconazole, itraconazole, fluconazole) Protease inhibitors Cimetidine Clarithromycin Cyclosporine Diltiazem Erythromycin Grapefruit juice Metoclopramide Nicardipine Verapamil
Decreased CNI level (CYP3A4 inducers)	Carbamazepine Phenytoin Phenobarbital Rifampicin St John's wort
Increased nephrotoxicity	Aminoglycosides Colchicine Fibrates NSAIDs
Hyperkalemia	ACE inhibitors A2RBs
Gum hyperplasia (with cyclosporine)	Nifedipine
Myopathy (with cyclosporine)	HMG-CoA reductase inhibitors

Note: combination of these agents (such as cyclosporine and sirolimus) will interact with each other.
CYP3A4, cytochrome P450 3A4; CNI: calcineurin inhibitor; NSAID: non-steroidal anti-inflammatory drug; ACE: angiotensin-converting enzyme; A2RB: angiotensin 2 receptor blockers; HMG-CoA: 3 hydroxy-3-methylglutaryl CoA.

the cytoplasmic unit of NF-AT (nuclear factor of activated T cells) and thus inhibits gene transcription of proteins such as IL-2 and interferon-γ. Inhibition of IL-2 blocks the formation of cytotoxic T cells and suppresses both T-cell activation and T-helper cell-dependent proliferation of B cells.

Table 2.4 Adverse effects of the calcineurin inhibitors (CNIs)

System	Adverse effects
Renal	Renal failure Hyperuricemia and gout Hyperkalemia Hypermagnesemia
Cardiovascular	Hypertension
Endocrine	Glucose intolerance and diabetes mellitus
Neurological	Headaches Migraine Tremor
Other	Hirsutism Gum hypertrophy

Note that some adverse effects are more common with one CNI than another.

Pharmacokinetics There are several preparations of cyclosporine currently available. The original preparation (Sandimmune) has been replaced largely by a microemulsion formulation (Neoral). Neoral is a preconcentrate formulation of cyclosporine which undergoes microemulsification in the presence of water, in the form of either a beverage or gastrointestinal fluid. This reduces intrapatient variability with a more consistent absorption profile and less effect from concomitant ingestion of food. Pharmacokinetic studies of Neoral indicate a greater correlation between trough concentrations and total drug exposure (as measured by area under the curve or AUC) than Sandimmune. Neoral therefore has greater predictability and consistency of cyclosporine exposure. In addition, there are now several generic formulations of cyclosporine available worldwide. It should be stressed that each formulation has a different pharmacologic profile and so they are not interchangeable. If a patient is switched from one formulation to another, levels and side effects should be closely monitored.

Cyclosporine is largely distributed outside the blood volume. In plasma approximately 90% is bound to plasma proteins, mostly lipoproteins. There is extensive biotransformation to approximately 15 metabolites and although no single major metabolic pathway has been identified there is significant cytochrome P450 3A4 (CYP3A4) activity. Excretion is largely in bile. There is significant variation in terminal half-life depending on the target population, varying from 6h in healthy individuals to 20h in patients with severe hepatic dysfunction.

Traditionally, therapeutic dose monitoring was done using trough levels, with the guide levels of 150–250ng/mL (whole blood levels measured by radioimmunoassay) for the first 3 months and then target levels of 100–150ng/mL. As the maximal effect on calcineurin inhibition correlates with the time of peak blood concentration, there has been a move to focus drug monitoring on the 2-hour post-dose level (C2 monitoring, rather than C0 monitoring). Studies have suggested a better outcome using C2 monitoring in the first 3 months after transplantation. Target levels at 2h lie between 0.8 and 1.2μg/mL in the first 3 months and 0.7–0.9μg/mL thereafter.

Pregnancy and lactation Cyclosporine is not teratogenic in animals. Epidemiological studies in humans have not identified teratogenicity, although there may be an associated increase in pre-term delivery. Offspring exposed to cyclosporine should be actively followed for evidence of drug toxicity. Cyclosporine is excreted in breast milk and mothers receiving treatment should not breastfeed because detrimental effects on the newborn cannot be excluded.

Tacrolimus

Licensed indications Prophylaxis of transplant rejection in liver, kidney, and heart allograft recipients.

Pharmacodynamics Tacrolimus accumulates in the cellular cytoplasm by binding to a cytosolic protein called FKBP12. The FKBP12–tacrolimus complex specifically and competitively binds to calcineurin, leading to a calcium-dependent inhibition of T-cell transduction pathways through suppression of synthesis of cytokines including IL-2. The formation of cytotoxic T cells is inhibited. T-cell activation and T-helper cell-dependent proliferation of B cells are suppressed.

Pharmacokinetics Tacrolimus is well absorbed throughout the gastrointestinal tract and intravenous administration is rarely required. After oral administration peak blood levels are seen within 1–3h. Studies in patients after liver transplantation have shown that steady-state concentrations are reached within 3 days in most patients. The rate and extent of absorption are maximal under fasting conditions. The presence of food in the gastrointestinal tract reduces the rate and extent of absorption and bioavailability is reduced most following administration after a high fat meal. In practice, patients should be advised to take the medication on an empty stomach either 1h before or 2–3h after, a meal.

In whole blood tacrolimus is highly bound to erythrocytes resulting in a whole blood to plasma ratio of 20:1. In plasma, more than 98% of the drug is bound to plasma proteins, mainly albumin and α_1-acid glycoprotein. Tacrolimus is widely metabolized in the liver by CYP3A4. There is also considerable metabolism in the intestinal wall. Several metabolites have been identified and only one of these has been shown in vitro to have immunosuppressive activity similar to tacrolimus. The others have either weak or no immunosuppressive activity. In the circulation, only one of the inactive metabolites is present at low concentrations. Excretion is in bile. In studies with ^{14}C-labelled tacrolimus, less than 1% of unchanged tacrolimus can be identified in urine and feces, indicating that tacrolimus is almost completely metabolized before elimination.

The starting dose is 0.1mg/kg per day in two divided doses. A strong correlation exists between drug exposure (as measured by the AUC) and whole blood trough levels, and most units aim for target trough whole blood levels of 10–15ng/mL in the first 3 months and between 5 and 10ng/mL thereafter. The half-life is long and variable in healthy individuals but is significantly shorter in transplant recipients (43h vs 12–16h). Increased clearance rates in transplant recipients contribute to the decreased half-life.

More recently, a modified-release formulation with an extended oral absorption profile has been developed for use as a single daily dose. Although the pharmacokinetics of the two preparations are broadly similar, there are some differences, so that close monitoring is recommended for the first few weeks if patients are switched from the twice-daily to the single-daily dosing regimen.

Pregnancy and lactation Tacrolimus is able to cross the placenta but the limited data available do not show an increased risk of adverse effects in the course and outcome of pregnancy in comparison with other immunosuppressive agents. Due to the need for treatment, tacrolimus can be considered in pregnant women when no safer alternative is available and where the benefit of treatment outweighs the risk to the fetus. There is a risk of premature delivery and the newborn is at risk of transient hyperkalemia after birth. The newborn should also be monitored for potential complications including effects on the kidney. Tacrolimus is excreted in breast milk and women should not breastfeed because detrimental effects on the newborn cannot be excluded.

Adverse effects Compared with cyclosporine, use of tacrolimus is associated with an increased risk of post-transplant diabetes mellitus. In children, cardiac hypertrophy has been reported.

Drugs that inhibit lymphocyte proliferation

Target of rapamycin inhibitors (sirolimus and everolimus)

Licensed indications Sirolimus is used in patients receiving a kidney transplant and everolimus is used in patents receiving either a kidney or heart transplant as prophylaxis of organ rejection in those with low-to-moderate immunological risk when receiving a renal transplant. It is recommended that sirolimus be used initially in combination with cyclosporine and corticosteroids, but may be continued as maintenance therapy with corticosteroids alone only if cyclosporine can be progressively withdrawn. Everolimus may be used for prophylaxis of organ rejection in kidney and heart transplantation

Pharmacodynamics Sirolimus and everolimus inhibit proliferation of both T and B lymphocytes by blocking calcium-dependent and calcium-independent intracellular signal transduction (Figure 2.3). Target of rapamycin (TOR) inhibitors bind to FKBP12 but, rather than inhibiting the calcineurin pathway, the TOR inhibitor–FKBP12 complex interacts with mTOR, a protein kinase that is integral to signal transduction. Inhibition of mTOR blocks synthesis of proteins required for cell cycle progression. As the drugs inhibit both T and B cells, antibody-mediated immunity is also affected. The TOR inhibitors also inhibit growth-factor-stimulated cell cycle progression of vascular smooth muscle cells at the G1 stage, and so may be of benefit in reducing the transplant vasculopathy seen in ischemic/reperfusion injury and chronic rejection.

Pharmacokinetics Both sirolimus and everolimus are rapidly, although relatively poorly, absorbed from the gut (oral bioavailability about 15%). Absorption is mediated via the counter-transporter activity of P-glycoprotein. Absorption is affected by concomitant ingestion of food and the patient should be advised to take the medicine consistently with or without food. Sirolimus is metabolized extensively through the CYP3A4 in the liver. There are seven major metabolites, none of which has significant immunosuppressive activity. Everolimus is broadly similar but has a shorter half-life. The half-life is long in healthy individuals (about 60 h for sirolimus and 28 h for everolimus) and longer in those with liver disease. Thus, steady state is reached in 6 days for sirolimus and 4 days for everolimus. Excretion is largely in the bile and little drug is excreted by the kidneys. Patients with liver disease may have impaired metabolism.

The recommended dose regimen for sirolimus is a loading dose of 6 mg followed by 2 mg daily, with the dose adjusted to maintain trough whole blood levels between 4 and 15 ng/mL. Higher trough levels are required in those on monotherapy. The drug should be taken consistently, at the same time of day, either with or without food. Sirolimus may be used in combination with cyclosporine (4 h after taking cyclosporine) and with corticosteroids. As cyclosporine is an inhibitor of CYP3A4, lower doses of sirolimus may be required by those taking both agents. For everolimus, the initial daily dose is 1.3–3.0 mg/day with target trough levels of 3–8 ng/ml.

Side effects Delayed wound healing arises from drug-induced inhibition of certain growth factors and tends to be more common in obese patients. Many units will delay introduction until 3 months post-transplantation. In trials of sirolimus in liver

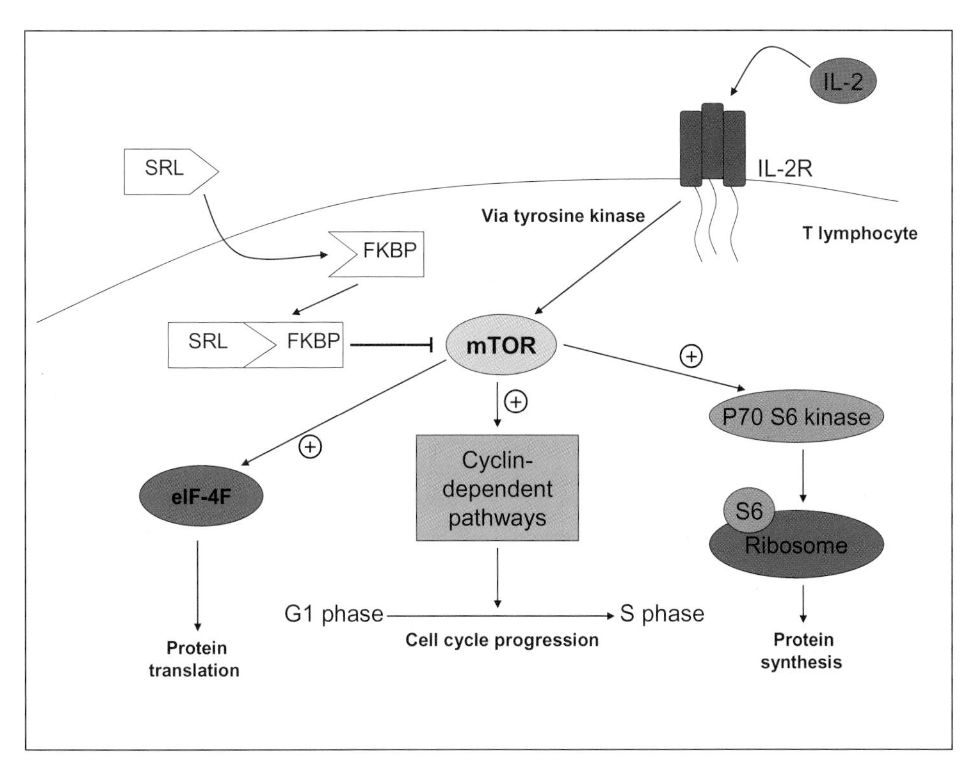

Figure 2.3 Mechanism of action of sirolimus. Sirolimus binds to the FK506-binding protein (FKBP); the complex that is formed then binds to the mammalian target of rapamycin (mTOR). This final complex inhibits pathways vital for cell cycle progression through a cyclin-dependent pathway, protein translation through eukaryotic initiation factor eIF-4F, and protein synthesis through the S6 protein kinase P70 S6 kinase. TOR1 inhibits proliferation of both T and B lymphocytes by blocking calcium-dependent and calcium-independent intracellular signal transduction. TOR1 binds to the FKBP12 but, rather than inhibiting the calcineurin pathway, the TOR1–FKBP12 complex interacts with mTOR, a protein kinase that is integral to signal transduction. Inhibition of mTOR blocks synthesis of proteins required for cell cycle progression, thus effectively blocking signal transduction. As TOR1 inhibits both T and B cells, antibody-mediated immunity is also affected. TOR1 also inhibits growth factor-stimulated cell cycle progression of vascular smooth muscle cells at the G1 stage, and so may be of benefit in reducing the transplant's vasculopathy seen in ischemic–reperfusion injury and chronic rejection.

transplantation, an increased incidence of hepatic artery thrombosis led to a 'black box' warning by the FDA for its use in this setting. New use of sirolimus has also been associated with failure to heal the tracheal anastomosis after lung transplantation. Hyperlipidemia, manifest as both hypercholesterolemia and hypertriglyceridemia, is common but often modified by co-administration of hydroxymethyl coenzyme A (HMG-CoA) reductase inhibitors and/or fibrates. Other common side effects include lymphocele, tachycardia, stomatitis, abdominal pain and diarrhea, anemia, leucopenia, thrombocytopenia, arthralgia, pneumonitis, acne, proteinuria, and urinary tract infections. Interstitial lung disease is a rare but potentially serious complication. Both drugs may exacerbate CNI-associated nephrotoxicity so renal function should be monitored regularly. Many transplant centers lower their target blood levels for the CNIs when they are used concomitantly with one of the TOR inhibitors.

Pregnancy and lactation In animal models, sirolimus has been associated with fetal toxicity manifested by increased mortality and reduced fetal weights. There are no human data from the use of sirolimus in pregnant women but it should not be used in pregnancy unless no other therapy is available. Effective contraception should be used while taking a TOR inhibitor and for at least 12 weeks after its cessation. In rats, sirolimus is excreted in breast milk and although no human data are available mothers taking sirolimus should be advised not to breastfeed.

Inhibitors of new nucleotide synthesis

Purine synthesis inhibitors (mycophenolate derivatives)

Indications These agents are approved for prophylaxis of rejection in combination with cyclosporine or corticosteroids in patients receiving liver, kidney, or cardiac allografts. Monotherapy with mycophenolate mofetil may be associated with chronic rejection so most will use the agent in conjunction with either a CNI or corticosteroids. Although not licensed for use with tacrolimus, the two agents are frequently used together.

Pharmacodynamics Use of mycophenolate derivatives exploits the fact that lymphocytes, unlike other cells, do not have a salvage pathway for synthesis of purines. Thus, mycophenolate inhibits T- and B-cell proliferation by inhibition of new purine synthesis by potent, selective, and reversible inhibition of the enzyme inosine monophosphate dehydrogenase (IMPDH). The effect of this is to block synthesis of the guanosine nucleotide. Without its incorporation into DNA, there is a cytostatic effect on lymphocytes, inhibiting mitogen- and alloantigen-induced stimulation as well as inhibiting antibody production, adhesion to endothelial cells, and, possibly, cell recruitment.

Pharmacokinetics Two preparations of mycophenolate are available: mycophenolate mofetil and enteric-coated mycophenolate sodium. Mycophenolate mofetil is an ester of mycophenolate and undergoes rapid and extensive absorption from the gastrointestinal tract and then complete presystemic metabolism to the active metabolite. Enteric-coated mycophenolate sodium is also extensively absorbed from the gastrointestinal tract and absorption of both formulations is not affected by concomitant ingestion of food. Mycophenolate is highly protein bound in plasma and, in conditions where there is reduced protein binding (e.g. uremia, hepatic failure, hypoalbuminemia, or concomitant use of drugs with high protein binding), patients are at increased risk of mycophenolate-related adverse effects.

Mycophenolate is metabolized by glucuronyl transferase in the liver to form mycophenolate glucuronide (MPAG). The majority of MPAG is excreted in the urine although a small proportion is excreted in the bile. MPAG excreted in the bile is deconjugated by gut flora and the resulting mycophenolate is reabsorbed to create a second peak of mycophenolate in blood that can be measured 6–8 h after dosing.

Clinically there is little to choose between the two preparations, although some suggest that gastrointestinal upset is less common with the enteric-coated formulation. The usual maintenance dose for enteric-coated mycophenolate sodium is 1440 mg/day and for mycophenolate mofetil is 2 g/day, both given in two or three divided doses. Mycophenolate mofetil is available in an intravenous formulation. Therapeutic drug monitoring is available but not used commonly. Patients should be monitored for neutropenia and the dose reduced or stopped if the absolute white count falls below 1.3×10^9/L.

Pregnancy and lactation Genotoxicity studies of mycophenolate in mouse models demonstrate a potential for chromosomal aberrations. This effect is clearly related to the pharmacodynamic mechanism of action. In animal models mycophenolate is excreted in breast milk. Human data are limited. However, the FDA recently classified these agents as category D (see Table 2.2) so that many transplant centers avoid the mycophenolate derivatives during pregnancy. When deemed necessary, effective contraception should be used before, during, and for 6 weeks after therapy.

Adverse effects Significant side effects include diarrhea, upper gastrointestinal disturbances. and myelosuppression, especially leukopenia and anemia.

Pyrimidine synthesis inhibitors (leflunomide)

Leflunomide is available for use in patients with rheumatoid arthritis. The agent has been used in transplantation, not so much because of its immunosuppressive properties, but because of putative benefit in controlling BK polyoma viral infection in transplanted kidneys. The active metabolite, A77172G, has a very long half-life (1–4 weeks). In those with arthritis, the loading dose is 100 mg daily for 3 days with a maintenance dose of 10–20 mg once daily. Side effects are few and include modest increase in blood pressure, mild gastrointestinal upset, reversible alopecia, leukopenia, and hepatitis. Stevens–Johnson syndrome may develop. Full blood count and liver function monitoring should be performed. FK778 is a synthetic malononitrilamide related to leflunomide and is currently being evaluated in allograft recipients.

Antimetabolites

Azathioprine

Indications Azathioprine is licensed to prolong survival in combination with glucocorticoids or other immunosuppressive agents in allograft recipients including those undergoing cardiac, kidney, or liver transplantation.

Pharmacodynamics Azathioprine is an imidazole derivative of 6-mercaptopurine (6MP) (an analogue of the purines, hypoxanthine and adenine). It is rapidly broken down in vivo by thiopurine methyl transferase (TPMT) to 6MP which rapidly crosses cell membranes. Once in the intracellular space, 6MP is further broken down into a number of purine thioanalogs including the main active metabolite thioinosine monophosphate. Although the exact mechanism of action remains unclear, it seems likely that a number of pathways for synthesis of nucleic acids are inhibited, thus preventing proliferation of cells involved in the determination and amplification of the immune response.

Pharmacokinetics Azathioprine may be given orally or as an intravenous injection and is well absorbed in the upper gastrointestinal tract. It undergoes rapid metabolism to 6MP and after intravenous injection the half-life is 6–28 min. The half-life of 6MP is similarly short at 38–114 min. Elimination is as 6-thiouric uric acid through the kidney.

Adverse effects Side effects of azathioprine include leukopenia (which may be significant in about 15%), hepatotoxicity (especially veno-occlusive disease), pancreatitis, pneumonitis, and megaloblastosis. After initiation of treatment, the white blood cell count should be monitored every 2 weeks and dose reduction instituted if the white count falls. Individuals with an inherited deficiency of TPMT may be unusually sensitive to the myelosuppressive effect of azathioprine and prone to developing rapid bone marrow suppression after starting treatment. Drug interactions are few but allopurinol (which competes for metabolism via xanthine oxidase) should be avoided because of the increased risk of bone marrow suppression.

Pregnancy and lactation Evidence of teratogenicity in humans is equivocal. There have been reports of preterm delivery and low birth weight following treatment with azathioprine, especially when it is given in combination with glucocorticoids. There have been extremely rare reports of physical abnormalities following treatment with azathioprine. 6MP has been shown in the breast milk of mothers who are breastfeeding, so mothers should be advised not to breastfeed.

Mizoribine

Indications Prophylaxis of acute rejection in kidney transplant recipients in combination with other immunosuppressive medication.

Pharmacodynamics The antimetabolite mizoribine is an imidazole nucleotide that blocks the purine biosynthesis pathway and thus inhibits T- and B-lymphocyte proliferation.

Pharmacokinetics Mizoribine is administered at a dose of 2 mg/kg per day.

Adverse effects Mizoribine is usually well tolerated but may cause hyperuricemia.

Cyclophosphamide

This is given orally or intravenously and, as a prodrug, requires hepatic metabolism to the active compound. A metabolite may induce a hemorrhagic cystitis.

Drugs that inhibit lymphocyte trafficking

FTY720

FTY720 is a potent agonist of the spingosine-1-phosphate receptor (SIPR). The effect of FTY720 is to sequester lymphocytes in the lymph nodes, away from the allograft and sites of inflammation. The agent also induces apoptosis in activated lymphocytes. More recently, it has been shown that FTY720 has anti-angiogenic properties, making it a potentially valuable agent in the immunosuppression of those transplanted for hepatocellular carcinoma. In contrast to conventional immunosuppressive agents, it does not affect the activation, proliferation, or effector functions of either B or T lymphocytes. In animal models, the agent is also effective in preventing the effects of ischemia/reperfusion injury. Preliminary studies in a variety of organ allograft recipients suggest that the agent is effective in maintaining graft function, at doses of 2.5–5 mg/day. Side effects include bradycardia because of the presence of the SIPR on atrial myocytes. Unfortunately, its development in transplantation has been suspended. However, the drug was recently approved for use in multiple sclerosis and therefore could re-emerge for off-label indications in the future.

Further reading

Augustine JJ, Bodziak KA, Hricik DE. Use of sirolimus in solid organ transplantation. *Drugs* 2007;**67**:369–91.

Bowman H, Lennard TW. Immunosuppressive drugs. *Br J Hosp Med.* 1992;**48**:570–9.

Campsen J, Zimmerman MA, Trotter JF, et al. Sirolimus and liver transplantation: clinical implications for hepatocellular carcinoma. *Exp Opin Pharmacother* 2007;**8**: 1275–82.

Cantarovich D, Vistoli F, Soulillou JP. Immunosuppression minimization in kidney transplantation. *Front Biosci* 2008;**13**:1413–32.

Ciancio G, Burke GW 3rd. Alemtuzumab (Campath-1H) in kidney transplantation. *Am J Transplant* 2008;**8**:15–20.

Danovitch G. Mycophenolate mofetil: a decade of clinical experience. *Transplantation* 2005;**80**:S272–4.

de Mattos AM, Olyaei AJ, Bennett WM. Pharmacology of immunosuppressive medications used in renal diseases and transplantation. *Am J Kidney Dis* 1996;**28**:631–67.

Grinyó JM, Cruzado JM. Mycophenolate mofetil and sirolimus combination in renal transplantation. *Am J Transplant* 2006;**6**:1991–9.

Gummert JF, Ikonen T, Morris RE. Newer immunosuppressive drugs: a review. *J Am Soc Nephrol* 1999; **10**:1366–80.

Haddad EM, McAlister VC, Renouf E, Malthaner R, Kjaer MS, Gluud LL. Cyclosporin versus tacrolimus for liver transplanted patients. *Cochrane Database Syst Rev* 2006;(4):CD005161.

Heisel O, Heisel R, Balshaw R, Keown P. New onset diabetes mellitus in patients receiving calcineurin inhibitors: a systematic review and meta-analysis. *Am J Transplant* 2004;**4**:583–95.

Hood KA, Zarembski DG. Mycophenolate mofetil: a unique immunosuppressive agent. *Am J Health Syst Pharm* 1997;**54**:285–94.

Kahan BD. Cyclosporine: the agent and its actions. *Transplant Proc* 1985;**17**:5S–18S.

Kapturczak MH, Meier-Kriesche HU, Kaplan B. Pharmacology of calcineurin antagonists. *Transplant Proc* 2004;**36**:25S–32S.

Kirk AD. Induction immunosuppression. *Transplantation* 2006;**8**:593–602.

MacGregor MS, Bradley JA. Overview of immunosuppressive therapy in organ transplantation. *Br J Hosp Med* 1995;**54**:276–84.

Morris PJ. Cyclosporine, FK-506 and other drugs in organ transplantation. *Curr Opin Immunol* 1991;**3**:748–51.

Mottershead M, Neuberger J. Daclizumab. *Exp Opin Biol Ther* 2007;**7**:1583–96.

Schiff J, Cole E, Cantarovich M. Therapeutic monitoring of calcineurin inhibitors for the nephrologist. *Clin J Am Soc Nephrol* 2007;**2**:374–84.

Shipkova M, Armstrong VW, Oellerich M, Wieland E. Mycophenolate mofetil in organ transplantation: focus on metabolism, safety and tolerability. *Exp Opin Drug Metab Toxicol* 2005;**1**:505–26.

Taylor AL, Watson CJ, Bradley JA. Immunosuppressive agents in solid organ transplantation: Mechanisms of action and therapeutic efficacy. *Crit Rev Oncol Hematol* 2005;**56**:23–46.

UK Renal Pharmacy Group. *The Renal Drug Handbook*. Oxford: Radcliffe Medical Press, 1999.

UK Renal Pharmacy Group. *The Renal Drug Handbook*, 2nd edn. Oxford: Radcliffe Medical Press, 2004.

Webster AC, Woodroffe RC, Taylor RS, Chapman JR, Craig JC. Tacrolimus versus ciclosporin as primary immunosuppression for kidney transplant recipients: meta-analysis and meta-regression of randomised trial data. *BMJ* 2005;**331**:810.

White DJ. Cyclosporin A. Clinical pharmacology and therapeutic potential. *Drugs* 1982;**24**:322–34.

Yabu JM, Vincenti F. Novel immunosuppression: small molecules and biologics. *Semin Nephrol* 2007;**27**: 479–86.

3 Medical management of the deceased donor in solid organ transplantation

John McCartney[1] *and Kenneth E Wood*[2]
[1]University of Wisconsin School of Medicine, Madison, Wisconsin, USA
[2]Trauma and Life Support Center, and Respiratory Care Medicine, University of Wisconsin School of Medicine, Wisconsin, USA

As waiting lists for each of the solid organs continue to lengthen, various strategies have emerged to combat the evolving dilemma of increased demand with a relatively stagnant supply. These include a spectrum of programs targeting the general population, ranging from public service initiatives designed to educate people about the dire need for organ donation to legislative programs aimed at simplifying processes for people to identify themselves as potential donors in the case of a catastrophic medical emergency. As surgical and medical techniques continue to advance, there has been ongoing re-evaluation of organ-specific donor criteria, attempting to optimize use of donors previously deemed unsuitable due to age or specific medical criteria. The last few years also have shown significant progress in the use of traditionally unacceptable classes of donors, such as those donating after cardiac death (DCD), as potential donation candidates. However, one of the largest and most readily available pools of potential organ donors, continually underappreciated in many hospitals, remain those patients who expire within their own intensive care units (ICUs). Many of these will have undergone extensive diagnostic and therapeutic evaluations, having never been recognized as reasonable candidates. When including the additional number of individuals who have been identified as potential candidates but sustain cardiovascular collapse and somatic cell death during the ensuing evaluation, before any actual procurement procedure, the number of missed donation opportunities is further increased.

For any patients who sustain a serious injury or illness, the initial approach focuses on attempts to restore them to their premorbid state. Whether the result of unexpected trauma in a previously healthy individual, or a new illness in the setting of someone with co-morbidities, each evaluation consists of the appropriate diagnostic studies and therapeutic interventions, provided in an efficient and expedited manner. At the time of initial presentation, either in the emergency room or shortly after arrival in the ICU, a small minority of patients will already have sustained a catastrophic injury to the central nervous system (CNS) and meet criteria for brain death. In this setting, candidacy for organ donation should be assessed immediately. If there is an absolute contraindication to their candidacy as a donor, or if the patient's representative refuses to consent to donation, life support should be withdrawn once the family has had an appropriate opportunity to gather and pay their respects.

A much larger portion of patients will present to critical care units with less severe levels of injury or illness. Each of these individuals will undergo the appropriate diagnostic evaluation specific to the unique circumstances and targeted therapeutic modalities will be initiated. Through advances in supportive care and monitoring techniques, it is now commonplace for individuals to survive illnesses that were historically thought to be fatal. Although these advances have yielded incredible results, a portion of

Primer on Transplantation, 3rd edition.
Edited by Donald Hricik.

these patients will still deteriorate and their inciting illness will ultimately prove to be fatal. Within the busy environment of a modern ICU, with complicated patient profiles and rapidly evolving hemodynamic derangements, it is crucial that appropriate surveillance protocols be employed to monitor those individuals who may represent potential organ donors.

For any individual, up until the point that a formal diagnosis of brain death has been declared, all aspects of patient care are focused on restoring the patient to the premorbid state. Utilizing pre-existing advanced directives, combined with serial discussions with family representatives when the patient is unable to adequately participate, an individualized care plan is formulated and then updated as changes to the patient's condition occur. The variable course for any individual patient through a catastrophic illness or injury must be recognized. It is crucial that appropriate surveillance and monitoring programs be well established in each center to identify those patients in whom evolving injury to the CNS is likely to proceed to brain death. Clinical triggers and notification of the local organ procurement organization (OPO) about those patients with a high likelihood of progression to brain death is a key component in any screening protocol. This assists the OPO and local transplant centers in the event that brain death is declared. It is crucial, during this entire process, that the needs of the individual patient and familial support are the focus. Establishing this framework assists with the ensuing discussions if the clinical situation deteriorates.

The bulk of this chapter deals with medical management of the brain-dead deceased donor. Non-heart-beating donors (i.e., DCDs) represent a growing proportion of deceased donors. Their management is addressed at the end of the chapter.

Declaration of brain death

Our understanding of brain death, from both an anatomical and a pathophysiologic perspective, has greatly evolved since the first description in 1959 by Mollaret and Goulon. *Le coma depasse*, literally termed "irreversible coma," represented a series of comatose patients with absent brain-stem reflexes, lack of respirations, and absence of electroencephalographic (EEG) activity. This description remains the mainstay of criteria for brain death as accepted both medically and legally today. Medical, legal, and bioethical issues related to declaration of brain death were first formally discussed through an ad hoc committee at Harvard Medical School in 1968 and further examined through the Conference of the Medical Royal Colleges and Faculties in the UK in 1976. In 1981, the President's Commission for the Study of Ethical Problems in Medicine and Biomedical and Behavioral Research published definitions clarifying specific criteria equating brain death with cardiovascular death.

During this same time period, the technical aspects of routine ICU care have evolved tremendously, making it possible to invasively support virtually every organ system. From advancements in hemodynamic monitoring and ventilator strategies to extracorporeal renal replacement therapy, the ability to maintain somatic cell function in the setting of severe neurologic compromise for indefinite periods of time is now possible. There is a much greater understanding of the physiologic changes that accompany severe brain injuries that lead to elevated intracranial pressures and ultimately herniation of the brain stem through the foramen ovale. The natural protective strategy is to maintain the perfusion of the CNS. In the setting of increased intracranial pressure, whether induced by hemorrhage, edema, a mass, or any other space-occupying process, the compensatory strategy is to elevate mean arterial pressure to maximize end-organ tissue perfusion. In this light, each of the pathophysiologic processes observed as a patient with catastrophic injury to the CNS evolves to actual brain death represents failed attempts at maintaining perfusion. Within this context, it is essential that each person participating in the care of patients within an ICU has a clear understanding of the criteria for the declaration of brain death. It is also important to note that there may be local variances in the declaration process. Information of both state and local requirements should be available in every ICU.

Briefly, the declaration of brain death requires detailed examination, demonstrating the loss of all brain function in the appropriate clinical setting without confounding variables. This begins with a detailed neurological examination of the comatose patient demonstrating loss of all reaction to painful stimuli in all four extremities. This is followed by careful examination for the loss of all brain-stem functions, including oculocephalic, vestibular, corneal, pupillary, and gag reflexes. This examination must occur in the appropriate clinical setting with an injury or illness pattern compatible with the degree of central nervous compromise encountered and appropriate radiographic findings. Equally important is the verification of any confounding variables that may interfere with the clinical examination. These include, but are not limited to, drug intoxications, severe electrolyte or endocrine disturbances, extreme temperature derangements, or the administration of sedatives, hypnotics, or neuromuscular paralyzing agents. There is no uniformly accepted standard for the qualifications of those performing this examination. In some locales, this examination must be repeated on two occasions with a certain waiting time between examinations. In others, two examinations performed at the same time by different qualified providers will suffice. Knowledge of accepted local practices is required.

Once confounding variables have been excluded, coma is established, and brain-stem function is absent, the next step involves performing an apnea test and assessing the patient's response to hypercapnia. An apnea test is performed by preoxygenating the individual on 100% FiO_2 (inspired oxygen fraction). A baseline arterial blood gas is then obtained and the patient is removed from mechanical ventilation. At some centers, the patient is maintained on 100% FiO_2 and continuous positive airway pressure (CPAP); at others, the patient is removed from the ventilatory circuit and an oxygen catheter is inserted through the endotracheal tube to the carina where 6–12 L of oxygen are delivered. In either protocol, it is essential that the patient does not receive any ventilatory support. The patient is then observed for any evidence of spontaneous respiratory effort. If there is any effort such as chest movement, the test is terminated and the patient, although severely injured, does not meet the criteria for brain death. Assuming that there are no signs of respiratory effort, after 8–10 min an arterial blood gas is obtained for reassessment of the gas tension of carbon dioxide (PCO_2). A PCO_2 > 8 kPa (>60 mmHg) demonstrates the patient's inability to respond to hypercapnia and is consistent with brain death. If the PCO_2 has not risen above 8 kPa (60 mmHg), the test should be repeated for an extended period of time. In the setting of an elevated baseline PCO_2, such as may be seen in underlying lung disease, a positive test is typically described as a rise of >4 kPa (20 mmHg) in PCO_2 above the baseline. If the patient develops hemodynamic instability or profound hypoxia during testing, typically defined as saturations <85% monitored by pulse oximetry, an arterial blood gas should be immediately obtained and the patient placed back on mechanical ventilation. If the above criteria are fulfilled, then the test is considered positive.

Key points 3.1 Elements of a positive apnea test in determination of brain death

Removal from respirator:

Continued administration of oxygen

Absence of chest movements

After 8–10 min, PCO_2 8 kPa (>60 mmHg) or >4 kPa (>20 mmHg) above baseline if previously hypercapnic

Patients who have a clinical examination consistent with brain death in the absence of any confounding issues and a positive apnea test are declared brain dead. The inability to perform any part of the physical examination such as a full cranial nerve examination due to facial injury or instability during apnea testing mandates a confirmatory test. There are four currently accepted confirmatory tests for the diagnosis of brain death and any of the four can be employed based on local resource availability and physician preference; they include an EEG demonstrating the absence of electrical activity, a technetium (^{99m}Tc) brain scan showing lack of uptake in the brain parenchyma (the "hollow skull" sign), transcranial Doppler sonography demonstrating lack of diastolic or reverberating flow, or cerebral angiography revealing lack of flow at the carotid bifurcation and circle of Willis. As discussed above, with very rare religious exceptions, it is now widely accepted that a formal declaration of brain death is equivalent to cardiovascular death. In the scenario where organ donation will not be pursued, the family should be given the opportunity to gather and pay their respects before the termination of life support, but, legally, the patient has already expired.

In the scenario where a patient is pronounced brain dead and a possible organ donor, care should be directed toward maintenance of the potentially transplantable organs. During the evaluation period, the basic axioms of critical care guide therapy. In many circumstances, the initial resuscitation of a potential donor involves correction of severe volume, acid–base, and electrolyte abnormalities that have evolved during the failed therapeutic attempts to combat an elevated intracranial pressure. It is not uncommon for patients to be markedly volume depleted and/or severely hypernatremic as a consequence of CNS-protective strategies such as use of mannitol or other osmotic diuretic agents. In many institutions, there is a natural tendency to diminish the intensity of support in this patient population. However, the need for aggressive ICU level monitoring and support is imperative to prevent hemodynamic collapse and cardiac arrest before organ procurement can be undertaken. This time period immediately after brain death is marked by intense hemodynamic instability related to the combined effects of the initial injury, the resuscitative effort, and the pathophysiologic effects of brain death. The processes leading to herniation of the brain, combined with the compensatory hemodynamic mechanisms that occur in an effort to maintain tissue perfusion, establish the framework of pathophysiology upon which the clinical care of the potential organ donor is based.

Consent for organ donation

To maximize the potential pool for organ donors, it is imperative that a uniform approach to consent exist for every person who expires. This is best accomplished through protocols using people trained in these discussions. As part of this process, it is crucial that families understand the definition of brain death. Although their loved one still has a palpable pulse and beating heart, he or she has expired, irrespective of any decisions re organ donation. Any decisions to participate in organ or tissue donation do not impact the timing of religious services or disfigure the body in a manner that precludes visitation and viewing customs. It is important to separate the process of brain death declaration from the request for organ donation in order to allow appropriate time for questions, grieving, and acceptance. There is tremendous variability in the conversion rate of potential donors to actual donors. Any protocol designed to improve this conversion must include components of surveillance to identify those patients likely to progress to brain death, a standardized protocol for the declaration of brain death, a uniform process of request for organ donation, and optimal medical management of all potential donors.

Case

A 21-year-old man sustained massive head trauma in a motor vehicle accident. Although his prognosis was grim at presentation, he initially exhibited spontaneous respirations precluding declaration of brain death. The bereaved family asked the nursing staff about possible organ donation but expressed concern about further mutilation of the body. A representative from the local organ procurement agency met with the family, spoke at length about the concept of brain death, and assured them that an organ procurement procedure would not interfere with viewing of the body or a funeral. Twelve hours later, the man was declared brain dead and the family consented to donation of all viable organs.

Physiology of brain death

Ischemia–reperfusion injury

The physiology of severe CNS injury, and the resultant pathology that is observed clinically is most consistent with ischemia-reperfusion injury. In the setting of elevated intracranial pressures, the rostral–caudal progression of ischemia resulting in herniation and brain death produces a predictable hemodynamic pattern. As the ischemia evolves to include the medulla oblongata, a profound autonomic surge of catecholamines develops in a final attempt to maintain cerebral perfusion pressures in the setting of increasing intracranial pressure. This catecholamine surge typically produces intense peripheral vasoconstriction and cardiac stimulation resulting in transient hypertension. After the subsequent brain-stem herniation and spinal denervation, there is deactivation of the sympathetic nervous system with the resultant vasodilation and reduced catecholamine levels. Unfortunately, this process results in a reduction in cardiac stimulation and hemodynamic instability. There is evolving evidence, as described below, that this process leads to an intense ischemia–reperfusion injury, with an associated inflammatory response and further endothelial injury. As this process evolves, the contribution of injury to the neuroendocrine structures within the CNS may further impact the hemodynamic instability that is frequently encountered.

Hypothalamic–pituitary axis

To understand the compensatory mechanisms that develop in the setting of a significant injury to the CNS, a basic knowledge of the underlying anatomic structures is required. This is particularly important when considering the specific components of the hypothalamic–pituitary axis which regulates control of virtually every component of the endocrine system. Anatomically, the hypothalamus is located at the base of the brain between the optic chiasma and the third ventricle. Through the pituitary stalk, a complicated portal vascular network connects the median eminence of the hypothalamus and the anterior portion of the pituitary gland, which lies immediately outside the dura in the sella turcica. The pituitary gland itself develops from two distinct embryologic tissues, the adenohypophysis, or anterior pituitary, and the neurohypophysis, or posterior pituitary. The anterior pituitary is derived from the embryologic oral cavity within Rathke's pouch, whereas the posterior pituitary is formed from neural ectoderm of the embryologic forebrain. Although these two structures combine during early development to form the complete pituitary gland, they continue to retain distinctly different innervations, blood supplies, and hormone production. In this way, they can be thought of as two different endocrine structures.

The blood supply to the hypothalamus arises from the superior hypophyseal artery. The anterior pituitary itself does not actually have a direct arterial supply, instead receiving blood flow from the hypothalamus through the intricate vascular network described previously. The posterior pituitary receives its arterial blood supply through the inferior hypophyseal artery. The venous drainage is also distinctly different, through the petrosal sinuses, and ultimately the internal jugular vein for the anterior system, and through the inferior hypophyseal vein for the posterior pituitary.

This dual blood supply serves to emphasize a stark contrast between the hormone products and regulatory processes of the anterior and posterior pituitary structures. The anterior pituitary gland is isolated from the systemic circulation, receiving blood flow exclusively through the low-pressure, portal vasculature. The median eminence of the hypothalamus is thus able to exert precise control over the anterior pituitary through release of small peptide regulatory hormones without significant dilution or degradation within the systemic circulation. The close proximity of these structures also allows high concentrations of these mediators with relatively little production in a pulsatile fashion. Conversely, hormone regulation of the posterior pituitary occurs through direct neuronal connections from the hypothalamus, originating in the supraoptic and paraventricular nuclei. Many hormones produced in the anterior pituitary, including growth hormone, luteinizing hormone, adrenocorticotropic hormone, thyroid-stimulating hormone (TSH), follicle-stimulating hormone, melanocyte-stimulating hormone, and endorphins. The two primary hormones derived from the posterior pituitary are vasopressin and oxytocin. In total, these various hormones represent virtually every aspect of the human endocrine system and account for much of normal homeostasis. Any injury to the hypothalamic–pituitary axis, whether directly due to trauma, vascular insult, or infection, or indirectly through elevated intracranial pressures, can disrupt both the formation and release of these various hormones.

There has been conflicting data about the extent to which dysfunction of the hypothalamic–pituitary axis affects the hemodynamic instability in potential organ donors. In animal models, which typically include a model of brain death in which a balloon inserted into the cranium is suddenly expanded, there have been multiple studies demonstrating a decline in both anterior and posterior pituitary hormone levels. In human studies, the decline in pituitary hormone levels has been more inconsistent, likely reflective of the heterogeneity of the injury patterns and variability in the timing from actual brain death to the declaration process. In addition, there is mixed evidence from both animal and human studies demonstrating improvement in hemodynamic parameters after hormone supplementation. There is significant experimental and clinical evidence of posterior dysfunction leading to vasopressin deficiency and diabetes insipidus. When this is manifest clinically by profound dilute diuresis in the setting of increased serum osmolarity, treatment with arginine vasopressin should be added to the regimen.

The issue of thyroid replacement in this setting has been the subject of debate. Although multiple studies have demonstrated low thyroxine (T_4) and TSH levels after brain death, in studies where reverse-triiodothyronine (rT_3) levels have been measured, the pattern is more consistent with "euthyroid sick syndrome." As T_4 has inotropic properties, it is not entirely clear whether the hemodynamic improvement after thyroid supplementation represents correction of endocrine dysfunction or simply augmented cardiac function. The role of adrenal insufficiency in potential organ donors and the effects of supplementation with exogenous glucocorticoids have also been controversial. Several studies have demonstrated improved hemodynamic parameters and improved conversion rates with utilization of hormonal replacement protocols. In potential organ donors with continued hemodynamic instability after appropriate volume replacement, it is reasonable to consider hormonal supplementation, typically consisting of a combination of T_4, glucocorticoids, and vasopressin.

Donor criteria

For each solid organ that can be transplanted, there are both general and organ-specific contraindications to donation. The absolute contraindications include a variety of infections, such as those with human immunodeficiency virus (HIV), prion-related diseases, human T-cell leukemia–lymphoma virus (HTLV), and systemic viral infections such as measles. Although bacteremia and fungemia will frequently preclude donation, they are not absolute contraindications and may be allowable in appropriate circumstances. Patients with active malignancies, with the exception of non-melanoma skin cancers and certain brain tumors, are not considered possible donors. In those with a history of malignancy, the duration of disease-free existence and cell type help determine possible candidacy.

The ideal donor for any organ is a previously healthy individual with an intense, abrupt, and isolated CNS injury with little systemic compromise. Such individuals constitute the vast minority of donors. Specific criteria for each organ system vary based on the organ in question. Arguably the organ system typically precluded due to specific donor criteria is the lung, representing the unique potential for injury or insult within the pulmonary system. With any significant CNS injury, there is the potential for aspiration due to difficulties with airway protection. In addition, in those potential donors with prolonged resuscitative efforts, there is potential for barotrauma, ventilator-associated infections, and iatrogenic complications that may all negatively impact the potential for donation. The ideal lung donor is aged less than 55 years, has a PaO_2/FiO_2 ratio > 300 on FiO_2 100% on 5 cmH_2O of PEEP (positive end-expiratory pressure), a clear chest radiograph with the absence of chest trauma, aspiration, purulent secretions, or malignancy, and a minimal smoking history. The appropriateness of these criteria has recently been challenged and attempts to increase the donor pool by expanding these criteria are under review. It is ultimately the responsibility of the OPO and directors of the transplant center to authorize the appropriateness of an individual donor.

Key points 3.2 Definition of an ideal lung donor

Aged <55 years

PaO_2/FiO_2 ratio of >300 on 5 cmH_2O of positive end-expiratory pressure

Clear chest radiograph

Smoking history <20 pack-years

Absence of:

Chest trauma

Aspiration

Purulent secretions

Malignancy

Cardiovascular management

Consistent with the approach to management of any critically ill patient, a fundamental understanding of the physiology of the pertinent illness provides the basis for optimal management strategies. Donor management necessitates an ongoing level of intensity;

however, it is imperative that the focus ultimately shifts from cerebral protective strategies to optimizing donor organs for transplantation. In effect, this is the simultaneous medical management of organs for eight potential recipients. Cardiovascular management is the cornerstone of donor management and facilitates donor somatic survivorship, which ensures that all organs can be procured. Similarly, optimal hemodynamic management and adequate perfusion pressures maintain all organs to be procured in the best possible condition. Lastly, the recently recognized inflammatory response of brain death related to ischemia–reperfusion injury is proposed to initiate the development of an immunologic continuum between the donor and recipient. Optimal hemodynamic management mitigates ongoing ischemia–reperfusion injury which can facilitate better graft function in the recipient.

Contributing factors

Cardiovascular and hemodynamic dysfunctions encountered during management of the potential organ donor represent a continuum of cardiovascular injury that starts with the initial neurologic insult to the brain. It has long been recognized that severe neurologic injury produces cardiac dysfunction. Recognizing that the magnitude of injury in the non-survivor of severe brain injury is likely greater than in survivors, it seems plausible to assume that the cardiovascular dysfunction is similarly more severe and compounded by the physiologic effects of brain death, including profound levels of vasodilation and endocrine dysfunction. A non-aggressive approach to hemodynamic stabilization or an inability to maintain coronary perfusion pressure gradients will contribute to the hemodynamic instability of the potential organ donor.

Neurocardiac injury patterns reported in patients with subarachnoid hemorrhage illustrate the effects related to the initial insult particularly well. In this population, the magnitude of the neurologic injury assessed by the Hunt–Hess score is a significant predictor of the extent of myocardial necrosis and echocardiographic abnormalities seen after the precipitating event. It appears that the mechanism of injury is related to excessive sympathetic stimulation and release of catecholamines. Systolic impairment has been reported in 10–28% of patients and diastolic dysfunction has been observed in 70% of patients with subarachnoid hemorrhage. It is important to recognize that a significant percentage of surviving patients with cardiac dysfunction will recover left ventricular systolic function over time. Unfortunately, echocardiographic evidence of left ventricular dysfunction often precludes procurement of the heart for transplantation.

The impact of brain death on cardiovascular function was first recognized in the early 1980s by the cardiovascular transplantation group in South Africa (28). When comparing hearts that were taken from healthy anesthetized baboons to hearts taken from brain-dead donors, the investigators noted that there was appreciable dysfunction in the brain-dead donor hearts. The investigators speculated that the significant dysfunction was related to the physiology of brain death and subsequently characterized the physiology of brain death through a series of elegant experiments. That physiology is characterized by an initial intense sympathetic surge, termed the "autonomic surge," reflecting a profound rise in circulating catecholamines as a compensatory response to maintain cerebral perfusion pressure gradients in the context of elevated intracranial pressure. This autonomic surge is associated with significant histopathologic changes in the myocardium, electrocardiographic changes indicative of ischemia, and functional impairment of cardiac contractility. The failure of the autonomic surge to maintain cerebral perfusion pressure gradients results in herniation with spinal cord ischemia, brain death, and resultant vasodilation.

Key points 3.3 Sequential physiologic events associated with severe central nervous system injury leading to brain death

- Autonomic surge that occurs in an effort to preserve cerebral perfusion
- Impaired cardiac contractility
- Herniation of the brain with spinal cord ischemia
- Brain death and profound vasodilation

The importance of the autonomic surge in human donors was recently illustrated in a study that reported significant improvement in donor myocardial function when the autonomic surge was aborted pharmacologically. Treatment with esmolol, uradipil, or nicardipine resulted in preservation of left ventricular ejection fraction and a higher rate of cardiac procurement. This study is cited solely to illustrate the potential impact of the catecholamine surge on the donor heart and not to advocate this as standard therapy.

The endocrine changes associated with brain death were first described by Novitzky and Cooper in a baboon model of brain death that results in a significant decrease in circulating thyroid hormones. Although well described in animal models, similar findings have been observed somewhat inconsistently in human organ donors. It has been proposed that the use of hormone resuscitation therapy consisting of thyroid hormone, steroids, insulin, and glucose facilitates the return of cardiac function and improves rates of procurement for all organs. Although frequently employed in donor management, hormone resuscitation therapy remains controversial and is discussed further.

To summarize, cardiovascular and hemodynamic management of the potential organ donor is complicated by the neurocardiac injury of the initial insult and the sequelae of physiologic events accompanying brain death. Optimal outcomes require aggressive management during the period immediately preceding brain death and in the period between brain death and declaration, and the securing of consent. The remainder of this section reviews a structured approach to the hemodynamic management of the potential organ donor.

Management algorithm

Figure 3.1 provides an overview of the cardiovascular and hemodynamic approach to the management of potential organ donors. All potential donors should be assessed for stability of mean arterial blood pressure, urine output, and extent of vasoactive support. Echocardiographic assessment of cardiac function is essential but interpretation of results depends critically on the timing of the studies as discussed below. In those potential organ donors achieving the stability thresholds identified in Figure 3.1, further cardiac assessment, sometimes including cardiac catheterization, should be undertaken if the donor is of suitable age and if procurement of the heart is being considered. As noted previously, many potential organ donors will have significant cardiac dysfunction. Echocardiographic studies performed immediately after brain death and before hemodynamic stabilization will likely reveal significant cardiac dysfunction.

The recent literature highlights the impact of echocardiographic assessment of left ventricular function on cardiac transplantation rates. In one study, 44% of potential heart donors did not have cardiac procurement. Echocardiographic abnormalities accounted for failure to procure hearts in 28% of cases and the odd ratio for failure of cardiac procurement increased by 1.4 for every 5% decrease in ejection fraction. It is important to emphasize that echocardiographic abnormalities do not always reflect histopathologic changes in the myocardium. In a recent echocardiographic study that evaluated 66 consecutive brain dead donors evaluated as heart donors, echocardiographic systolic dysfunction was evident in 42%. In those autopsied hearts that were not procured, there was a very poor correlation between the area of echocardiographic abnormality and the histopathology assessed at autopsy. Therefore, no heart should be excluded based on an initial echocardiogram. In a study that evaluated potential organ donors with ejection fractions <50% that were initially deemed not suitable for procurement, aggressive medical management was undertaken and resulted in 13 of 16 donors with an initial rejection procured with outcomes similar to ideal hearts.

Troponins are often used to evaluate cardiac suitability in potential organ donors because they are thought to reflect myocardial damage. Early studies strongly suggested that the presence of cardiac troponin concentrations was associated with significant cardiac dysfunction in the donor and caution was advocated about the use of donor hearts with elevated troponin levels. However, recent investigations have provided conflicting evidence. In a retrospective study that reviewed hearts accepted for transplantation, troponin levels were normal in 96 donors and elevated in 43 donors. This study reported that the recipients of hearts from donors with an elevated troponin level did not have a significant difference in the recipient need for circulatory support, nor was there any difference in short-term or longitudinal mortality. The authors concluded that minor troponin elevations were not associated with an

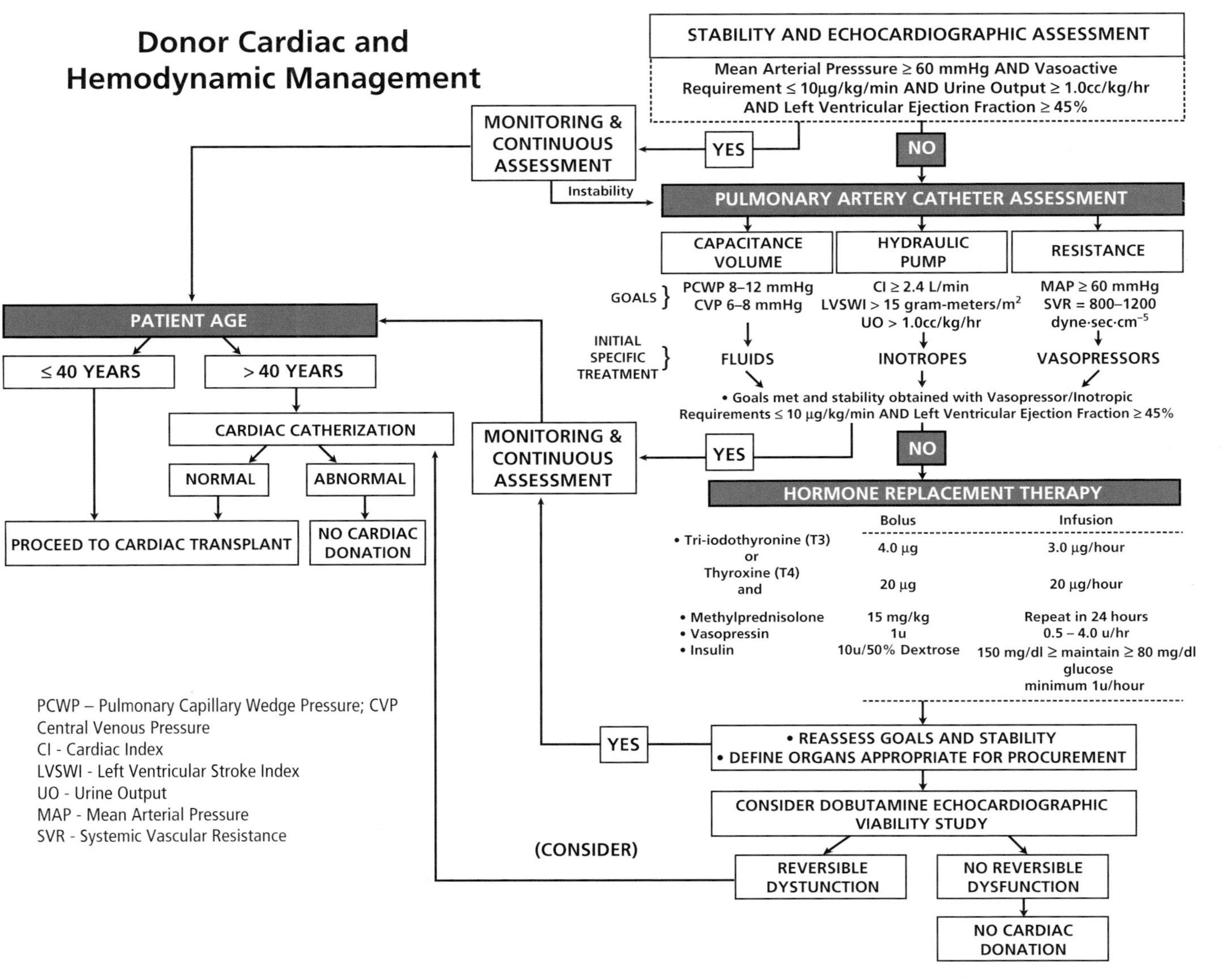

Figure 3.1 Algorithm for hemodynamic management of the deceased donor. Reproduced with permission of Massachusetts Medical Society.

increased risk of recipient mortality and suggested that potential heart donors should not be discarded based on troponin elevations alone.

Similar to the care of critically ill patients, an interdisciplinary approach employing the skills of intensivists, pulmonary and cardiac consultants, nurses, and respiratory therapists in concert with the OPO coordinator is strongly advocated. In one study, standardizing donor management through a protocol that relied on recommendations for general management, laboratory and diagnostic studies, and respiratory therapy during the continuum of referral, declaration, and consent resulted in a 10.3% increase per 100 donor organs recovered and a 3.3% increase in total organs per 100 donor organs transplanted. Similar dramatic improvements in the rates of organ procurement have been reported with the development of an organ donor management team dedicated to the aggressive management of potential organ donors. Utilizing an approach that consisted of early recognition of potential organ donor, a dedicated team involved in the medical management of the donor and aggressive resuscitation, the University of Southern California Trauma Intensive Care Team, reported that brain death-related complications had no effect on the number of organs donated. When comparing conventional donor management with an aggressive donor management team employing a standard protocol, multiple benefits were realized, including a significantly decreased number of donors lost from cardiovascular collapse and an increase in the number of organs recovered per donor.

Failure to achieve the stability thresholds identified in Figure 3.1 necessitates invasive monitoring to define the appropriateness of intravascular volume, cardiac function and the extent of vasodilation. The Canadian Counsel for Donation and Transplantation has recommended the following guiding principles for hemodynamic donor management:

- There should be clear recognition that intensivists characteristically titrate cardiovascular therapy to clinical, biochemical, and hemodynamic endpoints that ensure restoration and adequacy of intravascular volume without excess volume, and appropriate support of cardiac function and vascular tone to ensure optimal cardiac flow for organ perfusion.
- The use of vasoactive cardiovascular support assumes that intravascular volume has been adequately restored.
- Evaluation of cardiovascular function and hemodynamic status is a global measurement of multiple variables and no single measurement variable in isolation should dictate therapy.
- Escalation to include vasoactive support should be accompanied by an escalation in hemodynamic monitoring
- Key stability thresholds should serve as targets to guide therapy. However, rigid adherence to numbers should be balanced by the overall clinical evaluation of cardiovascular status similar to any other critically ill patient. Cardiovascular support should be based upon rational physiology with pure vasopressors (vasopressin, phenylephrine) distinguished from vasopressors with β agonists with inotropic action (norepinephrine, epinephrine).

As a consequence of therapies designed to minimize intracranial pressure elevations, the potential organ donor characteristically exhibits intravascular volume depletion, cardiac dysfunction, and vasodilation. Figure 3.2 depicts the differential diagnosis of hemodynamic instability in the potential organ donor. Hypovolemia is common secondary to the use of fluid restriction, diuretics, and mannitol. Diabetes insipidus and stress-induced hyperglycemic osmolar diuresis additionally contribute to decreased effective intravascular volume. These may be superimposed on the inadequate intravascular volume resuscitation, a capillary leak syndrome, or hypothermic diuresis. Cardiac dysfunction and vasodilation are usually coincident processes, primarily attributable to the brain death phenomenon, although other factors may contribute as depicted in Figure 3.2.

Fluid resuscitation

Fluid resuscitation should be based on an assessment of intravascular volume using measurement of either a central venous pressure (CVP) or pulmonary artery capillary wedge pressure (PCWP). Transfusion of packed red blood cells should be prescribed to maintain a hematocrit of at least 30% to promote oxygen delivery. Initial expansion of the intravascular volume when appropriate should be undertaken with 0.9% saline, even in the presence of hypernatremia. Subsequent to the correction of intravascular volume deficits and titration of fluid resuscitation to endpoints depicted in Figure 3.1, correction of hypernatremia should be undertaken using either Ringer's

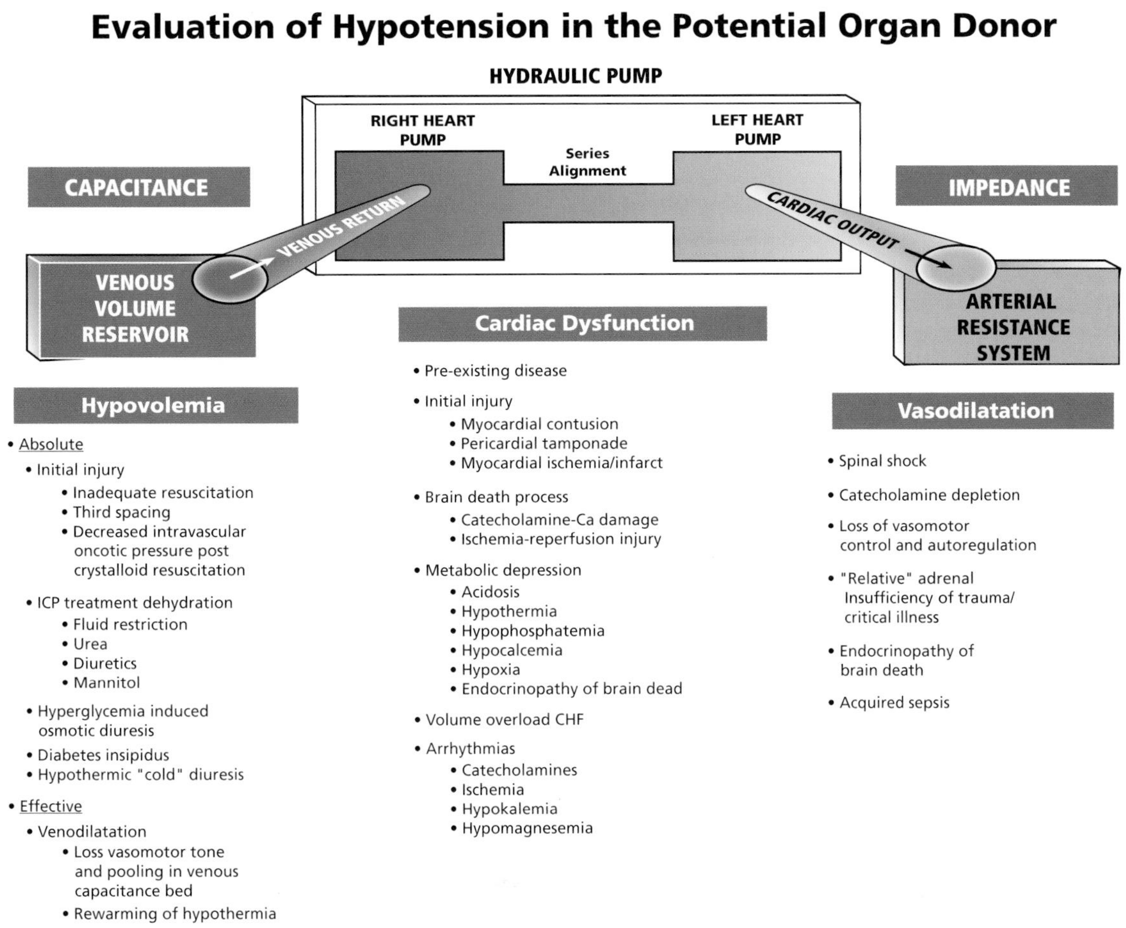

Evaluation of Hypotension in the Potential Organ Donor

HYDRAULIC PUMP

RIGHT HEART PUMP

Series Alignment

LEFT HEART PUMP

CAPACITANCE

VENOUS RETURN

VENOUS VOLUME RESERVOIR

CARDIAC OUTPUT

IMPEDANCE

ARTERIAL RESISTANCE SYSTEM

Hypovolemia

- Absolute
  - Initial injury
    - Inadequate resuscitation
    - Third spacing
    - Decreased intravascular oncotic pressure post crystalloid resuscitation
  - ICP treatment dehydration
    - Fluid restriction
    - Urea
    - Diuretics
    - Mannitol
  - Hyperglycemia induced osmotic diuresis
  - Diabetes insipidus
  - Hypothermic "cold" diuresis
- Effective
  - Venodilatation
    - Loss vasomotor tone and pooling in venous capacitance bed
    - Rewarming of hypothermia

Cardiac Dysfunction

- Pre-existing disease
- Initial injury
  - Myocardial contusion
  - Pericardial tamponade
  - Myocardial ischemia/infarct
- Brain death process
  - Catecholamine-Ca damage
  - Ischemia-reperfusion injury
- Metabolic depression
  - Acidosis
  - Hypothermia
  - Hypophosphatemia
  - Hypocalcemia
  - Hypoxia
  - Endocrinopathy of brain dead
- Volume overload CHF
- Arrhythmias
  - Catecholamines
  - Ischemia
  - Hypokalemia
  - Hypomagnesemia

Vasodilatation

- Spinal shock
- Catecholamine depletion
- Loss of vasomotor control and autoregulation
- "Relative" adrenal Insufficiency of trauma/critical illness
- Endocrinopathy of brain death
- Acquired sepsis

Figure 3.2 Pathophysiologic considerations in evaluating hypotension in a potential deceased donor. Reproduced with permission of Massachusetts Medical Society.

lactate solution or hypotonic saline. Given the frequent competing and antagonistic fluid resuscitation strategies related to lung and renal procurement, it is imperative to judiciously assess the adequacy of fluid resuscitation using endpoints of CVP or PCWP. Maintenance of renal function is facilitated by a more aggressive approach to volume resuscitation as case series have suggested that maintaining a urine output in excess of 100 mL/h in the hour before transplantation correlates with optimal postoperative renal function in the recipient. On the other hand, excessive fluid resuscitation against a background of brain death-induced changes in lung permeability may precipitate the accrual of extravascular lung water, jeopardizing lung suitability as the PaO_2/FiO_2 ratio becomes impaired and infiltrates appear on the chest radiograph. One of the most common reasons for failure to procure lungs is progressive pulmonary dysfunction consequent on excess resuscitation.

Vasoactive support

After the assessment of intravascular volume and titration of fluid resuscitation to the endpoints defined in Figure 3.1, many donors require vasoactive support. Previously, there was a reluctance to employ vasoactive support in the potential organ donor because of concerns that vasopressors might jeopardize organ function in the recipient. However, multiple recent series have reported negligible or non-existent associations between the level of vasoactive support in the donor and the outcome for the transplant recipient.

The putative adverse effects of catecholamines were most often reported in retrospective studies that provided inadequate details about assessment and normalization of intravascular volume. Indeed, recent investigations suggest that use of catecholamines may beneficially affect recipient renal function through their immunomodulatory effects on the inflammatory response. However, no firm recommendations regarding the specific vasoactive agent of choice can be made because randomized controlled trials are lacking. At this time, it would appear that therapy should be targeted and focused on the dominant physiologic abnormality. In cases of significant vasodilation, agents that promote vasoconstriction such as vasopressin, phenylephrine, or norepinephrine should be used. When the predominant physiologic abnormality is cardiac dysfunction, agents with greater inotropic support, such as dopamine or dobutamine, would be appropriate. Modulating and defining the specific combination of various agents are predicated upon variables derived from invasive monitoring or serial echocardiographic studies.

Hormone replacement therapy

Failure to achieve the predetermined thresholds identified in Figure 3.1 through the use of fluid resuscitation and vasoactive support warrants consideration for hormone replacement therapy (HRT). In the past, HRT was reserved for donors with ongoing hemodynamic instability. However, a recent large retrospective review of potential organ donors suggested that the combination of methylprednisolone, vasopressin, and thyroid hormone exerted a significant benefit for potential donors. The rate of organ procurement and corresponding organ transplantation was significantly higher in the HRT group. This same retrospective review concluded that cardiac recipient outcomes were dramatically improved by the use of HRT. It is important to recognize that these were retrospective and uncontrolled trials. HRT remains a controversial approach, which is best illustrated by the contrast in recommendations from two recent reviews of reported trials using HRT. One review concluded that routine administration of thyroid hormone in the management of potential organ donor was not warranted, although rescue replacement was deemed appropriate in some cases. In contrast, the review of Novitzky et al. (see Further reading) concluded that HRT results in dramatic improvement in cardiac function, enabling a greater rate of organ procurement. Insofar as there appear to be potential benefits and few adverse effects of HRT, it has become increasingly employed as a standard of practice in the early phases of organ donor management. Until randomized controlled trials provide guidance, it would seem appropriate to assess the need for HRT on a case-by-case basis.

Respiratory management

Respiratory management of the potential organ donor is frequently complicated by factors that result in lung procurement rates appreciably lower than those of other organs. Frequently, the pulmonary history of the patient is unknown and there may be underlying lung disease related to prior infections, occupational exposures, or use of tobacco that are not readily apparent on the presentation and initial evaluation of the donor. The causative event resulting in brain death, particularly when associated with trauma, is almost uniformly associated with aspiration and may be associated with pulmonary contusion. The period in the ICU further contributes to pulmonary dysfunction related to the complications of mechanical ventilation, including barotrauma, aspiration, hospital-acquired pneumonia, the effects of oxygen toxicity, and atelectasis.

The role of brain death in donor lung injury has traditionally been ascribed to neurogenic pulmonary edema. Consequent on the herniation process and the autonomic surge with high catecholamine levels, a blast injury to the pulmonary vasculature is proposed to initiate a transient massive hydrostatic pressure gradient that precipitates accumulation of alveolar fluid. Structural damage to the capillary endothelium similarly occurs secondary to the sympathetic activity. Recently, an intense inflammatory response has been described in which inflammatory cytokines activate endothelial cells to express adhesion molecules and mediate the production of interleukin-8 (IL-8). This neutrophil activator stimulates neutrophils and precipitates the release of reactive oxygen species and proteolytic enzymes that further enhance lung permeability.

The consequences of pulmonary donor inflammation have been well described by Fisher et al. (see

Further reading) in cases of non-traumatic brain death. Using open lung biopsy and bronchial alveolar lavage, they found that the concentration of neutrophils and IL-8 was dramatically higher in patients who sustained brain death compared with controls. Subsequent investigations correlated the extent of donor inflammation with recipient outcome and found a close correlation between the magnitude of the IL-8 expression and neutrophilic infiltration with graft function and recipient survival. This suggests that there is a preclinical injury to the lungs consequent on the brain death process and provides further evidence of the immunologic continuum between the donor and recipient.

The criteria for defining an "ideal" lung for transplantation were established early in the transplant era and have been criticized as arbitrary and capricious. These criteria generally include a PaO_2/FiO_2 ratio >300, a PEEP requirement <5 cmH_2O, a clear chest radiograph, age <55 years, tobacco use <20 pack-years, and the absence of trauma, surgery, aspiration secretions, malignancy, or infective-appearing secretions. Many lungs are precluded from procurement because of these stringent criteria. In a study that assessed lungs rejected for procurement because of pulmonary edema, the authors concluded that 41% of rejected lungs were potentially suitable for transplantation. Similar results were reported by Fisher et al. who compared the intensity of the inflammatory response in donors who were accepted to that of donors who were excluded by clinical criteria. Based on indices of inflammation; there was no difference between lungs that were accepted and those that were excluded, prompting the authors to conclude that the current selection criteria represented a very poor discriminator of pulmonary injury and that many lungs are unnecessarily excluded.

Although some lungs are able to maintain their ideal characteristics from brain death to procurement, many lungs are considered marginal. Marginality is traditionally defined as those lungs with a breech in the conventional criteria related to their baseline status, independent of problems acquired in the ICU. Lungs may also be characterized as marginal as a consequence of acquired and reversible processes in the ICU such as atelectasis, alveolar fluid accumulation, and aspiration. Newer respiratory and pulmonary management techniques have resulted in dramatic improvements in rates of lung procurement. In a study designed to maximize utilization of donor lungs for transplantation, Gabbay applied routine pulmonary and respiratory ICU management techniques consisting of manipulations of mechanical ventilation and PEEP, chest physiotherapy, ensuring appropriate fluid balance, and bronchoscopy in a pool of potential organ donors. In the population with an "unacceptable" PaO_2/FiO_2 ratio < 300, approximately 50% of the lungs were optimized and successfully procured. Marginal lungs constituted 57% of all transplantation preformed. The marginal and ideal lungs resulted in similar recipient outcomes, including postoperative gas exchange, ICU length of stay, and short- or medium-term mortality. Identical to an aggressive approach targeted at cardiac optimization of the potential donor, a structured and organized approach to managing the potential lung donor increases procurement of lungs.

Angel et al. (see Further reading) reported the impact of a lung transplantation donor management protocol on lung donation and recipient outcomes. Using a protocol strategy that included education and active donor management evaluation, the authors reported a dramatic increase in the rate of lung procurement. The educational initiative consisted of the transplant pulmonologist meeting with the OPO staff for training sessions on donor selection and management, emphasizing that all donors should be perceived as potential lung donors and that consent should be obtained for all organs. In addition, education was provided on donor management strategies. Active donor management consisted of ventilatory recruitment maneuvers, restriction of fluid administration, administration of diuretics, and implementation of techniques targeted at preventing aspiration. Alveolar recruitment was undertaken when the PaO_2/FiO_2 ratio was <300 or when pulmonary infiltrates, consistent with pulmonary edema or atelectasis, were present The alveolar recruitment strategy consisted of pressure control ventilation with an inspiratory pressure of 25 cmH_2O and a PEEP of 15 cmH_2O for 2 h.

After this period, the ventilatory mode was changed to a conventional volume control ventilation with a tidal volume of 10 mL/kg and a PEEP of 5 cmH_2O. Fluid balance was carefully monitored and a strategy, targeted at minimizing the use of crystalloid and adding diuretics to maintain a neutral to negative fluid balance, was incorporated into the protocol. The risk of aspiration was diminished by elevating the head of the bed 30° and inflating the balloon to the endotracheal tube to 25 cmH_2O. Bronchoscopy was performed on all patients to evaluate radiographically detected areas of pulmonary infiltrates, contusions, or aspiration. This management process was continued until lung procurement. Using this strategy, the rate of lung procurement was dramatically higher in the protocol period (25% compared with 11%). This represented an estimated risk ratio of 2.2 in favor of the protocol, with significantly more patients receiving transplants during this period (121 vs 53). Importantly, 54% of the actual lung donors had initially been considered poor donors and these donors provided 52% of the 121 lung transplants performed. Similar to the Gabby study, the type of donor was not associated with a significant decrease in recipient survivorship or any other clinical metric of recipient graft function. As this study illustrates, aggressive management of the potential organ donor has clearly been shown to result in increased rates of lung procurement and transplantation.

Case

A 43-year-old man was declared brain dead after a gunshot wound to the head. He required vasopressin for severe hypotension. The chest radiograph suggested pulmonary edema with atelectasis of the left lower lobe. A Swan–Ganz catheter was placed to monitor PCWP. Pressure control ventilation was instituted for 2 h with and inspiratory pressure of 25 cmH_2O and PEEP of 15 cmH_2O. Thereafter, volume control ventilation was resumed with PEEP of 5 cmH_2O. Bronchoscopy was performed and suggested no evidence of infection. The chest radiograph improved dramatically and organs were harvested for heart, lung, and kidney transplants.

Donation after cardiac death

Donation after cardiac death was previously referred to as non-heart-beating organ donation and was the only means available for organ procurement during the early period of transplantation in the USA. With the advent of uniformly accepted criteria for determination of brain death, many transplant centers stopped procuring organs from DCD donors and focused exclusively on the procurement of organs from brain-dead donors. Given the period of warm ischemia time that occurs in DCD, procurement from brain-dead donors was preferable because of improved organ function. Given the ongoing shortage of transplantable organs, there has been a resurgence in procurement from DCD donors. Currently, all OPOs are mandated from the federal government to work with their referring hospitals to establish formal DCD policies and protocols.

The issue of donation after cardiac death has been addressed by the Institute of Medicine which concluded that the procurement of organs from non-heart-beating donors is appropriate, effective, and an ethically accepted approach to secure transplantable organs. The Institute of Medicine stipulated that written protocols for the procedure should be openly available and transparent, that the process define separate responsibilities for the attending physician and transplant procurement physicians, that families be fully informed and offered the option of the withdrawal of life support, and that donors and families not suffer financial penalties. It was further suggested that the use of anticoagulants and vasodilators be used on a case-by-case basis and that the determination of death should be defined by cessation of cardiopulmonary function for at least 5 min by electrocardiographic and arterial pressure monitoring.

It is absolutely crucial that the decision to withdraw life-supporting therapy be made independent and before any initiation of discussions related to organ and tissue donation. Once the decision has been made to forego further life-sustaining therapy, it is appropriate to initiate the discussion and provide the family with the opportunity for donation after cardiac death. At this point, integrating the OPO into the discussion is appropriate. The overwhelming majority of DCD donors have a devastating neurologic injury although, occasionally, a subset of patients with non-neurologic injuries has become DCD donors. The withdrawal of support in the case of a DCD donor should be identical to the withdrawal process used for any other patient. Ensuring that the patient is comfortable, similar to the approach used in any other circumstance of withdraw care, is of paramount importance. The use of anticoagulants and vasodilators during this process should be made on a case-by-case basis with the family fully informed throughout the entire process. Throughout the withdrawal phase, blood pressure, oxygenation, and urine output are monitored in an effort to define the duration of warm ischemia. In general, the time from extubation/withdrawal of support that enables viable organs for transplantation is approximately 1 h. Further prolonged periods between extubation/withdrawal of therapy lead to hypotension and organ ischemia that effectively preclude the use of organs for transplantation. The withdrawal process may occur in the patient's room or the patient may be transferred to the operating room. Death is pronounced using cardiopulmonary criteria after a 5-min period of asystole and electrocardiographic silence. Organ recovery is subsequently initiated after pronouncement of death.

Further reading

Ad Hoc Committee of the Harvard Medical School to Examine the Definition of Brain Death. A definition of irreversible coma. *JAMA* 1968;**205**:337–40.

Angel LF, Levine DJ, Restrepo MI, et al. Impact of a lung transplantation donor-management protocol on lung donation and recipient outcomes. *Am J Respir Crit Care Med* 2006;**174**:710–6.

Audibert G, Charpentier C, Seguin-Devaux C, et al. Improvement of donor myocardial function after treatment of autonomic storm during brain death. *Transplantation* 2006;**82**:1031–6.

Avlonitis VS, Fisher AJ, Kirby JA, Dark JH. Pulmonary transplantation: The role of brain death in donor lung injury. *Transplantation* 2003;**75**:1928–33.

Banki N, Kopelnik A, Tung P, et al. Prospective analysis of prevalence, distribution, and rate of recovery of left ventricular systolic dysfunction in patients with subarachnoid hemorrhage. *J Neurosurg* 2006;**105**:15–20.

Banki NM, Zaroff JG. Neurogenic cardiac injury. *Curr Treat Options Cardiovasc Med* 2003;**5**:451–8.

Bittner HB, Kendall SW, Campbell KA, Montine TJ, Van Trigt P. A valid experimental brain death organ donor model. *J Heart Lung Transplant* 1995;**14**:308–17.

Chen EP, Bittner HB, Kendall SW, Van Trigt P. Hormonal and hemodynamic changes in a validated animal model of brain death. *Crit Care Med* 1996;**24**:1352–9.

Cooper DK, Novitzky D, Wicomb WN. Hormonal therapy in the brain-dead experimental animal. *Transplant Proc* 1988;**20**:51–4.

Cooper DK, Novitzky D, Wicomb WN. The pathophysiological effects of brain death on potential donor organs, with particular reference to the heart. *Ann R Coll Surg Engl* 1989;**71**:261–6.

Dujardin KS, McCully RB, Wijdicks EF, et al. Myocardial dysfunction associated with brain death: Clinical, echocardiographic, and pathologic features. *J Heart Lung Transplant* 2001;**20**:350–7.

Fisher AJ, Donnelly SC, Pritchard G, Dark JH, Corris PA. Objective assessment of criteria for selection of donor lungs suitable for transplantation. *Thorax* 2004;**59**:434–7.

Gabbay E, Williams TJ, Griffiths AP, et al. Maximizing the utilization of donor organs offered for lung transplantation. *Am J Respir Crit Care Med* 1999;**160**:265–71.

Goarin JP, Cohen S, Riou B, et al. The effects of triiodothyronine on hemodynamic status and cardiac function in potential heart donors. *Anesthesia Analg* 1996;**83**:41–7.

Gortmaker SL, Beasley CL, Sheehy E, et al. Improving the request process to increase family consent for organ donation. *J Transplant Coord* 1998;**8**:210–7.

Hing AJ, Hicks M, Garlick SR, et al. The effects of hormone resuscitation on cardiac function and hemodynamics in a porcine brain-dead organ donor model. *Am J Transplant* 2007;**7**:809–17.

Honorary Secretary of the Conference of Medical Royal Colleges and their Faculties in the United Kingdom. Diagnosis of brain death. Statement issued on 11 October 1976. *BMJ* 1976;**ii**:1187–8.

Howlett TA, Keogh AM, Perry L, Touzel R, Rees LH. Anterior and posterior pituitary function in brainstem-dead donors. A possible role for hormonal replacement therapy. *Transplantation* 1989;**47**:828–34.

Insitute of Medicine. *Non-heart-beating Organ Transplantation: Medical ethical issues in procurement.* Washington DC: National Academy Press, 1997.

Insitute of Medicine. *Non-heart-beating Organ Transplantation: Practice and protocols.* Washington DC: National Academy Press, 2000.

Khush KK, Menza RL, Babcock WD, Zaroff JG. Donor cardiac troponin i levels do not predict recipient survival after cardiac transplantation. *J Heart Lung Transplant* 2007;**26**:1048–53.

Kono T, Morita H, Kuroiwa T, Onaka H, Takatsuka H, Fujiwara A. Left ventricular wall motion abnormalities in patients with subarachnoid hemorrhage: Neurogenic stunned myocardium. *J Am Coll Cardiol* 1994;**24**:636–40.

Kopelnik A, Fisher L, Miss JC, et al. Prevalence and implications of diastolic dysfunction after subarachnoid hemorrhage. *Neurocrit Care* 2005;**3**:132–8.

Mariot J, Sadoune LO, Jacob F, et al. Hormone levels, hemodynamics, and metabolism in brain dead organ donors. *Transplant Proc* 1995;**27**:793–4.

Marshall R, Ahsan N, Dhillon S, Holman M, Yang HC. Adverse effect of donor vasopressor support on immediate and one-year kidney allograft function. *Surgery* 1996;**120**:663–5; discussion 666.

Mollaret P, Goulon M. [The depassed coma (preliminary memoir).] *Revue Neurologique* 1959;**101**:3–15.

Novitzky D, Cooper DK, Morrell D, Isaacs S. Change from aerobic to anaerobic metabolism after brain death, and reversal following triiodothyronine therapy. *Transplantation* 1988;**45**:32–6.

Novitzky D, Cooper DK, Rosendale JD, Kauffman HM. Hormonal therapy of the brain-dead organ donor: Experimental and clinical studies. *Transplantation* 2006;**82**:1396–401.

Novitzky D, Cooper DK. Results of hormonal therapy in human brain-dead potential organ donors. *Transplant Proc* 1988;**20**:59–62.

Pennefather SH, Bullock RE, Dark JH. The effect of fluid therapy on alveolar arterial oxygen gradient in brain-dead organ donors. *Transplantation* 1993;**56**:1418–22.

Powner DJ, Hendrich A, Lagler RG, Ng RH, Madden RL. Hormonal changes in brain dead patients. *Crit Care Med* 1990;**18**:702–8.

Powner DJ, Hernandez M. A review of thyroid hormone administration during adult donor care. *Progr Transplant* 2005;**15**:202–7.

President's Commission for the Study of Ethical Problems in Medicine and Biomedical and Behavioral Research. *A Report on the Medical, Legal and Ethical Issues in the Determination of Death*. 1981. Washington DC: US Government Printing Office.

Riou B, Dreux S, Roche S, et al. Circulating cardiac troponin t in potential heart transplant donors. *Circulation* 1995;**92**:409–14.

Rosendale JD, Chabalewski FL, McBride MA, et al. Increased transplanted organs from the use of a standardized donor management protocol. *Am J Transplant* 2002;**2**:761–8.

Rosendale JD, Kauffman HM, McBride MA, et al. Aggressive pharmacologic donor management results in more transplanted organs. *Transplantation* 2003;**75**:482–7.

Salim A, Martin M, Brown C, Belzberg H, Rhee P, Demetriades D. Complications of brain death: Frequency and impact on organ retrieval. *Am Surgeon* 2006;**72**:377–81.

Salim A, Martin M, Brown C, Rhee P, Demetriades D, Belzberg H. The effect of a protocol of aggressive donor management: Implications for the national organ donor shortage. *J Trauma* 2006;**61**:429–33; discussion 433–25.

Salim A, Vassiliu P, Velmahos GC, et al. The role of thyroid hormone administration in potential organ donors. *Arch Surg* 2001;**136**:1377–80.

Schnuelle P, Berger S, de Boer J, Persijn G, van der Woude FJ. Effects of catecholamine application to brain-dead donors on graft survival in solid organ transplantation. *Transplantation* 2001;**72**:455–63.

Schnuelle P, Lorenz D, Mueller A, Trede M, Van Der Woude FJ. Donor catecholamine use reduces acute allograft rejection and improves graft survival after cadaveric renal transplantation. *Kidney Int* 1999;**56**:738–46.

Wahlers T, Cremer J, Fieguth HG, et al. Donor heart-related variables and early mortality after heart transplantation. *J Heart Lung Transplant* 1991;**10**:22–7.

Ware LB, Wang Y, Fang X, et al. Assessment of lungs rejected for transplantation and implications for donor selection. *Lancet* 2002;**360**:619–20.

Wicomb WN, Cooper DK, Novitzky D. Impairment of renal slice function following brain death, with reversibility of injury by hormonal therapy. *Transplantation* 1986;**41**:29–33.

Williams MA, Lipsett PA, Rushton CH, et al. The physician's role in discussing organ donation with families. *Crit Care Med* 2003;**31**:1568–73.

Yamaoka Y, Taki Y, Gubernatis G, et al. Evaluation of the liver graft before procurement. Significance of arterial ketone body ratio in brain-dead patients. *Transplant Int* 1990;**3**:78–81.

Zaroff JG, Babcock WD, Shiboski SC, Solinger LL, Rosengard BR. Temporal changes in left ventricular systolic function in heart donors: Results of serial echocardiography. *J Heart Lung Transplant* 2003;**22**:383–8.

Zaroff JG, Babcock WD, Shiboski SC. The impact of left ventricular dysfunction on cardiac donor transplant rates. *J Heart Lung Transplant* 2003;**22**:334–7.

4 Infectious diseases in transplantation

Robin K Avery[1] *and Jay A Fishman*[2]

[1]The Cleveland Clinic and Cleveland Clinic Lerner College of Medicine, USA

[2]Massachusetts General Hospital and Harvard Medical School, Boston, Massachusetts, USA

Management of infection in the immunocompromised transplant recipient is complicated by a variety of factors. These include increased susceptibility to a spectrum of infectious pathogens, the difficulty of recognizing infectious syndromes in the face of diminished signs and symptoms of inflammation, an array of non-infectious etiologies of fever (including graft rejection and drug toxicity), and the frequency with which multiple processes coexist. At the same time, immunocompromised patients tolerate poorly any delays in appropriate antimicrobial therapies, increasing the urgency for an early, specific diagnosis. As anti-rejection therapies are largely aimed at suppression of T-lymphocyte functions, viral infections, in particular, are increased. These contribute to the risk for other opportunistic infections, including those due to *Pneumocystis* and *Aspergillus* species, and for cancers mediated by viral infections.

Risk of infection

The risk of infection in the transplant recipient is determined by the interaction of two factors:

1. Epidemiologic exposures of the patient including those unrecognized by the patient or distant in time – including the organisms and the virulence, intensity and timing of infectious exposures (Table 4.1)

2. The patient's net state of immunosuppression, including all the factors that contribute to the risk for infection such as the intensity and timing of exogenous immunosuppression, underlying conditions including metabolic disorders or neutropenia, the presence of vascular lines or other breaks in mucocutaneous barriers, and concomitant viral infections (Table 4.2).

Epidemiologic exposures

Knowledge of the details of an individual's epidemiologic history allows the clinician to establish a differential diagnosis for a given "infectious" presentation and to design the optimal preventive strategy for each patient. One aspect of this process relies on screening of the organ donor and the recipient (Tables 4.3 and 4.4). Key interventions that result from screening include empiric therapies for latent tuberculosis, *Strongyloides stercoralis* in patients from endemic regions, and patients who receive organs from donors discovered to have acute bacterial, viral, or fungal infections. Specific antiviral preventive strategies, notably for cytomegalovirus (CMV), are stratified according to individual risk for all transplant recipients.

Exposures of importance can be divided into four overlapping categories: donor- or recipient-derived infections, and community or nosocomial exposures.

Donor-derived infections

Infections that are derived from the donor tissues and cause invasive disease in the recipient are among the most important exposures in transplantation. Some of these are due to latent pathogens whereas

Primer on Transplantation, 3rd edition.

Table 4.1 Significant epidemiologic exposures relevant to transplantation

Donor derived	Nosocomial exposures
Viral	Methicillin-resistant staphylococci
Herpes group (cytomegalovirus, Epstein–Barr virus, human herpesviruses 6, 7, 8, herpes simplex virus)	Vancomycin-resistant enterococci (also linezolid and quinupristin–dalfopristin resistance)
Hepatitis viruses (notably B and C)	*Aspergillus* spp.
Retroviruses (HIV, HTLV-1 and -2)	*Candida* non-*albicans* strains
Others	**Community exposures**
Bacteria	Food and water borne (*Listeria monocytogenes*, *Salmonella* spp., *Cryptosporidium* spp., hepatitis A, *Campylobacter* spp.)
Gram-positive and Gram-negative bacteria (*Staphylococcus* spp, *Pseudomonas* spp., Enterobacteriaceae)	Respiratory viruses (respiratory syncytial virus [RSV], influenza, parainfluenza, adenovirus, metapneumovirus)
Mycobacteria (tuberculosis and non-tuberculous)	Common viruses – often with exposure to children (Coxsackie virus, parvovirus, polyomavirus, papillomavirus)
Nocardia asteroides	Atypical respiratory pathogens (*Legionella* spp., *Mycoplasma* spp., *Chlamydia* spp.)
Fungi	Geographic fungi and cryptococci, *Pneumocystis jiroveci*
Candida spp.	Parasites (often distant)
Aspergillus spp.	*Strongyloides stercoralis*
Endemic fungi (*Cryptococcus neoformans*)	*Leishmania spp*
Geographic fungi (*Histoplasma capsulatum*, *Coccidioides immitis*, *Blastomyces* spp.)	*Toxoplasma gondii*
Parasites	*Trypanosoma cruzi*
Toxoplasma gondii	
Trypanosoma cruzi	

Table 4.2 Factors contributing to the "net state of immunosuppression"

Factors
Immunosuppressive therapy: type, temporal sequence, intensity
Prior therapies (chemotherapy or antimicrobials)
Mucocutaneous barrier integrity (catheters, lines, drains)
Neutropenia, lymphopenia (often drug induced)
Underlying immune deficiency, e.g.,
Hypogammaglobulinemia
Systemic lupus, complement deficiencies
Metabolic conditions: uremia, malnutrition, diabetes, alcoholism/cirrhosis
Viral infection (cytomegalovirus, hepatitis B and C viruses, respiratory syncytial virus)
Immunosuppression (indirect effects of viral infection)
Graft rejection
Cancer/Cellular proliferation

Table 4.3 The pretransplant evaluation (consider the following)

Laboratory test	All patients	Patients with exposure in endemic area	Quantitative viral studies available (PCR)
Serologies			
CMV	✓		✓
HSV	✓		✓
VZV	✓		
EBV	✓		✓
HIV	✓		✓
HBV: HBsAg, HBcAb	✓		✓
Anti-HBs	✓		
HCV	✓		✓
Treponema pallidum (RPR)	✓		
Toxoplasma gondii	✓		
Strongyloides stercoralis		✓	
Leishmania spp		✓	
Trypanosoma cruzi		✓	Blood smear
Histoplasma capsulatum		✓	
Cryptococcus neoformans		✓	Cryptococcal antigen
Coccidioides immitis		✓	
Cultures, etc.			
Urinalysis and culture	✓		
Skin test: PPD	✓		
Chest radiograph (routine)	✓		
Stool ova and parasites (*Strongyloides*)		✓	
Urine ova and parasites/Cystoscopy		✓ (for kidneys)	(Schistosomiasis endemic areas)

See the text for abbreviations. PPD, purified protein derivative.

others are the result of bad timing – active infection transmitted at the time of transplantation. The subsequent activation of infection may reflect the intensity of immunosuppression and/or results from the allogeneic response (graft rejection), which can activate latent viral pathogens. Given the risk of transmission of infection from the organ donor to the recipient, certain infections should be considered relative contraindications to organ donation. As transplantation is, in general, semi-elective surgery, it is reasonable to avoid donation from individuals with unexplained fever, rash, neurologic syndromes, or other infectious syndromes. Some of the common criteria for exclusion of organ donors are listed in Table 4.4.

Recipient-derived exposures

Infections in this category are generally latent infections activated in the setting of immunosuppression. Thus, a careful history of travel and exposures can guide preventive strategies and empiric therapies. Notable among these infections are tuberculosis, strongyloidiasis, viral infections (herpes simplex and varicella-zoster), histoplasmosis, coccidioidiomycosis, hepatitis B or C, and HIV. Immunization status should be ascertained and updated in advance of transplantation (tetanus, hepatitis B, childhood vaccines, influenza, pneumococcal vaccine, varicella-zoster). Dietary habits should also be considered including the use of well water (cryptosporidia), uncooked meats (*Salmonella* and *Listeria* spp.),

Key points 4.1 Common forms of donor-derived infection

- Donors who are bacteremic or fungemic at the time of donation – these infections (staphylococci, pneumococci, *Candida* sp., *Salmonella* spp., *E. coli*) tend to "stick" to anastomotic sites (vascular, urinary) and may produce leaks or mycotic aneurysms as well as infection of fluid collections and abscesses
- Donors who are viremic (often asymptomatic) at the time of donation – including herpes simplex virus, West Nile virus, rabies, arboviruses, and the hepatitis viruses. Viremia may also occur during respiratory viral infections, which might allow transmission from extrapulmonary organs
- Latent viral infections transmitted with the graft including cytomegalovirus (CMV) and Epstein–Barr virus (EBV) that are associated with particular syndromes and morbidity in the immunocompromised population (discussed in text). The greatest risk is from primary infection – organ recipients who are seronegative (immunologically naïve) receiving grafts from seropositive donors
- Bacterial or fungal colonization (e.g., in the lung transplant donor), which can become an invasive infection in the recipient
- Late, latent infections including tuberculosis which may activate many years after the initial exposure. The treatment of disseminated mycobacterial infection is often complicated by drug interactions or toxicities in the transplant recipient

or unpasteurized dairy products (*Listeria* spp.). Asymptomatic *Strongyloides stercoralis* infection may activate more than 30 years after initial exposure due to the effects of immunosuppressive therapy. Such reactivation can result in either a hyperinfestation syndrome (characterized by hemorrhagic enterocolitis, hemorrhagic pneumonia, or both) or disseminated infection with accompanying Gram-negative bacteremia or meningitis.

Community exposures

Common exposures may be related to contaminated food and water ingestion, exposure to infected children or co-workers, or exposures resulting from hobbies (gardening), travel, or work. Respiratory virus infection caused by influenza, parainfluenza, respiratory syncytial virus (RSV), or adenoviruses, or by more atypical pathogens (herpes simplex virus [HSV], herpes zoster virus [HZV]) carry a risk for viral pneumonia and subsequent bacterial or fungal superinfection. Community (social or transfusion-associated) exposure to cytomegalovirus (CMV) and Epstein–Barr virus (EBV) may produce severe primary infection in the non-immune host. Recent and remote exposures to endemic, geographically restricted systemic mycoses (*Blastomyces dermatitidis*, *Coccidioides immitis*, and *Histoplasma capsulatum*) and *Mycobacterium tuberculosis* can result in localized pulmonary, systemic, or metastatic infection. Gastroenteritis due to *Salmonella* spp., *Yersinia* spp., or *Campylobacter jejuni* may result in more severe and prolonged diarrheal disease as well as the risk of bloodstream invasion and metastatic infection.

Case

A heart transplant recipient developed pulmonary nodules and was found on biopsy to have *Rhodococcus equi* infection. Although the patient owned no farm animals, she had walked through nearby fairgrounds where there were swirling hay dusts.

Nosocomial exposures

Nosocomial infections are of increasing importance because organisms with significant antimicrobial resistance predominate in many centers. These include vancomycin-, linezolid-, and quinupristin–dalfopristin-resistant enterococci, methicillin-resistant staphylococci, and fluconazole-resistant *Candida* spp. or *Aspergillus* spp. A single case of nosocomial aspergillus infection in a compromised host should be seen as an indication of a problem with infection control practices. Antimicrobial overuse and the emergence of an epidemic strain have resulted in increased rates of *Clostridium difficile* colitis. Outbreaks of infections due to *Legionella* spp. have been associated with hospital plumbing and contaminated water supplies or ventilation systems. Each nosocomial infection should be investigated to ascertain the source and prevent subsequent infections. Nosocomial spread of *Pneumocystis jiroveci* between immunocompromised patients has also been suggested by a variety of case series. Respiratory viral infections may be acquired from medical staff and should be considered among the causes of fever and respiratory decompensation in hospitalized or institutionalized, immunocompromised individuals.

Table 4.4 Infectious considerations in evaluation of deceased organ donors[a]

Viral infection or Viremia (untreated)
- Herpesviruses including acute Epstein–Barr virus (mononucleosis), herpes simplex, varicella-zoster, cytomegalovirus
- HIV infection (serologic or molecular assay or by history)
- Active measles, mumps, varicella-zoster virus, rubella infections
- Herpes simplex encephalitis or other encephalitis
- HTLV-I/-II (serologic and molecular assays difficult to interpret)
- Hepatitis A, B, or C
- Severe acute respiratory syndrome (SARS)
- West Nile virus infection; arbovirus infections (Eastern equine encephalitis virus, St Louis encephalitis, Japanese encephalitis virus, dengue, yellow fever) – active or diagnosed within 6 months
- Lymphocytic choriomeningitis virus (LCMV)
- Rabies
- JC polyomavirus virus infection
- Creutzfeldt–Jakob disease
- Active viral pneumonia: influenza, respiratory syncytial virus, adenovirus, parainfluenza virus, metapneumovirus infections (may be lung-specific)

Fungal infection (active/untreated)
- *Cryptococcus neoformans* or *Aspergillus* species infection of any site
- Systemic fungal infection including candidemia
- Active or history of infection due to *Histoplasma capsulatum* or *Coccidoides immitis* (may be lung-specific)

Central Nervous System infection
- Undiagnosed infection of central nervous system (e.g., encephalitis, meningitis)
- Untreated bacterial or viral meningoencephalitis (including tuberculosis)

Parasitic infection (untreated)
- *Trypanosoma cruzi*
- *Strongyloides stercoralis*
- *Toxoplasma gondii*
- *Leishmania* spp.
- *Babesia* spp.
- *Malaria* spp.
- *Ehrlichia* spp.

Pneumonia (untreated or undiagnosed) or bacteremia
- *Mycobacterium tuberculosis*, untreated disseminated non-tuberculous mycobacteria
- Meningococcal infection
- Bacteremia or sepsis syndrome
- Syphilis
- Lyme disease
- Rickettsial infection
- *Pneumocystis jiroveci*

Multisystem organ failure due to overwhelming sepsis, toxic shock syndrome

Untreated intra-abdominal infection (e.g., peritonitis or gangrenous bowel)

[a]Must be considered in the context of the individual donor and recipient. Undiagnosed infection may provide a greater infectious risk than incompletely treated donor-derived infection. Therapy may be continued in the recipient.

Table 4.5 Immunosuppression and specific infections

Anti-lymphocyte globulins (lytic) and alloimmune response: activation of latent (herpes)virus (CMV, EBV), fever, cytokines
Plasmapheresis: encapsulated bacteria
Co-stimulatory blockade: Unknown so far
Corticosteroids: bacteria, PCP, hepatitis B and C, fungal infection
Azathioprine: neutropenia, papillomavirus?
Mycophenolate mofetil: early bacterial infection, B cells, late CMV?
Calcineurin inhibitors (cyclosporine/tacrolimus): enhanced viral replication (absence of immunity), gingival infection, intracellular pathogens
Rapamycin: excess bacterial infections in combination with current agents, idiosyncratic pulmonary interstitial pneumonitis

CMV, cytomegalovirus; EBV, Epstein–Barr virus; PCP, *Pneumocystis jiroveci* pneumonia.

Net state of immunosuppression

The net state of immunosuppression is a measure of all of the factors contributing to the patient's risk for infection (see Table 4.2). Specific immunosuppressive agents are associated with increased risk for certain infections (Table 4.5). Combinations of these agents may enhance this risk or cause toxicity (e.g., nephrotoxicity) and may further enhance risk.

Key points 4.2 The most notable components of the "net state of immunosuppression"

- Immunosuppressive therapies, including the dose, duration, and sequence of these agents
- Technical problems from the transplant procedure, resulting in fluid collections or devitalized tissue
- Vascular access or dialysis catheters and surgical drainage catheters
- Critical illness requiring ICU care, broad-spectrum antimicrobial agents, prolonged intubation
- Renal and/or hepatic dysfunction and metabolic abnormalities including hyperglycemia
- Viral co-infection

With the proliferation of newer anti-rejection agents, longitudinal assessment of the immune status of the recipient has been of increasing interest. Monitoring relevant to infection risk can involve quantitation of particular types of cells (e.g., absolute lymphocyte count, CD4:CD8 ratio, and B-lymphocyte count) or measurement of immunoglobulin levels. More recently, functional assays have been developed that measure lymphocyte binding (e.g., tetramers) or cellular responses (e.g., interferon-γ release) in response to specific or non-specific antigenic stimuli and provide an assessment of cellular immune function. Genomic studies can characterize gene expression associated with a "state of rejection" or infection. Such tests ultimately may provide some quantitative measure of the net state of immunosuppression.

Timeline of infection

The risk factors for infection, epidemiology, and immune status are continuous variables over time. When immunosuppressive regimens are standardized, specific infections vary in a predictable pattern depending on the time elapsed since transplantation (Figure 4.1). This pattern is a reflection of most of the recipients in whom the intensity of immunosuppression generally is decreased over time and for whom other risk factors are reasonably common (surgery/hospitalization, immunosuppression, acute and chronic rejection, emergence of latent infections, and exposures to novel community infections). Although this concept is useful, at any given center the pattern may shift when immunosuppression is altered (e.g., substituting sirolimus for calcineurin inhibitors, use of co-stimulatory blockade instead of antithymocyte globulin, and minimization or withdrawal of corticosteroids). The risk of infection will be further altered by increases in the immunosuppression for treatment of graft rejection, intercurrent viral infection, neutropenia (drug toxicity), graft dysfunction, or significant epidemiologic exposures (travel or food).

The timeline reflects three overlapping periods of risk for infection:

1. The perioperative period to approximately 4 weeks after transplantation

2. The "opportunistic infection" period 1–6 months after transplantation (depending, for example, on the

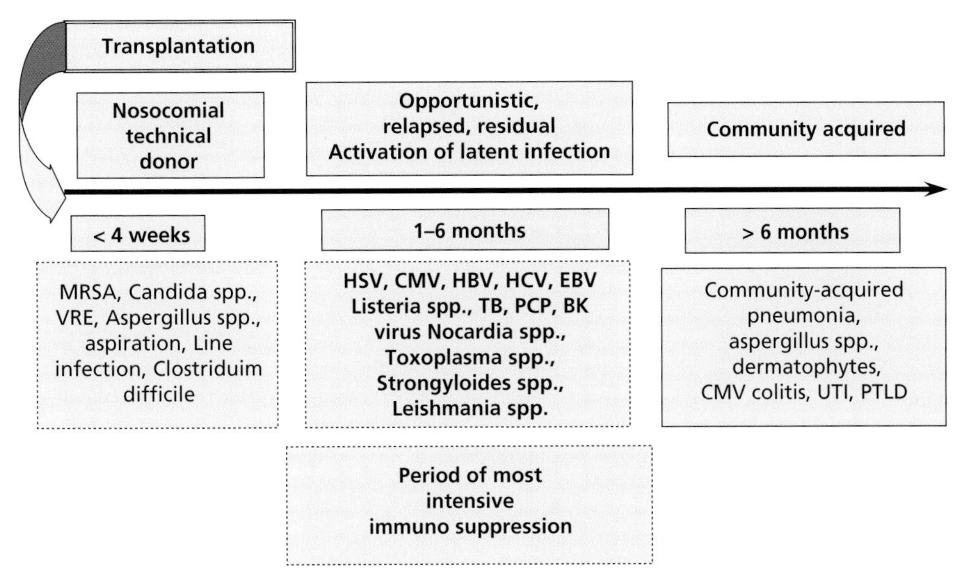

Figure 4.1 Timeline of post-transplant infections. CMV, cytomegalovirus; EBV, Epstein–Barr virus; HBV hepatitis B virus; HCV, hepatitis C virus; HSV, herpes simplex virus; MRSA, methicillin-resistant *Staphylococcus aureus*; PCP, *Pneumocystis jiroveci* pneumonia; PTLD, post-transplant lymphoproliferative disease; TB, tuberculosis; UTI, urinary tract infection; VRE, vancomycin-resistant enterococcus.

rapidity of taper of immune suppression and antibody-based "induction" therapies)
3. The period beyond 6 or 12 months after transplantation.
These periods reflect the changing major risk factors associated with infection: surgery and technical complications; intensive immunosuppression with viral activation; and community-acquired exposures and return to normal activities.

The timeline may be used in a variety of ways: to establish a differential diagnosis for the transplant patient suspected of having infection; as a clue to the presence of an excessive environmental hazard for the individual, either within the hospital or in the community; and as a guide to the design of preventative antimicrobial strategies. Infections occurring outside the usual period or of unusual severity suggest either excessive epidemiologic hazard or excessive immunosuppression.

Prevention of infection is linked to the risk for infection at various times after transplantation. Thus, the transplant recipient treated by plasmapheresis, or with hypogammaglobulinemia due to mycophenolate mofetil or azathioprine, requires enhanced protection against encapsulated bacteria (pneumococci, *Hemophilus influenzae*, meningococci) that may be provided by IgG replacement or trimethoprim–sulfamethoxazole. It should be noted that such strategies serve only to delay the onset of infection in the face of epidemiologic pressure. The use of preventive strategies (antimicrobial prophylaxis, vaccines) may only delay infection unless the intensity of immunosuppression is reduced or immunity develops.

Phase 1 (1–4 weeks post-transplant)

During the first month after transplantation, three types of infection occur:
1. The first type of infection is one that was present in the recipient before transplantation, was not eradicated, and emerges in the postoperative period. This may reflect, for example, untreated pneumonia or sinusitis, *C. difficile* colitis, or colonization with nosocomial pathogens. Control or eradication of such processes is an important part of preparation for transplantation.
2. The second type of early infection is transmitted from the infected donor to the recipient. This may be

nosocomially derived (resistant Gram-negative bacilli, *Staphylococcus aureus* or *Candida* spp.) due to either systemic infection in the donor (e.g., line infection) or contamination during the organ procurement process. Such patients are predisposed to abscesses around the allograft or to mycotic aneurysm at vascular suture lines. Donor-derived infections include tuberculosis (TB) or fungal (e.g., histoplasmosis) infections that emerge in the postoperative period before normal expectation. Recently, early donor-derived viral infections (lymphocytic choriomeningitis, rabies, West Nile virus) have also emerged in the first post-transplant month.

3. The third and most common type of infection in the early period is related to the complex surgical procedure of transplantation, and includes surgical wound infections, pneumonia (aspiration), bacteremia due to vascular catheters, urinary tract infections, or infected fluid collections at anastomotic sites, from bowel leaks, or of fluid collections. These infections are the result of nosocomial pathogens or endogenous flora and may be resistant to first-line antimicrobial agents. Given immune suppression, the signs of infection may be subtle and the severity or duration may be greater. *C. difficile* colitis is also common.

Notable by their absence in the first month after transplantation are opportunistic infections, even though the daily doses of immunosuppressive drugs are at their highest during this time. The implications of this observation are important: the net state of immunosuppression is not great enough to support the occurrence of opportunistic infections unless an exposure has been excessive. This observation suggests that it is not the daily dose of immunosuppressive drugs that is of importance but rather the sustained administration of these drugs (i.e., the "area under the curve") in determining the net state of immunosuppression. Thus, the occurrence of a single case of opportunistic infection in this period should trigger an epidemiologic investigation for an environmental hazard.

Phase 2 (1–6 months post-transplant)

Infection in the transplant recipient 1–6 months after transplantation has one of three causes:

1. Lingering infection from the postoperative period including relapsed *C. difficile* colitis, inadequately treated pneumonia, or infection related to a persistent technical problem (e.g., a urine or bile leak, lymphocele, hematoma).

2. Viral infections including CMV, HSV, shingles (varicella-zoster virus [VZV]), human herpesvirus 6 or 7, EBV, relapsed hepatitis (hepatitis B or C [HBV, HCV]). This group of viruses is unique because they induce life-long infection that is tissue associated (often transmitted with the allograft from seropositive donors or reactivated from past infection in the recipient). These viruses are also immunomodulating – systemically immunosuppressive (predisposing to opportunistic infection) – and, potentially, predispose to graft rejection. It is also notable that the herpes viruses are prominent due to the role of T-cell immune function in the control of these infections. Among the other viral pathogens of this period must be included BK polyomavirus in association with allograft dysfunction and community-acquired respiratory viruses (adenovirus, influenza, parainfluenza, RSV, metapneumovirus). The suppression of antibody production (e.g., using tacrolimus and mycophenolate mofetil or with lymphopenia) may predispose to other infections.

3. Opportunistic infection due to *Pneumocystis jiroveci*, *Listeria monocytogenes*, *Toxoplasma gondii*, *Nocardia* spp., *Aspergillus* spp. (Figure 4.2), and other agents. In this category are pathogens endemic to specific regions including paracoccidioidiomycosis or Chagas' disease in South America, histoplasmosis in midwestern USA, and strongyloidiasis in recipients from south-east Asia.

In this period, the stage is also set for the emergence of a subgroup of patients – the "chronic n'eer do well" – individuals who require higher than average immune suppression to maintain graft function or who have prolonged, untreated viral infections and other opportunistic infections – predicting long-term susceptibility to many other infections (discussed below in phase 3). Such individuals may merit prolonged (life-long) prophylaxis (antibacterial and/or antiviral) to prevent life-threatening infection.

Phase 3 (>6–12 months post-transplant)

Transplant recipients who are more than 6 months post-transplant can be divided into three groups in terms of infection risk:

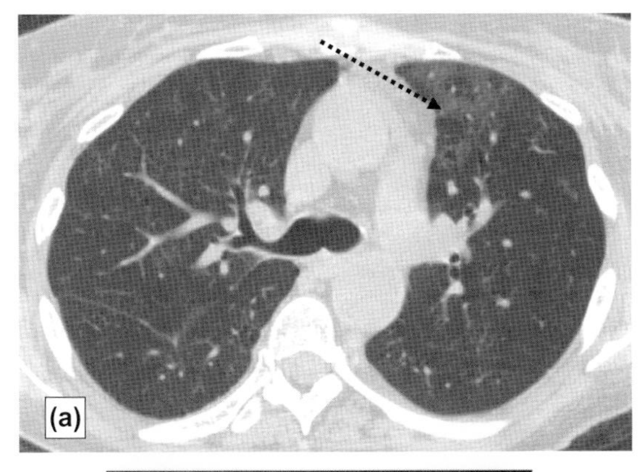

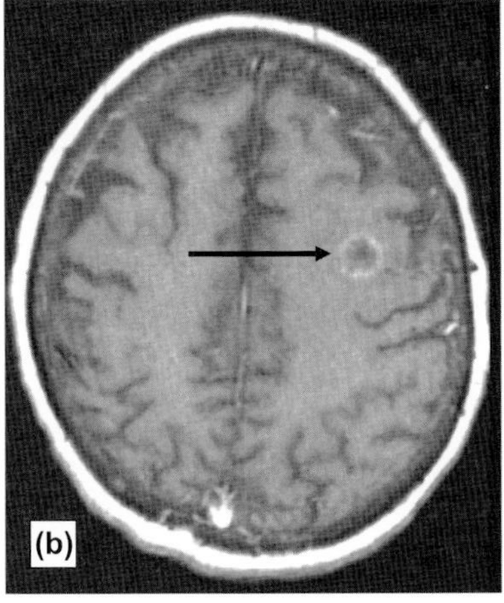

Figure 4.2 Liver transplant recipient with single colony of *Aspergillus fumigatus* in sputum and low-grade fever. She was otherwise asymptomatic. (a) Chest CT scan reveals patchy infiltrate (arrow). (b) Head CT scan reveals brain abscess (arrow) that was biopsied and grew *Aspergillus* sp. in culture.

1. The first group had a technically good procedure with satisfactory allograft function, tolerated reduction in immunosuppression, and lacked chronic viral infection. These patients resemble the general community in terms of infection risk, with community-acquired respiratory viruses constituting their major risk. Occasionally such patients will develop primary CMV infection (socially acquired) or infections related to underlying diseases (e.g., skin infections in diabetes).
2. The second group suffers the effects of persistent viral infections, which produces: – end-organ damage (e.g., BK polyomavirus nephropathy, cryoglobulinemia or cirrhosis from HCV) – malignancy (post-transplantation lymphoproliferative disease [PTLD] due to EBV, skin or anogenital cancer due to papillomaviruses).
3. The third group of patients is the "chronic ne'er do wells" who have less satisfactory allograft function and require more intensive immunosuppression. They are at risk for chronic viral infection and for opportunistic infections with *P. jiroveci*, *Listeria monocytogenes*, *Nocardia asteroides*, and *Cryptococcus neoformans*. Such patients require lifetime trimethoprim–sulfamethoxazole prophylaxis and are considered for antifungal prophylaxis. This group also develops the unusual infections of chronic immune deficiency such as *Nocardia, Rhodococcus, Cryptosporidium*, or *Microsporidium* spp., or invasive fungal pathogens (*Aspergillus* spp., or the families Zygomycetes, or Dematiaceae, or pigmented molds) (see Figure 4.2). Minimal signs of infection merit intensive evaluation in such high-risk individuals.

Pretransplant evaluation

Prospective donors and recipients undergo a panel of tests (see Table 4.3) to detect active or latent infections that may reactivate after transplantation. The specific organisms and conditions assayed are chosen by the Organ Procurement and Transplantation Network (OPTN) and are under review (a possible revised list is given in Table 4.4). These assays serve to establish the suitability of the donor or recipient and to stratify risk for common postoperative infections (e.g., CMV). Risk stratification is used to design appropriate post-transplant prophylactic strategies. Donor blood cultures are recommended if the donor has been hospitalized >72 h, and donor bronchial cultures for bacteria, fungi, and acid-fast bacilli (AFBs) are sent at the time of lung transplantation. A careful social and travel history may also provide clues to unsuspected exposures before seroconversion (e.g., HCV, HIV) or diagnosis (Chagas' disease).

Pre-transplant interventions in the recipient include updating of immunization status (Table 4.6) and initiation of treatment for strongyloides infection or latent TB. HBV immunization should be achieved in all recipients but may be especially important for

Table 4.6 Immunizations to consider before transplantation

Adult
Pneumococcal (if last dose >5 years ago)
Hepatitis B (if seronegative; consider accelerated or enhanced-potency series)
Td or Tdap booster (if last dose >5 years ago)
Varicella (if seronegative and >3 weeks before anticipated transplant)
Influenza – yearly, injected vaccine for both seasonal and novel H1N1 influenza
Completion of any unfinished pediatric vaccine series (see below)
Children
Diphtheria/tetanus/pertussis series
Hemophilus influenzae type b (Hib) series
Hepatitis B series
Conjugated or polysaccharide pneumococcal vaccine (see Guidelines)[a]
Varicella
Yearly influenza (injected vaccine, both seasonal and novel H1N1 influenza)
Meningococcal vaccine (adolescents or military recruits)
Live vaccines contraindicated in transplant recipients
Oral polio vaccine[b]
Varicella vaccine
Measles–mumps–rubella (MMR) vaccine
Smallpox vaccine
Oral typhoid vaccine[b]
Inhaled influenza vaccine (?await further data)

[a]Inactivated vaccines are acceptable.
[b]Oral polio is no longer used in the USA.

recipients of organs from HBV core-antibody-positive (HBsAg–, HBcAb+ [HBV surface antigen negative, HBV core antibody positive]) donors. Pretransplant cultures of colonizing respiratory organisms (such as *Pseudomonas* spp. in cystic fibrosis patients) are used to devise individualized peritransplant prophylaxis.

General principles in management of infectious syndromes

A number of concepts merit consideration in the management of infections in immunocompromised hosts:

- Diminished signs of infection are present in radiologic studies as well as in physical signs and symptoms. The use of computed tomography (CT) or magnetic resonance imaging (MRI) is essential for assessing the presence and nature of infectious and malignant processes.
- The "gold standard" for diagnosis is tissue histology. No radiologic finding is sufficiently diagnostic to obviate the need for this. Further, multiple simultaneous infections are common. Thus, invasive procedures to obtain pre-antimicrobial cultures or histology are a routine component of the initial evaluation of transplant recipients with infectious syndromes. Molecular assays are highly useful and

may be used to monitor the course of infection or therapy.

- Serologic tests (antibody assays) are useful in the pretransplant setting but are rarely of use for acute diagnosis after transplantation. Patients rarely seroconvert in a time frame useful for clinical diagnosis. Thus tests that detect proteins (e.g., enzyme-linked immunsorbance assay [ELISA], direct immunofluorescence for respiratory viruses) or nucleic acids (quantitative molecular assays) should be used.
- Antimicrobial resistance can be acquired during therapy and resistant organisms acquired during hospitalization. Sites at risk (ascites, blood clots, drains, lungs) must be sampled routinely to guide empiric therapy at times of clinical deterioration.
- Antimicrobial agents are of little use in the presence of undrained fluid collections, blood, or devitalized tissues. The use of antimicrobial agents in these settings merely delays clinical deterioration and promotes the acquisition of resistant microorganisms. Early and aggressive surgical debridement of such collections is essential for successful care.
- Resolution of infection is generally slower than in normal hosts. Thus, the course of therapy is usually longer and resolution must be documented – radiologically or via other assays.

Antimicrobial selection in the transplant recipient

There are four major principles of antimicrobial selection:

1. Obtain diagnostic samples for cultures and histology before initiating therapy
2. Initiate broad antimicrobial coverage with more focused therapy when culture results are available
3. Avoid agents with synergistic nephrotoxicity
4. Be aware of drug interactions (azoles, macrolides, rifampin).

Transplant recipients are susceptible to infections with a wide variety of pathogens. The clinical patterns at presentation are highly variable. Thus, specific microbiologic data are the key to ultimately successful therapy. To devise an early and empiric antimicrobial regimen, the timetable of infection, the net state of immunosuppression, center-specific antimicrobial susceptibility patterns, and environmental exposures can be utilized. After initial broad coverage, more focused coverage can be substituted when culture results are available. Unless no other choices are available, it is desirable to avoid nephrotoxic agents (aminoglycosides, amphotericin B, foscarnet) because their toxicity may be amplified in patients receiving cyclosporine or tacrolimus.

Drug interactions should always be considered. Macrolides (particularly clarithromycin and erythromycin) elevate levels of calcineurin inhibitors and can precipitate toxicity. Azithromycin can be used safely. Azole antifungals elevate levels of calcineurin inhibitors and sirolimus. Close monitoring of levels is required both when initiating and when discontinuing these agents. The transplantation center should always be informed when a macrolide or azole is started or stopped. Rifampin decreases calcineurin inhibitor levels and can precipitate rejection. If rifampin is necessary for treatment of TB or staphylococcal infection, discussion with the transplant team and careful monitoring are required.

Case

A heart transplant recipient developed symptoms of bronchitis and was started on clarithromycin at an urgent care center. The transplant team was unaware. Several days later he was admitted with a high cyclosporine level and a serum creatinine of 4.0 mg/dL from cyclosporine toxicity. Renal function improved when clarithromycin was discontinued and the cyclosporine level fell to the normal range.

Special considerations after transplantation

Postoperative infections

Postoperative infections are frequently related to technical complications of the transplantation itself, such as bleeding, urine leaks, or lymphoceles in kidney recipients, or bile leaks in liver recipients. Wound infections in abdominal transplant recipients may involve mixed pathogens, including enteric organisms such as enterococci and Gram-negative aerobes, *Candida* spp., and anaerobes (notably in people with diabetes) as well as skin-derived *Staphylococcus* spp. and streptococci. Although wound infections may complicate thoracic transplantation, heart or lung recipients often develop pneumonias and occasionally empyema. In heart recipients with prior ventricular-assist devices (VAD), preoperative VAD-related infections may persist (see below).

Antimicrobial resistance

In recent years, an increase in infections due to bacteria and yeasts carrying antimicrobial resistance has been observed. The challenge of these pathogens includes: development of newer antibiotic therapies; infection control measures including judicious use of antibiotics; and management of donor or recipient colonization.

Methicillin-resistant *Staphylococcus aureus* (MRSA) is a common cause of catheter-related bacteremias, wound infections, and ventilator-associated pneumonias, and is associated with a high mortality. Bacteremic seeding may occur, resulting in endocarditis, osteomyelitis, and septic thrombophlebitis with pulmonary emboli. In the immunocompromised host, recurrences after apparently successful therapy are more common than in the normal host. No intervention has consistently prevented post-transplant MRSA infections, although decreased colonization may be attempted in some patients with topical nasal application of mupirocin ointment with or without systemic antimicrobial therapy.

Vancomycin-resistant *Enterococcus faecium* and *faecalis* (VRE) infections are increasing among dialysis and liver transplant recipients and are associated with a high mortality. Such organisms are resistant to vancomycin and, in general, to ampicillin, with variable susceptibility to aminoglycosides (gentamicin) and macrolides (tetracycline). VRE infections are seen as a marker of the overall illness of the patient rather than as a direct causal factor in mortality. Invasive infections due to VRE generally occur in patients colonized with VRE. Thus far, there are no effective therapies to decolonize the gastrointestinal tract. Treatment of susceptible strains with gentamicin may be complicated by nephrotoxicity in transplant recipients receiving calcineurin inhibitors. In vitro susceptibility data (e.g., to chloramphenicol) may be misleading. Newer agents (e.g., linezolid, quinupristin–dalfopristin, daptomycin) have improved outcomes, but resistance to these agents is emerging also, side effects of therapy are common, and morbidity remains high. Multiresistant Gram-negative bacilli including *Pseudomonas* spp. and extended-spectrum β-lactamase-producing (ESBL) *E. coli* and *Klebsiella* spp., and carbapenemase-producing *Acinetobacter* and *Klebsiella* spp. may colonize patients after multiple courses of antimicrobial agents (e.g., recurrent pneumonia in cystic fibrosis or chronic cholangitis) or after prolonged ICU stays. Therapy must be guided by antimicrobial susceptibility patterns and documentation of the presence of invasive infection – colonization cannot be cleared in such patients and therapy may only breed further resistance. In the absence of the radiologic demonstration of pneumonia, cultures of colonized upper airways may be misleading in terms of the need for systemic antimicrobial therapy (e.g., sputum Gram stains without organisms or neutrophils). Adjunctive therapies may be added to standard antimicrobial agents including therapeutic bronchoscopic lavage, repletion of hypogammaglobulinemia, treatment of concomitant viral infections, or the use of inhaled colistin. When resistance to standard antipseudomonal drugs occurs, in vitro antimicrobial synergy studies may provide therapeutic alternatives.

Over half of the *Candida* spp. isolated in most US medical centers are now non-*albicans* strains. As a result, infections may be due to fluconazole-resistant yeast (e.g. many *C. glabrata* and all *C. krusei*). Assessment of fluconazole susceptibility should be performed for all yeasts isolated form sterile sites (blood, abdomen). Such isolates may be treated with echinocandins, later generation azoles (if susceptible), or amphotericin-based products.

Infections relating to vascular devices

Infections can be associated with temporary catheters, or indwelling access such as PICC lines or Hickman catheters. Four major forms of catheter-related infection include: exit site; tunnel infection (which requires catheter removal); bacteremia without external signs; and septic thrombophlebitis. Common pathogens include coagulase-negative staphylococci, *Staphylococcus aureus*, and occasionally Gram-negative bacteria and yeasts. Infections are generally managed by catheter removal and antibiotic therapy (although coagulase-negative staphylococcal infection can often be treated with the catheter in place.).

VADs may be in place for months and carry a high risk of infection. Often the drive-line exit site is the initial focus but may progress to bacteremia. Sequential infections with different pathogens are common. Resolution of the infection requires removal of the VAD at the time of transplantation plus ongoing post-transplant antibiotic therapy.

Pneumonia

Pneumonia in transplant recipients falls into three overlapping categories: nosocomial, community acquired, and opportunistic. In the early post-transplant period, transplant recipients may develop nosocomial pneumonias following aspiration or due to *S. aureus* and Gram-negative bacilli. The spectrum of pathogens is broader in the setting of lung transplantation, with prolonged hospitalization or with early graft dysfunction requiring intensive immune suppression (*Aspergillus* spp. and other fungi). Community-acquired respiratory viruses may be acquired (from staff or visitors) while hospitalized, be complicated by superinfection, and provoke lung rejection or progress to respiratory failure. These are often detected by rapid screens (e.g., nasal swab with immunofluorescence). At any time after discharge, pneumococci, and *Legionella*, *Mycoplasma*, and *Chlamydia* spp. may also cause infection. Opportunistic pathogens are most likely to cause pneumonia in the second post-transplant period when the patient is most highly immunosuppressed. Radiographic patterns, particularly on chest CT, are helpful. Nodular infiltrates, particularly if cavitating, suggest fungal or mycobacterial infection, or nocardiosis. The "halo sign" is suggestive of aspergillosis, but virtually any pattern may be seen with these infections. Rapid progression to multilobar pneumonia suggests organisms such as *Legionella* spp., *S. aureus*, or Gram-negative bacilli. Diffuse infiltrates suggest *Pneumocystis* spp. or viral infection. Pulmonary–CNS infections are most often observed with *Aspergillus* and *Nocardia* spp., cryptococci, members of Zygomycetes (*Mucor* spp. in the sinus and lung).

Transplant recipients with pneumonia merit urgent evaluation including history, physical examination, chest radiograph, blood and urine cultures, sputum for Gram stain, bacterial, fungal, and mycobacterial cultures, nasal swab for a respiratory viral panel, and consideration for early chest CT and bronchoscopy. Induced sputum examinations are most useful for the diagnosis of mycobacterial infection, pneumocystis pneumonia, and malignancy. Epidemiologic clues may suggest further studies including, urine for pneumococcal, legionella (pneumophila) and histoplasma antigens, serum cryptococcal antigen, galactomannan or β-glucan assays (less useful in transplant recipients than cancer patients). Antimicrobial therapy should not be delayed while awaiting culture data. Antimicrobial resistance patterns in the community and any prior antimicrobial therapies should be considered when selecting empiric therapies.

The history may provide useful clues to diagnosis: prior viral syndromes may suggest bacterial (staphylococci) or fungal (*Aspergillus* or *Pneumocystis* spp.) superinfection. The introduction of sirolimus may suggest non-infectious infiltrates. "Intolerance" of prophylaxis or marked hypoxemia may suggest pneumocystis infection. Travel to endemic areas may suggest histoplasma or coccidioides infections. Gardening may predispose to *Aspergillus* or *Nocardia* spp.; gastrointestinal syndromes are common with sepsis, pneumococcal infection, or legionellosis.

CT scans of the chest are useful when the chest radiograph is negative or when the radiographic findings are subtle or non-specific. CT defines the extent of the disease process and the selection of optimal invasive techniques to achieve microbiologic diagnosis. Atypical CT findings may suggest the presence of dual or sequential infections of the lungs which are common in transplant recipients. Expectorated sputum is often non-diagnostic. Bronchoalveolar lavage (BAL) is often helpful with a microbiologic panel including assays for *Pneumocystis jiroveci* pneumonia, bacteria, fungi, mycobacteria, *Legionella* spp., CMV, HSV, *Nocardia* spp., and respiratory viruses. Transbronchial biopsy is a useful tool in making an etiologic diagnosis and to distinguish colonization (or rejection in lung recipients) from invasive infection. In some cases when diagnosis is elusive, open-lung biopsy provides a larger tissue sample.

Nocardia spp.

Nocardia infection is most common in thoracic transplant recipients and may involve the lungs, CNS, and other sites. The classic radiographic pattern is pulmonary nodules with associated infiltrates. Trimethoprim–sulfamethoxazole prophylaxis, when given three times weekly or daily, provides partial but not complete protection. Therapy may include high-dose trimethoprim–sulfamethoxazole, imipenem, amikacin, linezolid, ceftriaxone, or combinations. Antimicrobial susceptibility testing is useful to guide therapy.

Legionella spp.
Legionella spp. can cause a rapidly progressive, multilobar pneumonia in transplant recipients. Nosocomial acquisition may occur from hospital water systems. The microbiology laboratory should be notified when *Legionella* sp. is suspected because it requires special stains and culture media. Therapy is generally with a macrolide (azithromycin) or quinolone.

Mycobacterial infection
TB is a major concern in endemic areas, where up to 15% of patients reactivate after transplantation with a mortality rate as high as 50%. Graft loss may result from rifampin-containing regimens (which lower calcineurin inhibitor levels and may lead to rejection). Pre-transplant PPD screening (or TB interferon-γ release assay) and isoniazid prophylaxis of latent TB infection can reduce these risks, and prophylaxis started pretransplantation can be completed post-transplantation. Recent results suggest that isoniazid is generally well tolerated in this population with careful monitoring for hepatotoxicity.

Non-tuberculous mycobacterial infection (NTBI) may cause pulmonary or disseminated disease, particularly in lung transplant recipients. NTBI is included in the differential diagnosis of diffuse lymphadenopathy with lymphoma and other malignancy, TB and nocardiosis, histoplasmosis, acute viral infections (CMV and EBV), toxoplasmosis, and others. Antimicrobial regimens containing three or more drugs for 12 months or longer are generally used in treatment.

Intra-abdominal infection and *Clostridium difficile*

Intra-abdominal infections are most common in the kidney, liver, pancreas, or intestinal transplant recipient and are often related to technical problems. The most common organisms include Gram-negative bacilli, enterococci, anaerobes, and *Candida* spp., but staphylococci may also be seen. Management usually involves drainage (CT guided or surgical) and pathogen-directed antibiotic therapy.

Underlying anatomic problems must also be addressed. Pancreatic leaks may require revision of the bowel or bladder anastomosis, whereas biliary strictures or leaks may require dilation, stenting, or revision. Necrotic tissues may need debridement (e.g., after hepatic artery thrombosis). Urinomas and lymphoceles may require repair or drainage. Serial CT scans may be useful in determining the duration of antimicrobial therapy.

C. difficile is a toxin-producing organism that causes pseudomembranous colitis, generally following antimicrobial therapy. Any agent may predispose to this infection, but prolonged or broad-spectrum antimicrobial therapy and clindamycin are most often associated with it. Recently, a relatively virulent strain of *C. difficile* has emerged that carries increased risk for toxic megacolon and the need for colectomy. Preventive measures include stringent infection control and prudent use of antibiotics. *C. difficile* should be suspected in any patient with abdominal dilation or pain, fever, and leukocytosis, with or without diarrhea. Therapy is with oral metronidazole or oral vancomycin, or intravenous metronidazole if ileus is present. Probiotic agents (e.g. *Lactobacillus acidophilus*) as an adjunctive measure have been reported in nonrandomized trials to be helpful in preventing recurrences. CMV colitis must be considered in the differential.

Urinary tract infections

Urinary tract infections are most common in the kidney or kidney–pancreas transplant recipient with altered ureteric drainage and in whom graft pyelonephritis may be accompanied by graft dysfunction and bacteremia. The most common pathogens associated with urinary tract infections are Gram-negative bacilli and enterococci, often with significant antimicrobial resistance. Ultrasonography is useful to rule out hydronephrosis and peritransplant collections.

Urinary tract candidiasis is common early post-transplantation and may lead to upper-tract infection and fungemia. In non-kidney recipients, recurrent urinary tract infections should prompt an evaluation for possible anatomic abnormalities or persistent foci. Graft pyelonephritis is a potentially life-threatening infection and requires prolonged therapy (≥3 weeks) with effective agents. Cure of infection must be documented before cessation of therapy.

Central nervous system disease

The presentation of fever and headache, seizure, altered mental status, or other signs of CNS infection in organ transplant recipients is a medical emergency. The presentation of CNS infection may be obscured

Table 4.7 Neurologic infectious syndromes in transplant recipients

Presentation	Common pathogens	Other considerations
Acute meningitis	*Listeria* spp.	Pneumococci, meningococci, bleed
Subacute-on-chronic meningitis	Cryptococci	TB, cancer (PTLD), HSV, *Nocardia*, *Histoplasma*, and *Coccidioides* spp., brain abscess
Focal neurologic deficit Seizure/cerebritis	*Aspergillus* spp.	*Nocardia* spp., cancer (EBV-PTLD), bacterial brain abscess, bleed/ischemic, toxoplasma, vasculitis
Dementia	PML (JC virus)	Toxic drug effects, demyelination, HSV, CMV

See text for abbreviations.

by immunosuppression; signs of associated meningeal inflammation may be absent and changes in the level of consciousness may be subtle. A differential diagnosis is developed based on the neurologic deficits, brain imaging studies, and the temporal development of disease (Table 4.7). All transplant recipients with CNS syndromes require imaging and lumbar puncture for Gram stain, cell count, differential, glucose and protein, cryptococcal antigen, polymerase chain reactions or PCRs (which may include HSV, HHV-6, VZV, CMV, EBV, and JC virus), VDRL, routine bacterial, fungal and mycobacterial cultures, and viral cultures. Ideally, a tube of cerebrospinal fluid (CSF) is saved for subsequent testing (e.g., toxoplasma antibodies or PCR, aspergillus PCR, others).

Four main patterns of CNS infection are recognized in transplant recipients (but are not mutually exclusive):

1. Acute meningitis, usually caused by *Listeria monocytogenes* or pneumococci, less often by HSV
2. Subacute-to-chronic meningitis (fever and headaches evolving over several days to weeks, sometimes with altered state of consciousness) usually caused by *Cryptococcus neoformans*, but also with systemic infection with *M. tuberculosis*, *Listeria* spp., *Histoplasma capsulatum*, *Nocardia asteroides*, *Strongyloides stercoralis*, *Coccidioides immitis*, HSV, and EBV-associated PTLD
3. Focal brain infection, presenting with seizures or focal neurologic abnormalities, caused by *L. monocytogenes*, *T. gondii*, or *N. asteroides*; occasionally nodular vasculitis with infarction due to CMV or VZV, and occasionally with EBV-associated PTLD, but most commonly due to metastatic *Aspergillus* spp. or other invasive fungal infection (often with lung infection)
4. Progressive dementia (± focal processes) related to progressive multifocal leukoencephalopathy (JC polyomavirus), or with other viral infections or the toxic effects of calcineurin inhibitors, often in combination with metabolic or other drug effects.

Viral infections

The impact of viral infections includes direct infectious syndromes, and indirect effects including increased risk for other opportunistic infections and, in general, an increased risk for graft rejection or malignancy. Most important viruses are now diagnosed using quantitative assays, primarily molecular amplification techniques (PCR or similar), or protein detection tests such as the CMV pp65 antigenemia assay. The treatment of viral infections is largely reliant on a reduction in the intensity of immunosuppression. Antiviral agents are not available or very effective for many pathogens, and viral clearance depends on the emergence of host immune function.

Cytomegalovirus

CMV, a member of the herpesvirus family, is common in the general population and remains latent throughout life. CMV can be transmitted from the donor to the recipient or reactivated in the seropositive recipient, particularly after intensification of immunosuppression. The donor seropositive and recipient seronegative (immunologically naïve) combination or "D+/R–" represents the highest risk category. Activation of CMV is stimulated by graft rejection, fever, and the use of depleting antilymphocyte antibodies among other factors. The clinical spectrum of CMV includes asymptomatic viremia, "CMV syndrome" (a flu-like illness with fevers, chills, myalgias, leukopenia, thrombocytopenia, and mildly elevated liver function tests), and tissue-invasive CMV (CMV pneumonitis, esophagitis, gastritis, colitis, hepatitis, retinitis, or other.) Symptomatic forms of CMV are generally associated with higher viral loads. CMV activation is often associated with activation of other viruses (human herpesviruses or HHV-6, -7, -8, or EBV), which is referred to as the "herpesvirus syndrome". CMV also predisposes to other opportunistic infections including those caused by *Aspergillus* and *Pneumocystis* spp., EBV-mediated lymphoma, accelerated atherogenesis after heart transplantation, and accelerated hepatitis C infection after liver transplantation. The diagnosis of CMV infection is by quantitative molecular assays or antigenemia assay. The molecular assays are more sensitive. Both may be negative in the face of invasive disease of the gastrointestinal tract or CNS.

The optimal approach to the prevention of CMV infection is controversial. The highest risk recipients (D+/R–) are generally treated for 3–6 months with antiviral prophylaxis (ganciclovir or valganciclovir, although CMV hyperimmune globulin and aciclovir and derivatives are also effective). Most of the lowest risk individuals (D–/R–) receive anti-HSV/VZV prophylaxis against cold sores and herpes zoster. The best approach to the seropositive recipient remains under investigation. The central question is whether prevention of asymptomatic viremia is useful. Recent analyses suggest that routine or "universal" prophylaxis is useful in reducing the risk for graft rejection as well as bacterial and fungal infections and PTLD. Prophylaxis is associated with higher drug costs and toxicities, and CMV infection may occur after the completion of prophylaxis (risk determined largely by the level of immunosuppression at that time). Preemptive therapy relies on serial monitoring and restricts antiviral therapy to those who develop viremia.

The treatment of CMV syndromes or invasive infection often includes a reduction in the intensity of immunosuppression with antiviral therapy. Traditionally, therapy for active CMV viremia was intravenous ganciclovir. A randomized trial of 3 weeks of intravenous ganciclovir versus oral valganciclovir therapy, followed by 4 weeks of oral valganciclovir, established the validity of treatment with oral valganciclovir in all but the most seriously ill patients. Regardless of the agent used, recurrences may occur. Ganciclovir-resistant CMV may develop, usually in the setting of the D+/R– combination, and particularly in the setting of subtherapeutic antiviral treatment (therapy or prophylaxis) and higher-intensity immunosuppression with higher viral loads. Alternative agents (e.g., foscarnet and cidofovir) are often nephrotoxic in combination with the calcineurin inhibitors (and have other toxicities) and the outcome of therapy for resistant CMV may be disappointing. Combination therapy using reduced-dose ganciclovir with foscarnet may be effective with reduced toxicity. Leflunomide has also been found to have a novel anti-CMV effect. CMV hyperimmune globulin may be used as an adjunct to therapy.

Herpes simplex virus and varicella-zoster virus

HSV may cause fever, malaise, and oropharyngeal or perineal ulcerations, especially in the early post-transplant period in patients not receiving CMV or other antiviral prophylaxis. HSV encephalitis (above) is one of the common forms of CNS infection in the immunocompromised host. Diagnosis of HSV encephalitis can be by viral cultures of CSF but more often is by HSV PCR from CSF.

VZV causes chickenpox (varicella), with reactivation from latency in neurons producing zoster (shingles). Primary chickenpox in the transplant recipient may cause pneumonia and fatal infection often due to bacterial or fungal superinfection. Pretransplant immunization of the seronegative candidate is desirable. Seropositive individuals (approximately 90% of adults) may reactivate VZV to develop zoster (shingles), which can be either dermatomal (localized) or disseminated (across multiple dermatomes or with systemic spread). Disseminated zoster may present with or without rash and skin pain, abdominal pain (cholangitis or hepatitis), pneumonitis, and/or CNS signs. Diagnosis is by viral culture of skin or other lesions, by immunofluorescence of slides prepared from active lesions, or Tzanck prep looking for multinucleated giant cells with viral inclusions. Therapy is generally with high-dose aciclovir or ganciclovir.

Epstein–Barr virus

EBV causes a variety of syndromes in the transplant recipient including fever and neutropenia, lymphocytosis, lymphadenopathy (i.e., "infectious mononucleosis"), splenomegaly, hepatitis, meningoencephalitis, and PTLD. The risk for these syndromes is greatest in seronegative recipients of seropositive organs (EBV D+/R–, especially in children), with intensive immunosuppression with antilymphocyte therapies or primary infection – often in adolescent recipients. As with all herpesvirus infections, viral replication is controlled in the normal host by virus-specific cytotoxic T lymphocytes. In the presence of immunosuppression, viral activation results in uncontrolled replication of EBV and B-lymphocyte infection with subsequent transformation of EBV-infected lymphocytes. EBV-associated PTLD is generally of B-cell origin but may be T-, NK-, or null-cell derived. Tumors may infiltrate the graft or CNS or present with mass lesions, pulmonary nodules, gastrointestinal or tonsillar bleeding, or lymphadenopathy.

The diagnosis of PTLD requires histopathology and studies for genetic rearrangements (immunoglobulin genes), cell phenotyping (CD20, monoclonality), and anatomic distribution. Low-grade forms of PTLD are polyclonal lymphoproliferative processes that may respond to cellular immunity stimulated by intensive reversal of immunosuppression (that risks graft rejection). With transformation to monoclonal malignancy, immune responsiveness disappears and alternate therapies (rituximab for CD20+ tumors, chemotherapy, surgery, or radiotherapy) are used. CNS disease is poorly responsive and generally requires radiotherapy. Prevention of PTLD is sometimes attempted with antiviral prophylaxis (ganciclovir and aciclovir) and monitoring of EBV DNA viral loads with reduction in immunosuppression early in the course of disease.

Other herpesviruses: HHV6, HHV7, HHV8

Other herpesviruses (HHV-6, -7, and -8) may reactivate after transplantation, or may be acquired from the donor (particularly HHV-8). HHV-6 and -7 are the causes of roseola in infants, and can cause post-transplant pneumonitis, hepatitis, meniningoencephalitis, and myelosuppression. HHV-8 (KSHV) is the cause of Kaposi's sarcoma. There is currently no specific antiviral therapy for HHV-8. HHV-6 may be treated with ganciclovir or foscarnet.

BK polyomavirus

BK virus (BKV) is a member of the polyomavirus family and is associated with ureteric obstruction and/or progressive allograft nephropathy (BKVAN) and graft loss in renal transplant recipients. This syndrome rarely affects extrarenal transplant recipients. A related virus, JC, causes progressive multifocal leukoencephalopathy (PML). BKV infection is common in adults with latent virus residing in the uroepithelium. After kidney transplantation, viral activation may occur producing interstitial nephritis and fibrosis with allograft nephropathy. BKVAN is most often associated with intensive immunosuppression, including pulse dose steroid therapy for rejection, and possibly renal ischemia–reperfusion injury. Diagnosis is made by histopathology in the setting of progressive renal allograft dysfunction, with intracytoplasmic and intranuclear inclusions demonstrated in uroepithelial cells, viral crystalline arrays by electron microscopy, or immunostaining for cross-reacting SV40 large T antigen. Molecular assays (quantitative BK DNA PCR) of blood and urine (quantitative BK RNA PCR) have also been used both to adjust immunosuppression and to monitor response to therapy.

There is no specific therapy for BKVAN. Patients may stabilize or improve with reduction of immunosuppression. Studies of low-dose cidofovir and intravenous polyclonal immune globulin have shown inconsistent benefit whereas leflunomide is under study for adjunctive therapy. Molecular screening (e.g., serum BKV quantitative PCR every 3 months for the first year or for any unexplained rise in serum creatinine) and early intervention (reduced immune suppression) is highly recommended. In the screening era, the incidence of graft loss due to BKVAN has markedly decreased.

Hepatitis

The management of hepatitis viruses is covered in detail in Chapter 10. In addition to the risk of recurrent disease after liver transplantation, hepatitis viruses may occur in non-hepatic transplant recipients, either as pre-existing infection in the recipient or as donor-acquired new infection. Hepatitis infection is often exacerbated in the setting of the treatment of graft rejection. Reactivation may be early and fulminant, or later and slowly progressive. Management issues are complex. It is worth noting that exacerbation of hepatitis may occur in the setting of concomitant viral infections such as CMV or EBV. The interaction between liver graft rejection and hepatitis remains to be defined. In HIV-infected individuals undergoing liver transplantation, hepatitis C may have a more rapid progression than in uninfected individuals even in the absence of detectable HIV.

Human papillomavirus

Human papillomavirus (HPV) is an increasing problem, particularly in long-term survivors of organ transplantation. Certain HPV types are associated with skin, cervical, and anal warts, and squamous cell cancers. Transplant recipients should undergo regular dermatologic examinations and should wear sun protection outdoors. Female recipients should have frequent screening pelvic exams and pap smears. Occasionally HPV may cause giant condylomatous lesions which can cause urethral or anal obstruction.

Parvovirus

Parvovirus B19, "fifth disease," is a common virus of childhood manifested by a "slapped-cheek" rash. Receptors for parvovirus are ubiquitous and present in the myocardium and on erythrocyte precursors. As a result, in immunocompromised hosts, parvovirus causes a variety of clinical syndromes including rash and fever, severe anemia unresponsive to erythropoietin, myocarditis, and pneumonitis. Serologic testing for parvovirus is often misleading and diagnosis should be made by quantitative DNA PCR for the virus. The treatment of choice is intravenous immunoglobulin (IVIG) with reduced immunosuppression. Multiple courses of therapy may be needed.

Case

A 37-year-old patient was admitted for a hemoglobin of 5.5 g/dL 6 months after a renal transplantation and despite erythropoietin therapy. Evaluation showed normal vitamin B_{12}, folate, and iron levels but a low reticulocyte count. Bone marrow biopsy showed giant pronormoblasts and serum DNA PCR assay was positive for parvovirus B19. The patient was treated with several doses of IVIG and recovered.

Community-acquired respiratory viruses

Influenza, parainfluenza, adenovirus, and RSV can all cause severe respiratory illness that may be complicated by superinfection (bacterial or fungal), enduring pulmonary dysfunction, or respiratory failure. All can be diagnosed in symptomatic individuals using rapid antigen detection assays (nasopharyngeal swabs) as well as cultures or molecular assays. Influenza and RSV are most common in the winter and early spring. These viruses are highly contagious, and require full respiratory isolation for hospitalized patients and contribute to bronchiolitis obliterans in lung transplant recipients. Yearly influenza immunization of transplant recipients is recommended, but immunization of healthcare workers and family members is also important. Recently, the novel H1N1 influenza virus has spread rapidly within the general population and poses a threat to immunocompromised patients. Immunization of all transplant recipients and candidates against seasonal and novel H1N1 influenza is recommended. As a result of increasing rates of resistance to antiviral agents in both seasonal and novel H1N1 influenza, it is recommended to follow the most recent treatment guidelines from the Centers for Disease Control and Prevention at www.cdc.gov/flu/professionals.

The use of aerosolized (and some intravenous) ribavirin has been described in patients with RSV or parainfluenza although there is no consensus on efficacy.

West Nile virus, rabies, lymphocytic choriomeningitis virus

West Nile virus (WNV) is a mosquito-borne flavivirus infection occurring in the summer and early fall. Transplant recipients are at increased risk of encephalitis, flaccid paralysis, and coma. There is no specific antiviral therapy. Transplant recipients should be given instructions on prevention (wearing insect repellent, staying inside at dawn or dusk when mosquitoes are feeding, clothes that cover arms and legs, eliminating standing water sources). In addition, organ donor-derived WNV infection has been described with fatal outcome. Screening recommendations for deceased organ donors are evolving.

Recent reports of fatal donor-transmitted rabies and lymphocytic choriomeningitis virus (LCM) represent highly unusual occurrences. Most rabies in the USA is bat associated. LCM is a rodent-associated virus that is endemic in rodents including mice and hamsters. In recent cases of donor-derived infections, concomitant CNS events may have masked development of diagnostic neurologic signs of infection. It is reasonable to exclude as donors individuals with unexplained and/or untreated encephalitis or neurologic disease.

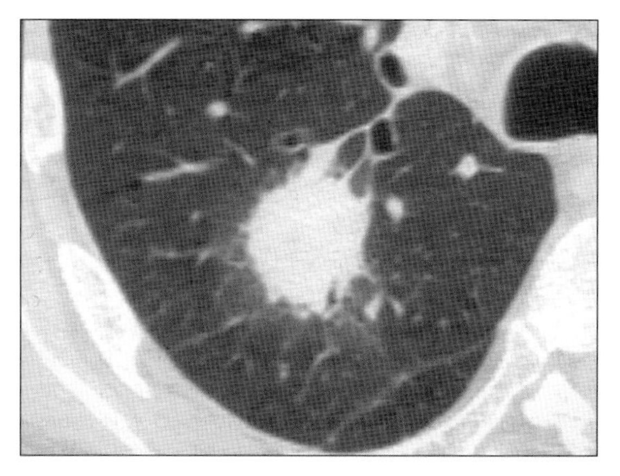

Figure 4.3 Kidney transplant recipient with cough and fever. Pulmonary nodule seen on chest CT scan read as "Likely *Aspergillus*" by radiologist. Biopsy demonstrated *Nocardia asteroides*.

Fungal infections

Risks for fungal infections are often organ specific and also relate to external environmental exposures. Prophylaxis may be considered in certain high-risk groups. Risks for fungal infections include prolonged intubation or intensive care unit (ICU) stays, extensive blood transfusions, significant metabolic or graft (pulmonary, hepatic, renal, or diabetes) dysfunction, and re-exploration in the early post-transplant period.

Yeast infections

Candida infections are often line or catheter related and are most common in liver, pancreas, and intestinal transplant recipients. Risk factors in addition to those above include exposures to multiple antibiotics, technical difficulties (pancreatic leak, enterotomies), and renal dysfunction. Prophylaxis with fluconazole or liposomal amphotericin B has been advocated for high-risk patients but practice varies.

Cryptococcosis is of greatest impact in the CNS but can also cause pneumonia and pulmonary nodules, cellulitis and nodular skin lesions, or disseminated disease. Cryptococcal meningitis may be associated with obstruction of the fourth ventricle, increased intracranial pressure, and the need for CSF shunting. Initial therapy is generally with amphotericin preparations, often with 5-flucytosine, with later conversion to fluconazole for maintenance. Note that *Cryptococcus* sp. is resistant to the echinocandins.

Mold infections

Mold infections often follow environmental (or nosocomial) exposures, beginning with colonization of the airways or sinuses, and followed by invasive infection. *Aspergillus* sp. is particularly common after lung transplantation. Pulmonary nodules, often with associated infiltrates, cavitation, and the "halo sign," are often hallmarks of fungal infection (Figures 4.2 and 4.3). Involvement of the sinuses, orbits, brain, and other sites may also occur. Mucor and rhizopus infection (members of the Zygomycetes) are less common but may be increasing with widespread use of voriconazole (to which they are resistant.) Non-aspergillus molds such as *Scedosporium* and *Paecilomyces* spp. are often resistant to multiple antifungal agents and are increasing in frequency. Culture and species identification with susceptibility testing are crucial to management of these life-threatening infections.

Endemic mycoses

Histoplasmosis, blastomycosis, and coccidioidomycosis are caused by dimorphic or "geographic" fungi. These organisms are yeasts at body temperature and molds at room temperature. They occur in geographically restricted areas, e.g. histoplasmosis in the midwest and coccidioidomycosis in the southwestern USA. Pretransplant screening for coccidioidomycosis is frequently performed by centers in the southwest USA. Past histoplasmosis is manifested by calcified lymph nodes and splenic calcifications. Disseminated infection may present with fever and pancytopenia, or gastrointestinal or splenic involvement. Fungal serologies may be falsely negative, and cultures or histology (e.g., of bone marrow or lung tissues) may be necessary for diagnosis. The histoplasma urinary antigen may be helpful. These fungi are susceptible to azole therapy and long-term therapy is required after transplantation.

Pneumocystis

Pneumocystis jiroveci causes a diffuse pneumonia (PCP as formerly known as *Pneumocystis carinii*) that presents with progressive dyspnea and hypoxemia out of proportion to physical findings. *Pneumocystis* sp. requires universal prophylaxis for at least the first 6–12 months after transplantation. In high-risk patients, such as lung transplant recipients or those with CMV or other chronic viral infections, lifelong prophylaxis may be indicated. Trimethoprim–sulfamethoxazole (TMP-SMX, either daily or three times weekly) is the drug of choice for prophylaxis. TMP-SMX also provides some prophylaxis against *Nocardia*, *Listeria*, and *Toxoplasma* spp. pulmonary, gastrointestinal, and urinary tract infections. Sulfa-allergic patients may receive atovaquone, aerosolized pentamidine, or dapsone for PCP prophylaxis. Breakthrough infections with PCP may be seen with inhaled pentamidine (upper lobes). Glucose-6-phosphate dehydrogenase (G6PD) screening should be obtained before using dapsone. TMP-SMX should be the drug of choice unless significant allergy or intolerance can be demonstrated.

Prevention of fungal infections

Environmental exposures are critical to the pathogenesis of fungal infections. Hospital or domiciliary construction causes aerosolization of fungal spores. Inpatients should wear masks when out of a filtered environment, especially when construction is occurring. Fungal colonization is more likely in patients with outdoor occupations or hobbies. Patients should be advised to avoid these activities for at least the first 6–12 months and should consult with their transplant clinician before resuming them.

Fungal prophylaxis or pre-emptive therapy remains controversial, but should be determined by the epidemiology of the geographic region and center, and based on any unique epidemiologic exposures. High-risk populations such as lung, pancreas, and some liver recipients are candidates for prophylaxis. Fluconazole and liposomal amphotericin have been used for liver or pancreas recipients; inhaled amphotericin or liposomal amphotericin, itraconazole, and voriconazole are used for lung transplant recipients, but practices vary. Interactions between azoles and calcineurin inhibitors or sirolimus must be carefully monitored. Most transplant recipients receive oral nystatin or clotrimazole in the first month for prevention of oral candidiasis.

Parasitic infections

Toxoplasma gondii is a protozoan parasite that is transmitted by eating undercooked meat or by contact with cat feces, and can reactivate in the transplant recipient. The organism encysts in skeletal and cardiac muscle and may be transmitted from a *Toxoplasma*-seropositive donor to a seronegative recipient of cardiac or other organs. Toxoplasmosis manifests as focal brain lesions, encephalitis, or pulmonary infiltrates. TMP-SMX (notably double strength daily) appears to prevent reactivation. However, some experts recommend pyrimethamine/clindamycin/leukovorin or atovaquone for early prophylaxis in D+/R– heart transplant recipients.

Trypanosoma cruzi causes Chagas' disease in endemic areas of Latin America. After an early febrile illness, cardiomyopathy, megacolon, or megaesophagus may occur years later. Donor-derived transmission has occurred, notably after heart transplantation. Screening should be considered for patients from endemic areas.

Strongyloides sp. is endemic in much of Asia, the tropics and southeastern USA. Infectious larvae penetrate skin and migrate to the intestine, where an autoinfection cycle may result in persistent infection for decades. When immunosuppression is initiated, disseminated infection may occur with a fatal outcome over 30 years after initial exposures. The parasite migrates widely and carries along enteric bacteria, resulting in diffuse pulmonary infiltrates, Gram-negative bacteremia, and meningitis. Pretransplant strongyloides serology (and therapy with ivermectin if positive) is recommended for any patient who has lived or traveled in an endemic area.

Case

A patient originally from southeast Asia underwent a renal transplant. Two months later, he presented with *E. coli* bacteremia and sepsis and progressed to respiratory and multiorgan failure. Strongyloides serology was positive. Despite therapy with ivermectin and broad-spectrum antibiotics, he died after a lengthy course.

Immunizations pre- and post-transplant

Vaccine-preventable diseases may cause severe complications in the transplant recipient (see Table 4.6). Vaccine efficacy is often suboptimal post-transplantation, and live vaccines are contraindicated. Anecdotal reports (e.g., regarding tetanus immunization post-transplantation) have raised concerns about triggering rejection, but larger studies have not documented increased rates of rejection in immunized transplant recipients. Live vaccines that are contraindicated in transplant recipients include varicella, measles–mumps–rubella (MMR), oral polio, oral typhoid, and smallpox vaccine (see Table 4.6). Inactivated polio and typhoid vaccines are acceptable. Household contacts of transplant recipients can receive MMR and varicella vaccine. Smallpox vaccine (vaccinia) can be transmitted by direct contact with the inoculation site and may cause severe vaccinia infection in the immunocompromised host. Covering the site with a bandage for 3 weeks after immunization and avoidance of direct contact can help to prevent transmission. The pretransplant evaluation should prompt re-evaluation of the candidate's vaccine status. Ideally vaccines should be administered before the onset of end-stage organ disease. If the patient is seronegative for hepatitis B, a three-dose HBV series should be given, as the patient may be offered a transplant from a HBcAb-positive donor. An enhanced-potency or accelerated regimen may be considered. Adults should receive pneumococcal vaccine and a tetanus–diphtheria booster pretransplant if not given in the last 5 years (see AST ID Guidelines for pediatric recommendations). The varicella-seronegative patient should receive varicella vaccine, but not if transplantation is anticipated within the next 3 weeks. Post-transplantation, yearly influenza immunization (both seasonal and novel H1N1 injected vaccines) and updating of the pneumococcal immunization every 5 years (or more frequently in high-risk cases) is recommended.

Further reading

American Society of Transplantation Infectious Disease Community of Practice. Guidelines for the prevention and management of infectious complications in solid organ transplantation. *Am J Transplant* 2009;**4**(suppl 9): 5–166.

Asberg A, Humar A, Rollag H, et al. Valganciclovir is non-inferior to intravenous ganciclovir for the treatment of cytomegalovirus disease in solid organ transplant recipients. *Am J Transplant* 2007;**7**:2106–13.

Avery RK, Michaels M. Update on immunization in solid organ transplant recipients: what clinicians need to know. *Am J Transplant* 2008;**8**:9–14.

Doucette K, Fishman JA. Nontuberculous mycobacterial infection in hematopoietic stem cell and solid organ transplant recipients. *Clin Infect Dis* 2004;**38**:1428–39.

Falagas ME, Snydman DR, Griffith J, Werner BG. Exposure to cytomegalovirus from the donated organ is a risk factor for bacteremia in orthotopic liver transplant recipients. Boston Center for Liver Transplantation CMVIG Study Group. *Clin Infect Dis* 1996;**23**:468–74.

Fishman JA, Rubin RH. Infection in organ-transplant recipients. *N Engl J Med* 1998;**338**:1741–51.

Fishman JA, Doran MT, Volpicelli SA, Cosimi AB, Flood JG, Rubin RH. Dosing of intravenous ganciclovir for the prophylaxis and treatment of cytomegalovirus infection in solid organ transplant recipients. *Transplantation* 2000; **69**:389–93.

Fishman JA. Infections in solid organ transplantation. *N Engl J Med* 2007;**357**:2601–14.

Fishman, JA. Transplantation for patients infected with human immunodeficiency virus: No longer experimental, but not yet routine. *J Infect Dis* 2003;**188**:1405–11.

Hadley S, Karchmer AW. Fungal infections in solid organ transplant recipients. *Infectious Dis Clin North Am* 1995;**9**:1045–74.

Kalil AC, Levitsky J, Lyden E, Stoner J, Freifeld AG. Meta-analysis: the efficacy of strategies to prevent organ disease by cytomegalovirus in solid organ transplant recipients. *Ann Intern Med* 2005;**143**: 870–80.

Kotton CN, Ryan ET, Fishman JA. Prevention of infection in adult travelers after solid organ transplantation. *Am J Transplant* 2005;**5**:8–14.

Limaye AP, Corey L, Koelle DM, Davis CL, Boeckh M. Emergence of ganciclovir-resistant cytomegalovirus disease among recipients of solid-organ transplants. *Lancet* 2000;**356**:645–9.

Lloveras J, Peterson PK, Simmons RL, et al. Mycobacterial infections in renal transplant recipients: seven cases and a review of the literature. *Arch Intern Med* 1982;**142**: 888–892.

Paya CV. Fungal infections in solid organ transplantation. *Clin Infect Dis* 1993;**16**:677.

Paya CV, Fung JJ, Nalesnik MA, et al. Epstein-Barr virus-induced posttransplant lymphoproliferative disorders. *ASTS/ASTP EBV-PTLD Task Force Transplantation* 1999;**68**:1517–25.

Paya C, Humar A, Dominguez E, et al. Efficacy and safety of valganciclovir vs oral ganciclovir for prevention of cytomegalovirus disease in solid organ transplant recipients. *Am J Transplant* 2004;**4**:611–20.

Preiksaitis JK, Brennan DC, Fishman JA, Allen U. Canadian Society of Transplantation workshop on cytomegalovirus management in solid organ transplantation: final report. *Am J Transplant* 2005;**5**:218–27.

Razonable RR, Rivero A, Rodriguez A, et al. Allograft rejection predicts the occurrence of late-onset cytomegalovirus (CMV) disease among CMV-mismatched solid organ transplant patients receiving prophylaxis with oral ganciclovir. *J Infectious Dis* 2001;**184**:1461–4.

Reinke P, Fietze E, Ode-Hakim S, et al. Late-acute renal allograft rejection and symptomless cytomegalovirus infection. *Lancet* 1994;**344**:1737–8.

Rodriguez M, Fishman JA. Prevention of infection due to *Pneumocystis* in HIV-negative patients. *Clin Micro Rev* 2004;**17**:770–82.

Scharpe J, Evenepoel P. Maes B, et al. Influenza vaccination is efficacious and safe in renal transplant patients. *Am J Transplant* 2007;**7**:1–6.

Sia IG, Wilson JA, Groettum CM, Espy MJ, Smith TF, Paya CV. Cytomegalovirus (CMV) DNA load predicts relapsing CMV infection after solid organ transplantation. *J Infectious Dis* 2000;**181**:717–20.

Singh N, Lortholary O, Alexander BD, et al. Antifungal management practices and evolution of infection in organ transplant recipients with *Cryptococcus neoformans* infection. *Transplantation* 2005;**80**:1033–9.

Wilck M, Fishman JA. The challenges of infection in transplantation: donor-derived infections. *Curr Opin Organ Transplant* 2005;**10**:301–6.

5 Management of the successful solid organ transplant recipient

Elizabeth A Kendrick and Connie L Davis
[1]University of Washington School of Medicine, Seattle, Washington, USA

Advances in early medical and surgical care of solid organ transplant recipients, and especially development of newer immunosuppressive drugs, have resulted in improved long-term patient and graft survival. Transplant recipients generally are followed closely by the transplant center in the early months after transplantation. Although the successful transplant recipient is in most cases "wedded" to the transplant center, a greater part of the long-term management of the patient falls upon non-transplant specialists and primary care physicians. These providers will be managing a growing number of transplant recipients and, often in consultation with the transplant center, will be responsible for managing transplant-related problems as well as overall primary care of the patient. Familiarity with common problems of organ transplant recipients is essential for the appropriate long-term care of these patients. Other chapters in this text provide overviews of management and follow-up of organ-specific issues. As discussed in these chapters, a major cause of graft loss is patient death, mostly as a result of cardiovascular events, infections, and cancer. Transplant recipients face an increased risk of morbidity from these problems partly as a result of side effects of long-term immunosuppressive drugs, so long-term management must include steps to decrease the risk and minimize the impact of these problems. The patient's transplant status and long-term immunosuppression may also impact routine primary care issues and standard recommended algorithms.

The timing of transferring a transplant recipient from the transplant center back to the referring physician and/or primary provider varies between transplant centers. In general, patients tend to be closely managed by the transplant center for at least 3–12 months. Most transplant centers provide a template for recommended laboratory monitoring and follow-up visits, but there is no single standard of practice. The most complete recommendations for transplant follow-up have been proposed for kidney transplant recipients. In 2000, the American Society of Transplantation (AST) published guidelines for early and long-term care of renal transplant recipients. In 2002, the European Renal Association published guidelines for follow-up of kidney transplant recipients beyond the first post-transplant year. International guidelines for the care of the kidney transplant recipient have just been published by the Kidney Disease: Improving Global Outcome (KDIGO) group. The goal of these guidelines is to help improve long-term outcomes of kidney transplant recipients and their allografts while minimizing complications. Standardized guidelines are not as well developed for recipients of other solid organ transplants, but existing guidelines for care of kidney transplant recipients provide a reasonable template for the care of these other patients. The AST's recommended frequency of and rationale for outpatient follow-up of renal transplant recipients are outlined in Table 5.1.

Early follow-up of transplant recipients emphasizes surveillance of allograft function, side effects of anti-rejection drugs, and complications of infectious

Primer on Transplantation, 3rd edition.
Edited by Donald Hricik.

Table 5.1 Recommended frequency and timing of outpatient visits for kidney transplant recipients

Time after transplantation	Interval for routine visits and laboratory monitoring[a]	Rationale
First 30 days	Two to three visits per week	Screen for acute rejection (high risk), postoperative complications, and adverse effects of immunosuppressive medications
1–3 months	Once per week (children) Every 1–3 weeks (adults)	Screen for acute rejection (high risk), opportunistic infections, adverse effects of immunosuppressive medications, and adherence (especially children)
4–12 months	Every 2–4 weeks (children) Every 4–8 weeks (adults)	Screen for acute rejection (moderate risk), opportunistic infections, adverse effects of immunosuppressive medications, adherence (especially children), and growth and development (children)
>12 months	Every month (children), every 2–4 months (adults)	Screen for graft dysfunction
	Every 3–6 months	Screen for graft dysfunction, cardiovascular disease risk, cancer, adverse effects of immunosuppressive medications, general health maintenance, adherence, and growth and development (children)

[a]Visits may be for laboratory tests only or may include contact with transplant nurses, coordinators, and/or physicians, as deemed necessary by either the patient or caregivers.
Adapted from Kasiske BL, Vazquez MA, Harmon WE, et al. Recommendations for the outpatient surveillance of renal transplant recipients. American Society of Transplantation. *J Am Soc Nephrol* 2000;**11**:S1–86.

diseases. Beyond 1 year, stability of graft function remains a primary concern, although the causes of acute and chronic graft dysfunction become more varied. Long-term transplant recipients with stable graft function remain at risk for medical complications, often related to chronic immunosuppression. Such complications may contribute to ongoing morbidity, mortality, and impaired quality of life. Table 5.2 outlines common problems encountered in transplant recipients as well as primary care management issues important in this group of patients. It is probably fair to say that the state of chronic immunosuppression and side effects of anti-rejection drugs are responsible for the lion's share of post-transplant problems, sometimes magnifying pre-existing disorders. The primary care provider will generally play the major role in managing stable transplant recipients beyond the first post-transplant year, whereas the transplant center may play a supporting role, seeing patients as infrequently as once a year. However, optimal management of these transplant recipients requires effective communication between the community physician and the transplant center. Table 5.3 lists those situations that require the specialized expertise of the transplant center.

Common symptoms or abnormalities occurring in transplant recipients

Cosmetic issues

Cosmetic problems resulting from immunosuppressive drugs occur commonly in transplant recipients. Chronic use of corticosteroids can cause a cushingoid appearance and dermatologic alterations, including acne. Weight gain is common, usually blamed on steroids, and is discussed later. These complaints can respond to steroid minimization, but this should be done in concert with the transplant center to avoid risking rejection of the graft. Acne usually responds to topical agents such as benzoyl peroxide or antibiotic therapy. Topical erythromycin or clindamycin, or systemic erythromycin, has been used with good results. Systemic macrolide antibiotics interact with the metabolism of the calcineurin inhibitors, so alternative therapy may be preferable. Patients with severe acne may benefit from evaluation by a dermatologist. Acne may be more common with use of cyclosporine than with tacrolimus. Rarely, severe acne has been reported with use of rapamycin and can respond to withdrawal of the drug.

Table 5.2 Common medical problems present in transplant recipients and monitoring recommendation for primary care issue

Problem	Recommendation
Cardiovascular problems	
Increased risk of coronary artery disease and cardiac dysfunction	Attention to modifiable risk factors
Increased risk of peripheral vascular disease	Importance of smoking cessation
Hypertension	Periodic screening tests in high risk patients (e.g., cardiac stress test with nuclear imaging or stress echo)
Increased infection risk	Fever in transplant recipients requires consideration of wide differential of etiology; regular dental care
Increased cancer risk	
Lymphoma	Patients require regular dermatologic and gynecologic screening
Squamous and basal cell carcinoma	Periodic laboratory testing for screening
Cervical and vulvar carcinoma	
Metabolic disorders	
Hyperlipidemia	Drug interactions with lipid-lowering drugs
Obesity	Monitor body mass index, diet, and exercise
New-onset diabetes	
Hyperuricemia	
Hyperkalemia	
Hypomagnesemia	
Hypophosphatemia	
Hematologic abnormalities	
Anemia	May require consultation with transplant center to rule out infection, decide on adjustment of immunosuppressive drugs
Leukopenia	
Thrombocytopenia	
Chronic kidney disease	Monitor kidney function and screen for proteinuria; may benefit by referral to nephrology
Metabolic bone disease	
Osteoporosis	Screen high-risk patients for decreased bone density
Avascular necrosis	May be ongoing problem in former end-stage renal disease patients; screen for vitamin D deficiency
Hyperparathyroidism	
Cosmetic problems	May benefit from adjustment of immunosuppression in consultation with transplant center
Pregnancy	Discuss use of contraceptive measures; desire for pregnancy should be discussed
Depression	Screening and consideration for treatment with transplant center
Non-adherence to medications	Regular assessment of adherence
Drug interactions	Educate patient re discussing initiation of new medications with primary physician knowledgeable with interactions

Table 5.3 Situations requiring consultation with the transplant center

Major changes in the immunosuppressive drug regimen
Difficulty with medication insurance coverage; nearing 36 months after transplantation in a patient not eligible for continued Medicare coverage
Patient non-adherence to immunosuppressive drug therapy
Suspicion of acute or chronic allograft rejection; acute or chronic dysfunction of the graft not explained
Suspected or diagnosed cancer
Unremitting or unexplained febrile illness
Swelling or pain of a renal graft; gross hematuria or new-onset proteinuria
Unexplained or persistent leucopenia or thrombocytopenia
Acute hospitalization
Renal transplant recipient returning to dialysis or to be considered for another transplantation
Patient enrolled in a clinical trial

Adapted from Howard AD. Long-term posttransplantation care: the expanding role of community nephrologists. *Am J Kidney Dis* 2006;47(4 suppl 2):S111–24.

Cosmetic complaints attributable to the calcineurin inhibitors (CNIs) are also common. Cyclosporine can cause hirsutism which can be particularly troublesome to female patients. Usually this problem can be managed by periodic hair removal or bleaching. Conversely, some patients on tacrolimus complain of hair loss. In most patients this abates over time, but, in an occasional patient, alopecia may be severe. The use of mycophenolic acid derivatives may contribute to hair loss. Cyclosporine use is also associated with gingival hyperplasia which is occasionally severe, interfering with oral intake or increasing the risk of oral infections. This problem appears to be more pronounced in patients taking non-dihydropyridine calcium channel blockers or phenytoin. These drugs should be discontinued or changed to alternative therapy if possible. Some patients benefit from chronic antibiotic therapy to reduce gum inflammation, but, in severe cases, gingivectomy may be required. Switching from cyclosporine to tacrolimus is often effective, but should be done under the direction of the transplant center.

Case

A 50-year-old man with end-stage liver disease resulting from hepatitis C received a deceased donor liver transplant 1 year earlier. Maintenance immunosuppression included cyclosporine, prednisone, and mycophenolate mofetil. His hypertension was well controlled on metoprolol, nifedipine, and furosemide. In the past 6 months he developed bleeding gums. Examination revealed severe gingival hyperplasia. Nifedipine was discontinued but there was no improvement 2 months later. After consultation with the patient's transplant center, tacrolimus was begun as a substitute for cyclosporine. Over the next 4 months, the gingival hyperplasia resolved.

Hematologic abnormalities

Disorders of red blood cells

Anemia is probably more common in renal transplant recipients than in other solid organ transplant recipients because there is not infrequently an element of renal dysfunction and defective erythropoeitin production. A significant proportion of these patients may be iron deficient, especially in the early post-transplant period, and may require iron supplementation. Beyond the first post-transplant year, 20–30% of patients remain anemic from some combination of impaired renal function, impaired erythropoeitin production, and/or the effects of antiproliferative immunosuppressants (i.e., target of rapamycin [TOR] inhibitors, mycophenolic acid derivatives, and azathioprine) that directly effect proliferation of red cell precursors or impair the action of erythropoeitin. Correction of anemia theoretically may improve the patient's quality of life and reduce cardiovascular risk.

Anemia is also not uncommon in non-renal transplant recipients, and is particularly prevalent in the presence of renal impairment. Anemia has been associated with the use of angiotensin-converting enzyme inhibitors (ACEIs) or angiotensin receptor blockers (ARBs), but has mainly been reported in renal transplant recipients. This effect appears to be due to an inhibitory effect of these drugs on erythroid precursors. Aplastic anemia due to parvovirus B19 infection has been reported and can respond to intravenous immunoglobulin infusion. Polymerase chain reaction (PCR) testing of the serum or bone marrow for parvovirus DNA is usually required to make the diagnosis. An uncommon cause of anemia, usually associated with thrombocytopenia as well, is the hemolytic–uremic syndrome which rarely complicates the use of CNIs and possibly sirolimus.

Key points 5.1 Causes of anemia in solid organ transplantation

- Impaired renal function
- Iron deficiency
- Antiproliferative immunosuppressants
- Angiotensin-converting enzyme inhibitors or angiotensin receptor blockers
- Parvovirus infection

A reported 10–20% of renal transplant recipients may manifest polycythemia or post-transplant erythrocytosis (PTE), usually defined by a hematocrit >51%, Secondary causes such as chronic lung disease, sleep apnea, or stenosis of the renal transplant artery or native renal mass should be excluded. The mechanisms for PTE, although not completely defined, may be related to increased sensitivity of red cell precursors to erythropoietin, possibly involving angiotensin receptors on these cells. Treatment may be required if the patient has symptoms such as malaise, lethargy, or headache, and to avoid thromboembolic events, which can occur in up to 30% of patients. PTE often responds to treatment with ACEIs or ARBs. Those patients who do not respond to these medications may require intermittent phlebotomy. In some patients PTE resolves spontaneously. Treatment should be considered if the hematocrit is consistently >55%.

Leukopenia and thrombocytopenia

Leukopenia and thrombocytopenia seen in transplant recipients are most often drug related. The antiproliferative agents can all affect cell lines, and significant leukopenia or thrombocytopenia may necessitate dose reduction or, sometimes, temporary or even permanent discontinuation of these drugs. Many other drugs commonly administered to transplant recipients can contribute to leukopenia and thrombocytopenia. Some of the anti-lymphocyte antibodies administered as induction therapy or for treatment of acute rejection (e.g., rabbit antithymocyte globulin, OKT3, alemtuzumab) result in lymphopenia that can persist for many months or years. Leukopenia is common with antiviral drugs such as ganciclovir or valganciclovir, and may mandate reduction in dose. Many other antimicrobial drugs, including trimethoprim–sulfamethoxazole, can lower white blood cell or platelet counts idiosyncratically. Finally, leukopenia or pancytopenia may occur in the setting of viral infections, especially infection with cytomegalovirus (CMV). Evaluation of persistent leukopenia or thrombocytopenia of unclear etiology may require extensive infectious disease and hematologic evaluations, possibly including bone marrow biopsy, cultures, or radiologic imaging studies to exclude occult opportunistic infection or hematologic malignancy.

Case

A 40-year-old woman received a kidney transplant from a deceased donor 1 month earlier. She had a 5-day course of rabbit anti-thymocyte globulin followed by maintenance therapy with tacrolimus, and mycophenolate mofetil. She exhibited immediate allograft function and steroids were stopped on postoperative day 5. Before transplantation, the patient tested negative for antibodies to CMV, but the donor was positive, and a 6-month course of valganciclovir (900 mg/day) was prescribed. Routine laboratory test performed 6 weeks after transplantation showed a white blood cell count (WBC) of

1100/mm^3 and a chart review showed that there had been a gradual decline in the count during the previous 3 weeks. Valganciclovir was temporarily held. Three days later, the WBC count was 1600/mm^3. Mycophenolate dose was decreased from 1000 mg twice daily to 750 mg twice daily. Four days later, WBC the increased to 2600/mm^3. Valganciclovir was renewed at a dose of 450 mg/day.

Adjustments in immunosuppression medications for leukopenia or thrombocytopenia should be done in consultation with the transplant center. Drug-related blood dyscrasias may take several weeks to improve despite adjustment or discontinuation of the putative drug. Severe neutropenia as defined by an absolute neutrophil count of <1000/mm^3 can increase the risk of bacteremia and granulocyte colony-stimulating factor (G-CSF) may be beneficial on a short-term basis.

Gastrointestinal problems

Most transplant centers have adopted protocols that include the use of histamine blockers (H_2-receptor blocker) or proton-pump inhibitors (PPIs) to prevent upper gastrointestinal complications (e.g., peptic ulcers or gastric erosions) in the early post-transplant period, particularly in patients treated with high doses of corticosteroids in the perioperative period. Patients on chronic low-dose steroids (e.g., <10 mg/day) should have a lower risk of upper gastrointestinal complications, so that these prophylactic drugs are often discontinued weeks or months later when the steroids have been tapered. Complaints of dyspepsia are often initially managed by switching to a PPI if the patient is on an H_2-receptor blocker, or increasing the dosage of the PPI. Persistent symptoms of dyspepsia should prompt further investigation such as upper endoscopy and search for specific etiologies, including infectious forms of esophagitis or gastritis resulting from *Candida* spp., CMV, or other herpesviruses.

Diarrhea can occur in as many as 50% of transplant recipients. Anti-rejection drugs such as the mycophenolic acid derivatives and tacrolimus are often causative agents. Patients may be taking oral magnesium or phosphorous supplements which can contribute to this problem as well. For the most part, diarrhea is mild and transient. Persistent symptoms usually respond to drug dosage modification. Diarrhea can be caused by elevated serum levels of tacrolimus, and conversely the shorter gastrointestinal transit time in the presence of diarrhea can decrease enteric metabolism of the drug and raise serum levels. Diarrhea in transplant recipients receiving mycophenolic acid derivatives can occasionally be associated with histologic alterations in the colonic mucosa and sometimes resemble those seen in Crohn's disease.

Despite the significant association of diarrhea with certain drugs, these patients should also undergo evaluation for possible infectious etiologies. Table 5.4 lists potential infectious etiologies for diarrhea as well as the diagnostic tests required. Figure 5.1 shows an algorithm for diagnosis and management of diarrhea in transplant recipients derived from the DIDACT study by Maes et al. (see Further reading). Using this schema, this group was able to determine the specific etiology of diarrhea and to provide a cure in approximately 85% of patients. Notably, this approach is based on the premise that reduction of immunosuppression may increase the risk of graft rejection so that other etiologies should be considered and treated before lowering the doses of suspected immunosuppressants. In practice, this algorithm is sometimes reversed with empiric reduction of mycophenolic acid derivatives. Using this practice, further studies should be entertained if diarrhea does not resolve. Moreover, efforts should be made to titrate the dose of immunosuppressants back to baseline once the diarrhea resolves.

Case

A 35-year-old man with type 1 diabetes mellitus received a live donor kidney transplant from his wife 10 years ago. His allograft function had been excellent with a baseline serum creatinine concentration of 1.2 mg/dL. Maintenance immunosuppression consisted of tacrolimus, enteric-coated mycophenolic acid, and alternate-day prednisone. The patient had severe gastroparesis, and 3 weeks ago his primary care physician prescribed erythromycin in an effort to improve gastric emptying. He called his transplant center requesting a second opinion about management of nausea and vomiting. Routine blood tests revealed: blood urea nitrogen (BUN) 65 mg/dL, serum creatinine 4.8 mg/dL, and trough FK506 level 31 ng/mL (target levels had been 5–8 ng/mL). Tacrolimus and erythromycin were both discontinued and serum creatinine returned to baseline within 5 days.

Table 5.4 Potential infectious causes of diarrhea in immunosuppressed transplant recipients

Organism	Diagnostic test
Bacterial	
Salmonella spp.	Stool for expanded enteric pathogens culture
Shigella spp.	
E. coli	
Vibrio spp.	
Aeromonas spp.	
Camphylobacter spp.	
Mycobacterium complex	Acid-fast bacilli culture
Clostridium difficile toxin	Send stool for toxin detection
Viral	
Cytomegalovirus	Serum viral polymerase chain reaction
Adenovirus	
Enterovirus	Stool shedding may not be pathogenic; may require colonic biopsy to document tissue invasion
Rotavirus	
Parasitic	
Isospora belli	Stool for ova and parasites
Cryptosporidia	May require more than one specimen for diagnosis
Microsporidia	
Pneumocystis jiroveci	Cryptosporidia, microsporidia, *Isospora* spp. require specific orders
Balantidium coli	
Giardia spp.	Antigen testing
Fungal	
Candida spp.	Stool culture and direct exam
Cryptococci	
Aspergillus spp.	

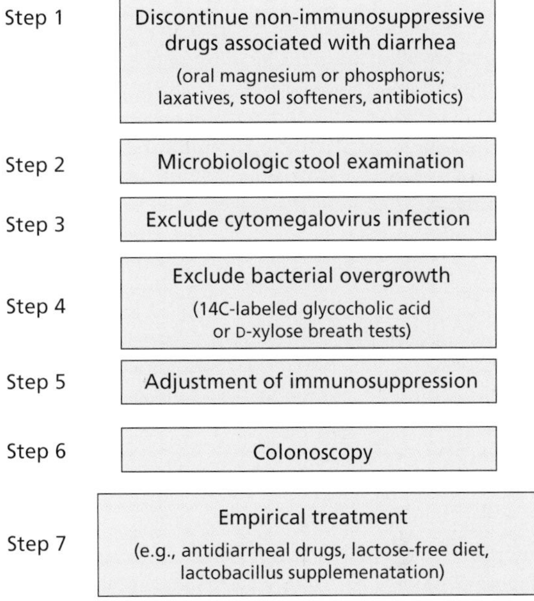

Figure 5.1 Diagnostic flowchart for evaluation of causative factor of severe diarrhea in transplant recipients. (Adapted with permission from Maes B, Haday K, de Moor B, et al. Severe diarrhea in renal transplant patients: Results of the DIDACT study. *Am J Transplant* 2006;6:1466–72.)

Fever

The cause of a fever in an immunosuppressed patient may not be readily evident and may present a diagnostic puzzle. Infections are the most common cause of fever in these patients, but common infections may present in an atypical fashion so these patients are at higher risk for atypical or opportunistic infections. Sometimes, neoplasms such as lymphoma can present as fever of unknown origin. A careful physical examination and detailed laboratory and radiologic evaluation are often necessary to correctly diagnose and manage the patient. A standardized approach to evaluation of the persistently febrile transplant recipient is essential. Blood and urine cultures should be performed and a chest radiograph should be obtained even if there are no significant pulmonary symptoms. Obtaining a urinalysis and urine culture is especially important in kidney transplant recipients because graft pyelonephritis may be present without localizing symptoms. Stool studies or nasal and throat cultures may be helpful if symptoms are present. Additional radiologic studies such as sinus radiographs, and chest and/or abdominal computed tomography (CT) can be done if there are localizing symptoms or if unexplained fever persists. Viral studies, especially for CMV or Epstein–Barr virus (EBV) infection should always be considered. Patients can manifest common community acquired infections; however, lack of clinical response to initial empiric treatment will likely require more intensive evaluation, as discussed in great detail in Chapter 4.

Common metabolic abnormalities

Hyperuricemia and gout

Hyperuricemia is a common metabolic problem in transplant recipients and often results from the use of CNIs that impair renal uric acid secretion. Tacrolimus may be associated with less risk of hyperuricemia than cyclosporine. Impaired renal function, use of diuretics, and the metabolic syndrome can contribute to this problem. Gout has been reported in as many as 10–20% of transplant recipients, can cause significant disability and impaired quality of life, and again is more common in patients receiving cyclosporine than in those receiving tacrolimus. Attention to diet is important but may not be sufficient to significantly reduce hyperuricemia. Allopurinol can be effective, but should not be used in conjunction with azathioprine because of bone marrow suppression. Allopurinol can be used safely with the mycophenolic acid derivatives. Some antihypertensive drugs, namely amlodipine and losartan, are reported to have a uricosuric effect that may be helpful in some patients. Acute gouty flares can respond to increased doses of oral steroids or colchicine. Colchicine may be poorly tolerated due to the increased likelihood of diarrhea when used with immunosuppressant drugs. In addition, metabolic interactions between colchicine and immunosuppressant drugs, in particular cyclosporine, can increase the risk of other symptoms of drug toxicity due to colchicine such as myopathy. Due to their deleterious effects on intrarenal hemodynamics, non-steroidal anti-inflammatory drugs (NSAIDs) should be avoided, especially in renal transplant recipients or non-renal transplant recipients with impaired renal function. However, if there is nothing else that relieves the pain, a short-course NSAID may be used while monitoring kidney function and blood pressure.

Electrolyte abnormalities

Electrolyte imbalances are common in solid organ transplant recipients. In kidney recipients, they are often related to renal tubular dysfunctions that reflect expected abnormalities in a transplanted kidney, compounded by some effects of immunosuppressants. Both tacrolimus and cyclosporine can cause impairment of potassium secretion in the distal tubule similar to that seen in type IV renal tubular acidosis. These patients are commonly on other drugs (e.g., ACEIs, ARBs, β blockers) that also can cause elevated serum potassium via a variety of mechanisms. Clinically significant hyperkalemia usually responds to dietary potassium restriction, drug dosage modification or discontinuation. The addition of diuretics or use of the exchange resin, Kayexalate, may be helpful. Kayexalate should be used cautiously in patients with significant gastrointestinal problems such as motility disorders. Florinef is sometimes used to manage persistent hyperkalemia, but may exacerbate pre-existing hypertension or cause symptomatic extracellular volume excess. Moreover, the long-term effects of using an aldosterone agonist on the myocardium and kidney are not known, but there is concern that such agents could promote cardiac hypertrophy or fibrosis in both organs.

Proximal tubular dysfunction can lead to urinary magnesium and phosphorus wasting. manifesting as hypomagnesemia or hypophosphatemia. Renal magnesium wasting is a side effect of the CNIs perhaps as a result of drug-induced decreases in the apical membrane channel that regulates magnesium uptake. Hypophosphatemia is most typically observed in kidney transplant recipients early after transplantation. It is most often seen in patients with rapid normalization of the glomerular filtration rate, and may result as a consequence of persistently elevated levels of parathyroid hormone or other phosphatonins such as FGF-23. Correcting low serum phosphorus through increased dietary intake is generally much easier than correcting hypomagnesemia. Oral replacement of either electrolyte can be limited by diarrhea.

Hyperlipidemia

Immunosuppressive drugs frequently contribute to dyslipidemia. Transplant recipients treated with CNIs and corticosteroids often have adverse risk lipid profiles with elevated concentrations of low-density lipoproteins (LDLs) and reduced concentrations of high-density lipoproteins (HDLs). Sirolimus can cause moderate-to-severe hypercholesterolemia and hypertriglyceridemia. Hyperlipidemia may contribute to the elevated cardiovascular risk profile already present in many transplant recipients. Numerous studies have shown that lipid-lowering drugs can be effective in improving abnormal lipid profiles with an acceptable safety profile.

The majority of studies examining lipid-lowering therapy in transplant recipients use hydroxymethylglutaryl coenzyme A (HMG-CoA) reductase inhibitors, or "statins," as the therapeutic agent. All statins appear to be effective in lowering LDLs and total cholesterol (TC) and there is little evidence to support recommending one over another. Each of atorvastatin, simvastatin, pravastatin, and fluvastatin has been used in studies of kidney transplant recipients. In general, these agents can decrease TC by 20–30%, and LDL-cholesterol by 35–40%. They are less effective in raising HDL-cholesterol or for treating hypertriglyceridemia, although atorvastatin may have some effect in lowering triglycerides. Recently, in a large, multicenter, randomized, placebo control trial (ALERT study), fluvastatin effectively lowered LDL-cholesterol to a goal of <100 mg/dL, but more importantly demonstrated a 30% decreased risk in fatal and non-fatal cardiac events.

Small short-term studies in liver transplant recipients have demonstrated the efficacy and relative safety of using statins in this population. However, long-term outcome studies in liver transplant recipients are lacking. The use of these drugs in liver patients may be more problematic in the presence of liver allograft dysfunction. The benefit of lipid-lowering therapy has been better defined in cardiac transplantation. In this setting, early use of statins after transplantation has been shown to be effective in controlling hyperlipidemia and decreasing the risk of cardiac allograft vasculopathy. Specifically, pravastatin and simvastatin have been used to this end in randomized trials, and an approximately 20% difference in 4-year survival rate has been shown in patients who received statins. Rates of cardiac allograft vasculopathy were nearly half those of non-treated patients. Cardiac allograft vasculopathy is now recognized to be a manifestation of chronic rejection, and it is believed that statins may be acting by immunomodulatory effects separate from their lipid-lowering effects. The statins may have beneficial effects on mediators that improve endothelial function or that suppress cytokine and natural killer cell activation. Indeed, older studies suggested that the statins exert an immunosuppressive effect in heart and lung transplant recipients. Evidence that statins have similar effects in other organ transplant recipients is lacking.

Certain safety issues should be considered when using statins or other lipid-lowering drugs in transplant recipients (Table 5.5). Hepatic metabolism and excretion of statins are affected by concurrent use of CNIs, thereby increasing the risk of rhabdomyolysis, a rare complication in the general population. This interaction can dramatically increase the blood levels of the statins, whereas converse changes in CNI metabolism in general are not clinically significant. When statins are prescribed to transplant recipients, the lowest dose possible should be used to initiate therapy. One must also be cognizant of other drugs (verapamil, azole antifungals, macrolides, proteinase inhibitors used for HIV infection) that can increase CNI levels and further magnify the risk of statin-induced rhabdomyolysis or liver toxicity. These adverse effects do not necessarily occur early in the course of therapy, and may occur after the drug has been used for a prolonged period. Individual statins may differ with respect to the risk of adverse effects. The extent to which metabolism is affected also varies among the available agents.

Atorvastatin, pravastatin, and fluvastatin appear to be the least myotoxic. Liver function tests and transaminases should be monitored while the patient is on the drug. In the setting of cardiac transplantation, in which statin use is more universal, it has been recommended that creatine phosphokinase (CPK) levels be monitored, even in the absence of symptoms, every 2–3 months after the transplantation, especially when the drug is titrated. In the absence of symptoms, elevations of CPK more than five times the upper limit of normal warrant discontinuation of the drug for some period of time. Less severe elevations warrant consideration of decreasing the dosage of the drug, stopping it, or changing to a different statin that is less likely to have this effect. Whenever a patient presents with significant new muscular complaints, the statin should be stopped at least temporarily and the CPK measured. Fibrates also may cause myotoxicity, most often when they are used in combination with a statin. Fibrates as well as omega-3 fatty acids are generally more effective in controlling hypertriglyceridemia. Cholestyramine may interfere with gastrointestinal absorption of immunosuppressive drugs, although the clinical impact of this appears to be low.

Table 5.5 Use of lipid-lowering drugs in transplant recipients

Type of lipid-lowering drug	Cytochrome P450 3A4 interaction	Dosage adjustment for renal function	Recommended initial daily dosing in mg	Special considerations in transplant recipients
Statins				Higher risk of myositis and rhabdomyolysis when used with CNI
Lovastatin (Mevacor)	Yes	Yes	10–20	
Simvastatin (Zocor)	Yes	Yes	5–10	
Pravastatin (Pravachol)	No	Yes[a]	10	
Atorvastatin (Lipitor)	Yes		5–10	
Fluvastatin (Lescol)	No		10–20	
Rosuvastatin (Crestor)	No		5–10	
Fibric acid derivatives				Increased risk of rhabdomyolysis when used in combination with statins (particularly with gemfibrozil)
Gemfibrozil (Lopid)	Inconsistent inhibition of other CYP isoenzymes	Yes[b]	600	
Fenofibrate (Tricor)		Yes	67	
Bezafibrate		Yes	200	
Clofibrate		Yes	500	
Ciprofibrate		Unknown	200	
Bile acid sequestrants	N/A	N/A		May exacerbate GI complaints due to other required transplant drugs; may interfere with GI absorption of immunosuppressive medications
Cholestyramine (Questran)			4–24 g/day	
Colestipol (Colestid)			5–30 g/day	
Nicotinic acid	None	Significant renal clearance	50–100 mg two to three times a day	Potentiates risk of myopathy when used with statins
Omega-3 fatty acids (fish oil)	None	None	Most studies have used 6–9 g/day	May cause GI upset; most report fishy aftertaste; can inhibit platelet function and increase risk of bleeding; can increase LDL and worsen DM control

[a]Dose reduction recommended for severe renal dysfunction with estimated creatinine clearance of <30 mL/min per 1.73 m^2.
[b]Use of fibrates should be avoided for glomerular filtration rate <15 mL/min per 1.73 m^2.
CNI, calcineurin inhibitor; CYP, cytochrome P450; DM, diabetes mellitus; GI, gastrointestinal; LDL, low-density lipoprotein.

Obesity

Weight gain leading to obesity is a common problem after solid organ transplantation. Corticosteroid use as part of the immunosuppression protocol has usually been viewed as the culprit, but, with the current widespread use of steroid-free regimens, it has become evident that significant weight gain can occur, even with complete avoidance of steroids. Whether other anti-rejection drugs contribute to weight gain is not clear. Improved appetite due to an improved sense of well-being after transplantation is a likely factor. Patients who are overweight pretransplantation have a higher risk of weight gain post-transplantation. Excessive weight gain increases the risk for post-transplant diabetes mellitus (PTDM), hypertension, and hyperlipidemia, thus contributing to overall cardiovascular risk. Despite well-defined adverse metabolic and cardiovascular complications related to obesity, the existing literature is conflicted as to whether obesity impacts transplant graft function and patient survival. Reports of the effect of obesity in renal transplant recipients are fairly evenly split in supporting or not supporting a negative effect on patient and graft survival. An unequivocal negative effect has not been demonstrated in other solid organ recipients, apart from the possible complication of hepatosteatosis in liver transplant recipients and insulin resistance with the development type 2 diabetes mellitus in pancreas transplant recipients.

Successful treatment or avoidance of obesity in the transplant recipient can be challenging, as it is in the general population. Weight loss interventions have not been well studied in the transplant population. Some centers have reported that intensive and individualized dietary advice in the early post-transplant period is successful in preventing subsequent weight gain. Dietary management and establishment of a regular exercise program should receive continued emphasis in the ongoing care of these patients. Effective medications to aid with weight loss are limited. Pharmacologic agents that interfere with fat absorption as a means to lose weight, such as orlistat, have been used with some success in the transplant setting. Unfortunately the resulting fat malabsorption can interfere significantly with the gastrointestinal absorption of many anti-rejection drugs, particularly the CNIs. A significant decrease in the serum levels of these drugs has been reported and in some cases and has precipitated acute rejection. Surgical weight loss procedures, including gastric bypass and gastric banding, have been performed in this population with reported success in many patients. Intestinal bypass procedures resulting in malabsorption would be expected to impact levels and dosages of immunosuppressive drugs.

Post-transplant diabetes mellitus

The development of new-onset type 2 diabetes mellitus has become a significant cause of morbidity in patients after solid organ transplantation. Most patients who develop diabetes mellitus will do so within the first 3 years after transplant, although reports have shown a continued increased incidence for up to 10 years. Up to 10% of patients may require treatment for PTDM in the first year after transplantation. By 10 years, 20% have PTDM and even more patients exhibit impaired glucose tolerance (IGT). Those patients who develop PTDM are at risk for diabetic complications (nephropathy, neuropathy, and retinopathy) in the same time frame expected for people with diabetes in the non-transplant setting. Patients with IGT often manifest this in the setting of metabolic syndrome and, similar to those with overt PTDM, have a higher risk for cardiovascular events as well as for progression to frank diabetes mellitus.

Early reports describing PTDM were flawed by variations in the definition of the disorder, most often based on the need for treatment with insulin. It is now apparent that some patients have less overt abnormalities in glucose metabolism and may be missed by this definition. Therefore, the diagnosis of IGT or diabetes mellitus should be based on criteria outlined by the World Health Organization (WHO).

The increased incidence of abnormal glucose metabolism is associated with the use of the corticosteroids and the CNIs. Both β-cell dysfunction causing impaired insulin release and insulin resistance have been found with the use CNIs. Tacrolimus appears to have a higher diabetogenic effect than cyclosporine. There are some reports showing improved glucose metabolism in patients with PTDM who were switched from tacrolimus to cyclosporine. The incidence of PTDM may be decreased with steroid avoidance or early steroid withdrawal. Late steroid withdrawal appears to be less helpful. In some patients, hyperglycemia is transient and associated only with higher steroid dosages used at the time of the transplantation or for treatment of rejection. Factors that increase the risk of PTDM include older age, obesity, significant weight gain after transplantation, family history of type 2 diabetes mellitus, a history pregnancy-induced diabetes, and African-American or Hispanic ethnicity. There is also greater association of PTDM with chronic hepatitis C infection and, in some reports, adult polycystic kidney disease.

Key points 5.2 Risk factors for new-onset diabetes mellitus after transplantation

Older age

Obesity

African-American or Hispanic ethnicity

Family history of diabetes mellitus

Recent guidelines have recommended screening for abnormal glucose metabolism once weekly for the first month after transplantation using fasting plasma glucose (FPG) and at 3, 6, and 12 months thereafter. Impaired FPG can be further evaluated by an oral glucose tolerance test (OGTT). Measurement of glycated hemoglobin (HbA1c) is generally not useful in the early post-transplant setting because anemia and the high red blood cell turnover typically occur early after transplantation. It is of more use in the ongoing monitoring and treatment of chronic PTDM. The diagnosis of PTDM should lead to treatment. Non-pharmacologic therapy including dietary modification, exercise, and weight loss should be emphasized initially. This is equally important in those with IGT. Even moderate amounts of weight loss can significantly improve glucose tolerance.

All oral hypoglycemic agents have been found to be safe and effective in the treatment of PTDM. However, use of metformin can be limited by impairment of renal function. Many patients with PTDM require insulin therapy. There may be a role for reassessing the immunosuppressive drug regimen in patients with PTDM or IGT, but this should be done only in close concert with the transplant center to avoid precipitating graft dysfunction due to inadequate immunosuppression. Corticosteroid and CNI dosages should be minimized as much as possible. IGT has been shown to be lessened, with lower tacrolimus levels in particular. There may be a role for switching a patient from tacrolimus to cyclosporine or withdrawing the CNI altogether because this has been shown to improve glucose tolerance in some patients, although careful follow-up for the onset of rejection is needed. The goal for treatment is to achieve normal or near-normal glycemia with an HbA1c <7.0%. Less well-controlled PTDM can exacerbate lipid abnormalities and increase the risk of long-term complications. Long-term management of transplant recipients with PTDM should include appropriate screening for retinal complications, neuropathy, and detection of diabetic kidney disease.

Renal disease in transplant recipients

Impairment of renal graft function in kidney transplant recipients has many potential etiologies and can be multifactorial. The evaluation, causes and treatment of renal allograft dysfunction are discussed in Chapter 7. In other solid organ transplant recipients, chronic renal failure after transplantation is becoming an increasing problem, especially as the lifespan of such patients has improved. Chronic nephrotoxicity of CNIs appears to be the major cause of chronic renal failure or chronic kidney disease (CKD), but diabetic nephropathy or glomerulonephritis related to chronic viral hepatitis may also contribute. Among non-renal organ transplant recipients, liver transplant recipients have the highest incidence of CKD, perhaps related to a high rate of renal function abnormalities present before transplantation (including hepatorenal syndrome) and the likely occurrence of hepatitis C-related renal disease in patients who are persistently positive for hepatitis C after transplantation.

Figure 5.2 shows the reported cumulative incidence of CKD in non-renal solid organ transplant recipients in the USA as defined by need for dialysis or a kidney transplant. Among liver transplant recipients, there is an almost 25% incidence of advanced renal failure by 10 years after transplantation. As a group, solid organ transplant recipients who have developed end-stage renal disease (ESRD) represent a growing proportion of the kidney transplant waiting list. In general, these patients appear to do well with kidney transplantation, and prior non-renal transplantation

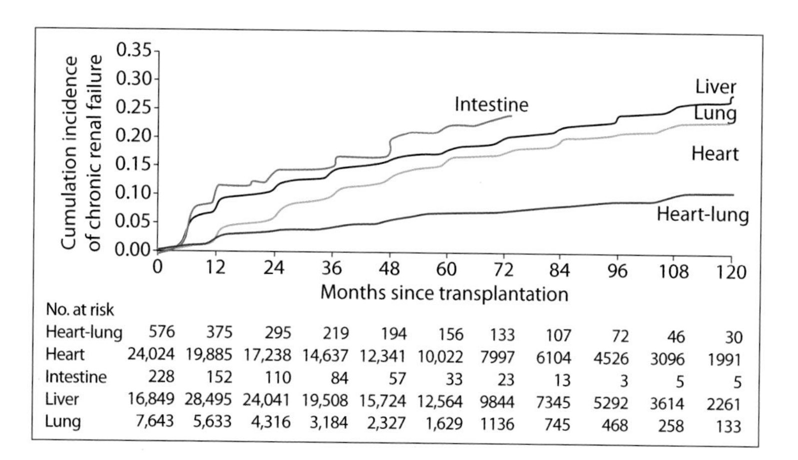

No. at risk											
Heart-lung	576	375	295	219	194	156	133	107	72	46	30
Heart	24,024	19,885	17,238	14,637	12,341	10,022	7997	6104	4526	3096	1991
Intestine	228	152	110	84	57	33	23	13	3	5	5
Liver	16,849	28,495	24,041	19,508	15,724	12,564	9844	7345	5292	3614	2261
Lung	7,643	5,633	4,316	3,184	2,327	1,629	1136	745	468	258	133

Figure 5.2 Cumulative incidence of chronic renal failure among 69 321 people who received non-renal organ transplants in the USA between January 1, 1990 and December 31, 2000. (Used with permission from Ojo AO, Held PJ, Port FK, et al. Chronic renal failure after transplantation of a nonrenal organ. *N Engl J Med* 2003;**349**:931–40.)

does not exclude them from consideration. As is true in general for patients with ESRD due to primary kidney disease, these patients appear to have better outcomes if they receive a kidney transplant compared with remaining on dialysis.

Solid organ transplant recipients with significant renal function abnormalities should be referred to a nephrologist for evaluation. The presence of significant proteinuria may require a native kidney biopsy to define the cause of kidney disease because this is not typical of CKD due to CNIs. Dosages of CNIs should be minimized as much as possible, but this does not always result in improvement or stabilization of renal function. Conversion from CNIs to sirolimus has met with mixed results and recent evidence indicating that sirolimus can increase urine protein excretion provides a concern in some patients. Non-specific measures such as tight blood pressure control, particularly with the use of ACEIs or ARBs in patients with proteinuria, may be of benefit to slow progression of kidney failure.

Cancer in organ transplant recipients

That transplant recipients are at higher risk for certain cancers, specifically non-melanoma skin cancers, lymphoma, and Kaposi's sarcoma, has been well established. Recently, studies using large established databases, specifically of kidney transplant recipients, have shown that these patients are also at higher risk for many other tumors. The risk of common tumors such as colon, lung, prostate, and breast cancer are roughly twofold higher than that of the general population. The risk for some other tumors is even more pronounced: a threefold increased risk for testicular and bladder cancer and a 15-fold increase in the risk of kidney cancer. Whether other non-renal solid organ transplant recipients are also at higher risk for cancers that have not historically been linked to immunosuppression is not known. It is important to note that dialysis patients waiting on the transplant list also have an elevated risk for development of a variety of neoplasms, suggesting that "uremia" itself may impart a risk of cancer. For kidney transplant recipients, it has been estimated that cancer risk is equivalent to non-transplanted individuals who are 20–30 years older. These findings raise important questions about whether standard guidelines for cancer screening and prevention apply to the transplant population. To say the least, the role of screening for malignancy in transplant recipients is a matter of controversy. It is generally accepted that transplant recipients should receive cancer screening appropriate for age and genetic or hereditary risk factors as outlined by the American Cancer Society. However, in individual cases, the benefit of the screening procedure must be weighed against the cost and considered in the context of the patient's overall life expectancy.

Transplant candidates with pre-existing malignancies require a disease-free waiting period before undergoing transplantation to minimize the risk of future recurrence. The length of waiting time varies according to the natural history and recurrence rates of the specific tumor. This issue is more fully discussed in Chapters 7 and 10. A major concern in these patients is that immunosuppression may increase the risk of recurrence by affecting the growth of residual tumor or previously dormant metastases. Although there are no extensive data to address this concern, one registry study did suggest a high recurrence rate greater than 26% in cases of bladder cancer, sarcoma, melanoma, and myeloma, and a history of symptomatic renal cell cancer. Moderately elevated rates of recurrence (11–25%) were seen in previous cases of Wilms' tumor, and cancers of the uterus, colon, prostate, and breast. Recurrence rates less than 10% occurred in patients with prior cancers of the cervix, testicles, or thyroid. Incidentally found renal cell cancer and previously treated lymphoma also seem to recur infrequently. Cancers known to be affected by immunosuppression, such as non-melanoma skin cancers and Kaposi's sarcoma, as discussed below, have a significant risk of recurrence. The risk of recurrence in liver transplant recipients previously treated for hepatocellular carcinoma or other hepatobiliary neoplasms is discussed in Chapter 10.

The cancers traditionally associated with the use of immunosuppression are skin cancers, lymphoma, and Kaposi's sarcoma. Increased replication of specific viruses known to be associated with the generation of these tumors may be related to suppression of innate immunity. Human papillomavirus has a strong association with squamous cell carcinoma (SCC), EBV with PTLD, and humanherpes virus 8 (HHV-8) with Kaposi's sarcoma. A guiding principle in the management of these specific tumors as well as any cancer after transplantation is minimization of immunosuppression. This should be done with guidance from the transplant center. Sirolimus is putatively anti-neoplastic and, in some settings, the transplant center may opt to convert a patient to this agent.

Skin cancer

SCC is the most common type of skin cancer seen in transplant recipients. This is a reversal of the pattern seen in the general population, in whom basal cell carcinoma (BCC) is much more common. The risk of a transplant recipient having an SCC has been estimated to be 65–100 times that of the general population. The incidence of SCC increases with duration of time after transplantation and with cumulative immunosuppression. There are reports of a higher incidence of SCC in recipients of heart transplants compared with other organ transplant recipients such as kidneys, but this is probably related to the greater immunosuppression that those patients receive. The highest incidence has been reported in Australia, where 43% of patients develop SCC at 10 years post-transplantation. However, the incidence is still very high in northern climes where skin cancer has occurred in 19% of patients studied in the UK. The occurrence of BCC is also increased, but not as dramatically.

SCCs and BCCs occur in transplant recipients about 30 years earlier than expected for someone in the general population with similar sun exposure. These cancers, especially SCCs, tend to be much more aggressive in transplant recipients, with greater local invasion, higher tendency for multiple locations, and higher risk of recurrence. Metastatic disease in SCC is almost unheard of in the general population, but occurs in 7–8% in transplant recipients. Short-term patient survival is very poor in the presence of metastases disease (1-year survival rate of 39% reported with distant metastases).

Early detection is the key to avoiding complications related to skin cancer. White transplant recipients should undergo a full body skin examination every 1–2 years. Most skin cancers will occur in sun-exposed skin; however, a significant number can involve the trunk. Thus, areas of the body that are normally not exposed need to be examined as well. Patients should be counseled on self-examination, especially if they are at high risk based on previous cancers or actinic keratoses. All patients should be counseled about the risk of sun exposure and the importance of using sunscreen. Use of UVB/UVA sunscreen with a sun protection factor of 15 or greater on all sun-exposed skin on a daily basis is recommended, as is the use of hats and other protective clothing. Not uncommonly, the lips and ears are sites of skin cancer, and these areas may not get adequate protection. White individuals with a history of skin cancer before transplantation are at particularly high risk and should be followed more closely, as should patients who have subsequently developed cancer after their transplant. Non-white recipients are probably at negligible risk and do not require such intensive screening.

If detected early, SCCs and BCCs can generally be treated adequately with local excision. Mohs' micrographic surgery may be required for lesions where tissue conservation is required, such as the face and scalp. More advanced lesions can require more extensive excision and possibly local node dissection. Premalignant lesions (actinic keratoses) should be treated aggressively. Modalities include cryosurgery, topical 5-fluorouracil, and curettage. Warts are not uncommon in transplant recipients and are sometimes difficult to differentiate from cancers or actinic keratoses, and may require biopsy. In patients with recurrent skin cancers, reduction of immunosuppression should be considered. This should be done together with a transplant center to avoid placing the patient at risk for allograft rejection. The extent to which immunosuppression should be decreased is related to the severity of the cancer and risk of mortality, as well the life-sustaining nature of the transplanted organ. Table 5.6 outlines consensus recommendations for

Table 5.6 Expert consensus on reduction of immunosuppression for specific skin cancer scenarios

Skin cancer scenario[b]	Level of reduction of immunosuppression to consider[a]		
	Kidney allograft	Heart allograft	Liver allograft
1. No history of actinic keratosis or skin cancer	None[c]	None[c]	None[c]
2. History of actinic keratosis (no risk of mortality; marker for increased skin cancer risk in future)	None	None[c]	None[c]
3. History of one or more NMSC per year (negligible risk of mortality, one or fewer minor surgical procedure per year; patients handle this with ease; warning sign of possible future skin cancers)	Mild	None	Mild[c]
4. History of 2–5 NMSCs per year (0·5% risk of mortality over 3 years, minor–moderate surgical procedure two to five times per year; patients can usually handle this, but it starts to bother them; likelihood of numerous future skin cancers)	Mild[c]	Mild	Mild
5. History of 6–10 NMSCs per year (1% risk of mortality over 3 years, minor–moderate surgical procedure 6–10 times per year; patients can usually handle this, but it bothers them; high likelihood of numerous future skin cancers)	Mild[c]	Mild[c]	Mild
6. History of 11–25 NMSCs per year (2% risk of mortality over 3 years, minor–moderate surgical procedure 11–25 times per year; this level of morbidity causes moderate distress and moderate disfigurement; depression may begin; high likelihood of severe future skin cancers)	Mild[c]	Mild[c]	Mild
7. History of > 25 NMSCs per year (5% risk of mortality over 3 years, moderate–severe surgical procedure >25 times per year; this level of morbidity causes severe distress and disfigurement; patients question whether transplant was worth it; depression is common; high likelihood of severe and possibly life-threatening future skin cancers)	Moderate	Mild	Moderate
8. Individual high-risk skin cancer: 1% mortality over 3 years (average-risk SCC; cutaneous and oral KS; stage IA melanoma[d])	Mild[c]	None	Mild
9. Individual high-risk skin cancer: 5% mortality over 3 years (moderate-risk SCC; stage IB melanoma[d])	Mild	Mild	Mild

(Continued)

Table 5.6 (*Continued*)

Skin cancer scenario[b]	Level of reduction of immunosuppression to consider[a]		
	Kidney allograft	Heart allograft	Liver allograft
10. Individual high-risk skin cancer: 10% mortality over 3 years (high-risk SCC; early Merkel's cell carcinoma; stage IIA melanoma[d])	Moderate	Mild	Moderate
11. Individual high-risk skin cancer: 25% mortality over 3 years (very high-risk SCC; stage IIB melanoma[d])	Moderate	Mild	Moderate
12. Individual high-risk skin cancer: 50% mortality over 3 years (metastatic SCC; stage IIC/III melanoma[d]; aggressive Merkel's cell carcinoma; visceral KS)	Severe[c]	Moderate	Moderate
13. Individual high-risk skin cancer: 90% mortality over 3 years (untreatable metastatic SCC; stage IV melanoma[d]; metastatic Merkel's cell carcinoma)	Severe[c]	Severe	Severe

KS, Kaposi's sarcoma; NMSC, non-melanoma skin cancer; SCC, squamous cell carcinoma.
[a]Appropriate level of reduction of immunosuppression should be individualized on the basis of specific patient- and tumor-related data.
[b]Estimates of mortality risk are derived from data in immunocompetent patients; risk may be higher in immunosuppressed patients.
[c]Unaminous opinion.
[d]Melanoma staging derived from the American Joint Commission on Cancer.
Used with permission from Otley CC, Berg D, Ulrich C, et al. Reduction of immunosuppression for transplant-associated skin cancer: expert consensus survey. *Br J Dermatol* 2006;**154**:395–400.

reduction of immunosuppression depending on organ transplant type. as made by an expert group of dermatologists experienced in managing skin cancers in transplant recipients. Results of retrospective studies suggest that sirolimus may have an anti-tumor effect for skin cancer and some centers consider conversion to this drug in patients with multiple SCCs or BCCs.

Lymphoma

PTLD has been reported to occur in 1–8% of transplant recipients. The incidence of PTLD seems to be higher in non-renal transplant patients, probably related to increased amount of overall immunosuppression. Most PTLDs are of B-cell origin and are often associated with reactivation or primary infection with EBV. PTLD can occur as early as the first year after transplantation or as late as 10 years or more afterwards. It can involve any organ in the body, including the allograft. It most commonly involves the lymphoid tissues, central nervous system, and bowel. It can present as unexplained fever, weight loss, or graft dysfunction. Transplant recipients at highest risk for PTLD are those without prior exposure to EBV (i.e., having negative antibody testing before transplantation) who receive an organ from an EBV-positive donor. Other risk factors include cytomegalovirus (CMV) infection and the use of lymphocyte-depleting antibodies for induction therapy or treatment of acute rejection.

Initial treatment for PTLD involves decreasing immunosuppression. Some patients may respond to this measure alone, although generally other therapy is required. In kidney transplant recipients, complete discontinuation of immunosuppression should be considered when the PTLD is severe or extensive because the patient can return to dialysis if the organ is rejected. Significant reductions of immunosuppression can be more problematic in other organ transplant recipients whose organs are more life sustaining (e.g., heart or lung). Not surprisingly, survival is better if response is seen with immunosuppression minimization alone. Patients with localized disease may respond well to surgery and local radiation. Remission of disease with systemic chemotherapy regimens occurs in as many as 75% of patients who did not respond to decreased immunosuppression alone. However, there may be significant problems with toxicity including bone marrow suppression, sepsis, and cardiotoxicity. Despite the association of PTLD with certain herpes viruses, a beneficial response to antiviral therapy has not been shown consistently. Some groups have used interferon-α or intravenous immunoglobulin with reported success in a small number of patients. A number of reports have shown a fairly good rate of remission with the use of the humanized anti-CD20 monoclonal antibody, rituximab – at least in patients whose tumors are CD20 positive.

Case

A 56-year-old man with a history of end-stage liver disease due to chronic hepatitis B infection underwent liver transplantation. He received induction immunosuppression using basiliximab and subsequently was maintained on tacrolimus, azathioprine, and prednisone. Pretransplant IgG antibody testing for CMV and EBV were positive. Prednisone was discontinued within the first month after transplantation. His liver graft function was excellent and serial protocol liver biopsies did not show rejection or recurrent disease. Two years after transplantation, he noticed a right submandibular mass. Needle aspiration performed by one of his local physicians to rule out infection was unrevealing. It was felt that it might be related to a dental infection. After a root canal and course of antibiotics, the mass continued to enlarge. An excisional biopsy was performed: pathology was consistent with a diffuse large B-cell lymphoma. The cells were positive for CD20 and CD45 markers and negative for CD3. *In situ* hybridization for EBV was negative. Before planned therapy with rituximab could be initiated, he began having episodes of bradycardia, hypotension, and syncope. Imaging showed a sizable mass in the right neck and submandibular region impinging on the carotid artery. He underwent urgent radiation therapy with significant regression of the mass. Immunosuppression was discontinued with the exception of dexamethasone. He then received 4-weekly doses of rituximab. Follow-up CT including of the neck, chest, abdomen, and pelvis was negative for evidence of residual disease. Immunosuppression was reinitiated with low-dose sirolimus. Several months later he complained of progressive low back pain. CT showed a retroperitoneal mass as well as a right axillary mass. Pathology on excisional biopsy of a right axillary node was consistent with recurrent B-cell lymphoma. Chemotherapy was initiated using CHOP (cyclophosphamide–hydroxydaunorubicin–Oncovin [vincristine]–prednisone) and rituximab. Immunosuppression for the liver transplant was completely discontinued. His disease regressed and 2 years later he is still in remission. His liver graft function remains excellent off immunosuppression and he has not had any episodes of rejection.

Cardiovascular disease

Cardiovascular disease contributes to a significant proportion of the morbidity and mortality encountered after solid organ transplantation. This is most evident in and has been most extensively studied in recipients of kidney transplants, but has been shown to occur in other solid organ recipients as well. The presence of "traditional" cardiovascular risk factors, such as advanced age, diabetes, smoking, and hyperlipidemia, can mean that these patients come to transplantation with pre-existing cardiovascular disease. Patients with CKD have a risk of cardiovascular disease that is elevated beyond that accounted for by these traditional factors. Left ventricular (LV) hypertrophy is present in most patients with advanced CKD and may be associated with non-ischemic LV dysfunction. Chronic volume overload, hypertension, and the effects of hyperparathyroidism on myocardial fibrosis are putative causes of cardiovascular disease in the presence of CKD. Hyperphosphatemia and elevated calcium–phosphorus products are associated with high incidence of vascular calcifications, particularly in the coronary arteries. However, the exact relationship between these calcifications and the higher risk for coronary events has not been completely defined. The chronic inflammatory state associated with ESRD and chronic dialysis may play a role. Recipients of other solid organ transplants may not have the same burden of disease, but side effects of immunosuppression may put them at risk for development of cardiovascular problems after transplantation. As noted above, the CNIs, corticosteroids, and the TOR inhibitors each has variable effects on the development of hyperlipidemia, hypertension, and glucose intolerance – each of which may increase the risk of cardiovascular disease. In both renal and non-renal solid organ transplant recipients, the development of CKD resulting from the nephrotoxicity of CNIs has become an increasing problem and itself increases the risk of cardiovascular disease.

Renal transplantation decreases the risk of cardiovascular events such as myocardial infarction or stroke when compared with equivalent patients remaining on dialysis. However, the risk of cardiovascular events remains elevated two to three times that of age- and sex-matched controls in the general population. A similar risk of ischemic cardiac events and for cardiovascular deaths has been shown in liver transplant recipients, although this has not been as extensively investigated in this population.

Recipients of solid organ transplants have been shown to have an improved outcome when existing coronary artery disease is managed aggressively. Myocardial perfusion imaging, in conjunction with stratification of patients based on risk factors, can help identify patients who warrant further evaluation with coronary angiography. Abnormal myocardial perfusion testing can identify patients who are at high risk for future cardiovascular events. Patients who are aggressively managed, either with coronary artery bypass grafting or percutaneous transluminal coronary angioplasty, appear to have an acceptable rate of complications and outcomes similar to those of non-transplant patients. Available studies do not consistently show a difference in outcome of operative versus percutaneous treatment modalities, although morbidity and mortality are obviously higher with surgical intervention. There may be a higher risk of postoperative infections due to chronic immunosuppression, but this does not appear to cause long-term morbidity. Small studies have shown 1- to 2-year patient survival rates between 85% and 90% in patients who undergo these procedures; 5- and 10-year survival rates are approximately 65% and 40%, respectively.

Patients with significant impairment of renal function, usually defined as a serum creatinine concentration ≥2.0 mg/day, are at risk for acute renal failure with the use of contrast agents. The risk can be minimized with intravenous hydration and possibly with adjunctive use of *N*-acetylcysteine. Acute renal failure after exposure to radiocontrast is sometimes, albeit rarely, irreversible, and may precipitate return to chronic hemodialysis. Temporary discontinuation of ACEIs, ARBs, and diuretics should be considered and some centers routinely recommend holding one or two doses of the patient's CNI before administration of contrast.

Although there is ample evidence documenting risk factors for cardiovascular disease in transplant recipients, there is less evidence documenting the benefit of aggressive risk management. Nevertheless, it seems reasonable to extrapolate from studies done in the non-transplant population documenting benefits of aggressive risk factor modification in those without overt evidence of cardiovascular disease.

Hypertension

The vast majority of renal transplant recipients are hypertensive, even in the presence of good renal graft function. Hypertension also is reported in up to half of liver transplant recipients. In kidney transplant recipients, many factors contribute to the pathophysiology of hypertension, including elevated blood pressure before transplantation, the presence of diseased native kidneys, and, uncommonly, renal artery stenosis involving the transplanted graft. CNIs and corticosteroids also contribute to the pathophysiology of post-transplant hypertension. Renal vasoconstriction due to CNIs, and sodium and water retention due to corticosteroids, are putative mechanisms. Patients are less likely to have hypertension if their immunosuppressive drug regimen does not include a CNI. In addition to being a risk factor for cardiovascular disease, hypertension may contribute to the progression of CKD. Kidney transplant recipients with uncontrolled hypertension have a twofold risk of graft failure. Proteinuria in association with hypertension increases the risk for progression of renal dysfunction in the general population and probably has the same effect in kidney transplant recipients.

Transplant recipients should be treated for hypertension according to the most recent recommendations of the Joint National Committee on Prevention, Detection, and Treatment of High Blood Pressure (JNC 7). Blood pressure should be kept below the defined cutoff for hypertension, <140/90 mmHg. However, both cardiovascular risk and progression of renal dysfunction continue to decline with tighter goals of blood pressure control. As most transplant recipients are considered to have increased cardiovascular risk, including some degree of renal impairment, current recommendations are for target blood pressure <130/80 mmHg as outlined by both JNC 7 and the Kidney Disease Outcomes Quality Initiative (K/DOQI). For those patients who have significant proteinuria (defined by >1 g/day), a blood pressure <125/75 mmHg is a reasonable target.

All classes of antihypertensive agents are effective in treating hypertension in the transplant recipient, although more than one drug is usually required. The choice of agent may be guided by other comorbidities, such as the use of β blockers in cardiac disease, or ACEIs or ARBs in the presence of proteinuria and/or diabetic renal disease. There may be other effects of a drug apart from blood pressure control that may influence choice of an agent (e.g., use of ACEIs in patients with concomitant polycythemia). Pharmacologic interactions between some antihypertensive agents and anti-rejection drugs should always be kept in mind.

Case

A 38-year-old male kidney transplant recipient has exhibited a gradual rise in hematocrit to a recent value of 58%. He has hypertension that has been well controlled on amlodipine and doxazosin. Losartan was substituted for doxazosin. Hematocrit gradually decreased to 44% over the next 6 weeks and blood pressure remained well-controlled.

Calcium channel blockers including dihydropyridine (DHP, e.g., nifedipine and amlodipine) and non-dihydropyridine (NDHP, e.g., diltiazem and verapamil) agents are used effectively in transplant recipients. These agents may mitigate CNI nephrotoxicity by reversing renal vasoconstriction caused by these immunosuppressants. NDHP drugs may also have an antiproteinuric effect which is not seen with DHP agents. NDHP drugs may interfere with the hepatic metabolism of CNIs, often requiring downward dosage adjustments of these drugs. In fact, NDHPs are sometimes used to intentionally decrease the dose and the cost of the CNIs. DHP-type calcium channel blockers often cause peripheral edema that can significantly affect quality of life and may require additional treatment with diuretics. In addition, there is a higher incidence and severity of gingival hyperplasia associated with cyclosporine when used together with DHP calcium channel blockers.

There are several theoretical advantages to using ACEIs or ARBs in transplant recipients. This has been most extensively studied in renal transplant recipients. These agents can decrease proteinuria by 50% or more by their action to decrease intraglomerular pressure as well as their separate effects on glomerular permselectivity. The use of these agents in both diabetic and non-diabetic patients with CKD and proteinuria has been shown to slow the rate of decline of renal function. Studies have also shown that these agents can ameliorate the upregulation of transforming growth factor-β (TGF-β) by CNIs. TGF-β is associated with the tubulointerstitial fibrosis and arteriolopathy that is the hallmark on chronic CNI nephrotoxicity. They may also diminish renal damage mediated by aldosterone.

Despite these theoretical benefits, retrospective studies have provided conflicting data regarding the influence of angiotensin inhibitors on patient or graft survival in kidney transplant recipients. Large randomized trials are lacking. Moreover, the theoretical benefits of these agents must be balanced against potential side effects, some of which are unique to transplant recipients. Use of these antihypertensive drugs may be limited by their tendency to cause hyperkalemia, especially in patients treated with CNIs. Dietary restriction and the use of diuretics in combination with these drugs may alleviate this problem. A small rise in serum creatinine would be expected with use of these drugs due to their effect in decreasing intraglomerular pressure. More significant elevations in creatinine may be seen if they are used with diuretics because of relative intravascular volume depletion. In kidney transplant recipients, a more significant rise in creatinine concentration can be seen in the presence of stenosis of the renal transplant artery and should prompt evaluation with appropriate imaging studies. Finally, ACEIs and ARBs can cause significant, albeit reversible, anemia in a substantial minority of kidney transplant recipients.

Other classes of antihypertensive drugs are useful to control hypertension in transplant recipients, but potential side effects are relevant in this population. β Blockers may contribute to hyperkalemia. Diuretics may contribute to lipid abnormalities, hyperuricemia, and transient renal dysfunction from volume depletion. α Blockers and other vasodilators may cause edema. These problems can adversely affect quality of life.

Bone disease

Bone disease is common in transplant recipients and multiple factors are involved in its pathogenesis. These factors vary depending on the organ transplanted. In kidney transplant recipients, osteopenia can be influenced by heredity, gender, exercise habits, the presence of diabetes mellitus, and, most importantly, pre-existing renal osteodystrophy. Nutritional factors and chronic liver disease may contribute to pre-existing bone disease in liver transplant recipients. In addition, a number of drugs, including the CNIs and corticosteroids contribute to the pathophysiology of osteopenia. Indeed, as bone density as measured by DXA (dual-energy X-ray absorptiometry) scans decreases by an average of a third in the first 6 months after transplantation, use of high doses of corticosteroids in the early post-transplant period has been incriminated historically as a major culprit. However, many studies have shown that post-transplant osteopenia can be severe, even in patients treated with steroid-free protocols.

A significant number of transplant recipients may lose enough bone mass to become "osteoporotic," thereby increasing the risk for fractures. However, fractures resulting from osteoporosis usually involve the lumbar spine or the hip. Fractures in transplant recipients just as frequently include the non-axial skeleton (especially the feet), supporting the hypothesis that post-transplant bone disease is not a simple form of osteoporosis. Fractures represent a major cause of morbidity and occasional mortality in transplant recipients. Reported fracture rates after transplantation vary from 5% to 35%, much of it occurring in the first year. Fracture risk has been estimated to be between 50 and 100 times higher than that of the normal population.

Numerous studies have shown that bisphosphonates are effective at preventing bone loss when used early after transplantation. They also may help to improve bone density when used late in the setting of established bone loss. Despite this positive effect on bone density, the benefit of these agents in preventing fractures remains a subject of debate. Moreover, there is a concern that these agents may lead to adynamic bone disease when used for prolonged periods of time, at least in kidney transplant recipients. Even so, based on studies showing decreased fracture risk in the non-transplant population, these agents are currently widely prescribed to transplant recipients considered to be at high risk for bone fractures. Several different treatment regimens have been shown to improve bone density in these patients, including daily or weekly oral therapy, or even intermittent intravenous administration.

Other treatment strategies should be considered. Vitamin D replacement alone, either in the form of activated 1,25-dihydroxy-vitamin D (calcitriol), cholecalciferol, or ergocalciferol, when compared head to head with bisphosphonates, is less effective in preserving bone density, but probably better than no therapy. There may be additional benefit to combined therapy. Adequate calcium intake of 1000–1500 mg/day of elemental calcium is recommended and patients should be given oral calcium supplements if dietary intake is not sufficient. Regular weight-bearing exercise should be encouraged. Male patients should be screened for hypogonadism and cautious consideration given to hormone replacement therapy in postmenopausal or amenorrheic women. Thyroid and parathyroid dysfunction should be ruled out.

Screening with DXA bone densitometry can help to identify patients with established bone loss who might benefit from therapy. Optimally, this should occur before transplantation or shortly thereafter in order to decide which patients would benefit from therapy early during the time of greatest bone loss. Some transplant programs screen all patients, but others reserve screening for patients deemed to at particularly high risk (e.g. postmenopausal women). Some programs have standardized protocols using bisphosphonates in the first 1–2 years after transplantation. Patients with known osteoporosis or osteopenia or those at risk who have not previously been screened should be evaluated later in their transplant follow-up according to recommendations established for the general population.

Avascular necrosis

Transplant recipients are at risk for the development of avascular necrosis (AVN), a bone disorder generally associated with use of corticosteroids. The femoral head is the area most commonly involved, although AVN in the talus, lunate, scaphoid, patella, and humeral head has been reported. Many patients may have more than one joint involved. Overall, the incidence of AVN in transplant recipients appears to be low at around 4–6%, but has been reported to be as high as 40%. Differences in the reported incidence may reflect length of follow-up and the imaging modality used for evaluation. Plain radiographs notoriously lack sensitivity and MRI has emerged as the imaging modality of choice. The risk of AVN has probably decreased over time as a consequence of low-dose steroid or steroid-free regimens. Once established, it is difficult to say whether minimization or discontinuation of steroids is of benefit. AVN can result in significant disability and diminished quality of life for the transplant recipient. Patients may eventually require replacement of the affected joint. Less severe disease may be managed conservatively with bed rest and partial weight bearing. Some patients may benefit by osteotomy or core decompression as a joint-saving technique. The best approach is to avoid the complication by minimizing corticosteroid use as much as possible.

Key points 5.3 Most common skeletal sites for avascular necrosis

Femoral head

Talus

Lunate

Scaphoid

Patella

Humeral head

Hyperparathyroidism

Renal transplant recipients often exhibit persistent secondary hyperparathyroidism or may even develop tertiary hyperparathyroidism related to overactivity of the parathyroid gland which develops routinely in patients with ESRD. Secondary hyperparathyroidism may persist for many months after transplantation and is critically dependent on the level of renal function obtained by transplantation. There is emerging evidence that screening for and correcting 25-hydroxyvitamin D deficiency can be helpful in resolution of this problem. Hypercalcemia may signal tertiary hyperparathyroidism that may not respond to medical therapy and may eventually require surgical parathyroidectomy. The role of cinacalcet in managing such patients is uncertain and requires further study.

Other significant primary care issues in transplant recipients

Reproduction and sexual function

Disturbances in the hypothalamic–pituitary axis related to chronic illness cause infertility and sexual dysfunction in many patients before solid organ transplantation. Sexual dysfunction has been extensively described in patients with CKD and in those with cirrhosis. Menstrual irregularities associated with anovulation occur in women. Most men have low testosterone levels, report erectile dysfunction and decreased libido, and can have impaired spermatogenesis. In general, these disturbances tend to improve in patients who receive a well-functioning organ, but the outcomes are less than uniform. Low testosterone levels have been reported to persist in up to 20% of heart transplant recipients. In the renal transplant population, erectile dysfunction (ED) can persist in as many as 30–50% of men. Age-related changes or comorbidities such as diabetic neuropathy may contribute. Use of certain drugs for common problems in transplant recipients can be associated with ED (e.g. treatment with β blockers, calcium channel blockers, or antidepressants). There are many reports to demonstrate improvement in ED with treatment with sildenafil or its congeners in kidney transplant recipients. Sildenafil is metabolized by the same hepatic pathway as the CNIs and in theory could decrease the serum levels of these drugs. However, small studies of this drug in kidney transplant recipients have failed to find any difference in drug exposure, possibly related to the intermittent nature of usage. There is little available information about the benefit of testosterone replacement in the transplant population. Indeed, the benefit of testosterone replacement in the general male population is uncertain, and must be balanced against significant adverse effects such as sleep apnea, polycythemia, adverse lipid profile, and an increased risk of prostatic disease.

With the possible exception of an association between low testosterone levels and use of corticosteroids, most immunosuppressant medications do not seem to affect sexual function or fertility in males. Although reports are limited, children fathered by transplant recipients do not seem to have a higher incidence of birth defects. The one exception is the TOR inhibitors, which appear to adversely affect spermatogeneis and sperm function quite regularly. Discontinuation of this class of agents may be necessary in male patients wishing to father children.

There is extensive information about pregnancy after solid organ transplantation. As fertility seems to return quickly to age-appropriate levels in female transplant recipients, it is important that an adequate method of contraception is initiated in female recipients of child-bearing age. Transplant status as such should not dictate the choice of contraception measure, although comorbidities in individual patients may limit the use of oral contraceptives. The presence of hypertension, lipid abnormalities, or liver dysfunction may be a relative contraindication to use of these agents. Some but not all transplant professionals feel that contraception using intrauterine devices may be ineffective because this method relies on the inflammatory reaction set up by the device, and this inflammation may be reduced by immunosuppression medications. Female transplant recipients desiring pregnancy should be counseled that it is certainly a feasible option, but, as detailed below, the women need to be fully aware of the risks involved.

The National Transplantation Pregnancy Registry has reported the outcome of over 1600 pregnancies in over 1000 female transplant recipients in the USA. Approximately 75% have occurred in kidney recipients, 15% in liver transplant recipients, and approximately 5% each in heart and combined kidney–pancreas transplant recipients. Only a handful have been reported after lung or other combined organ transplants. Recommendations as to the optimal timing of pregnancy are listed in Table 5.7.

Historical registry analyses suggest poorer fetal outcomes with shorter transplant-to-conception time intervals, and this forms the basis for recommending a waiting period of 1–2 years after transplantation before conceiving. In addition, a trend toward more acute rejection episodes has been observed with earlier conceptions. However, a more recent report demonstrated equivalent outcomes for both pregnancy and long-term graft function in a group of renal transplant recipients who became pregnant <1 year after transplantation compared with those >1 year. Therefore, although it is preferable that patients wait at least 1 year after transplantation to ensure optimum graft function and lowest risk of rejection, pregnancies occurring before that time frame do not necessarily mandate recommendation for termination. Most anti-rejection drugs are safe to continue during pregnancy. There is a long track record of safety for cyclosporine, azathioprine, prednisone, and more recently tacrolimus during pregnancy. Overall, there is a higher incidence of low-for-birth-weight infants and prematurity, but no evidence of higher risk of birth defects. Interestingly, azathioprine carries a Food and Drug Administration pregnancy rating of "D," although the literature supports its relative safety during pregnancy in transplant recipients and those treated for autoimmune diseases. A higher incidence of structural abnormalities in newborns has been reported with mycophenolate mofetil exposure during pregnancy and therefore it also carries a pregnancy rating of "D." Although it may be wise to discontinue mycophenolate mofetil either before desired conception or early after pregnancy is detected, the wisdom of this strategy must always be balanced against the risk to the allograft and the mother. There is little experience with the use of sirolimus during pregnancy. Studies in animals have shown some teratogenic potential. Among the handful of women who were reported to the national registry and who were receiving sirolimus at the time of conception, the drug was most often discontinued during the first trimes-

Table 5.7 Optimal circumstances for pregnancy in solid organ transplant patients

More than 1 year post-transplantation
Good graft function with no evidence of rejection
No rejection episodes have occurred for 1 year before conception
For kidney transplant recipients: creatinine concentration stable at ≤1.5 mg/dL; no significant proteinuria (<500 mg/day)
Immunosuppression at nadir and stable dosing

ter. No structural defects were reported. There are only a few case reports of successful outcome of pregnancies for patients in whom sirolimus was continued throughout the entire pregnancy. Consideration also needs to be given to the other drugs that may have teratogenic potential and require discontinuation before conception, such as ACEIs and possibly statins. There is theoretical potential risk of immunosuppressive drug exposure to the infant who is breastfed by a mother who is an organ transplant recipient. Traditionally, breastfeeding has been discouraged because of this risk.

Pregnant transplant recipients should receive prenatal care by an experienced high-risk obstetrician who communicates regularly with the transplant center. These patients are at higher risk for medical complications during pregnancy and require close follow-up. Many patients will require treatment for hypertension during the pregnancy. The incidence of pre-eclampsia appears to be higher, especially in kidney transplant recipients in whom it has been reported in a third of patients. Pre-existing hypertension and/or proteinuria can make it difficult to diagnose superimposed pre-eclampsia. There is a significant incidence of pregnancy-induced diabetes mellitus in transplant recipients. Obstetric risks include intrauterine growth retardation, low-for-birth-weight infants, higher risk of premature birth, and higher incidence of need for delivery by cesarean section. Cesarean section should be performed for obstetric indications alone. In kidney and/or pancreas graft recipients requiring cesarean section, it may be desirable to have the transplant surgeon available to avoid injury to the grafts because of their location.

Dosages of immunosuppressive drugs needed to maintain adequate drug sometimes must be increased due to an increase in volume of distribution, especially during the second and third trimesters. This is particularly true of the CNIs. Drug levels should be followed closely to avoid inadequate exposure that could increase the risk of rejection. Treatment of rejection episodes should be based on standard practice for the non-pregnant transplant recipient. High doses of corticosteroids are generally tolerated well with no appreciable risk to the fetus, and are generally used as first-line agents. Experience with the use of anti-lymphocyte antibodies for the treatment of acute rejection during pregnancy has been limited but IgG does cross the placenta.

Case

A 24-year-old woman is being seen at follow-up for her kidney transplant 2 years ago. She has a history of spina bifida and ESRD due to cloacal extrophy and reflux. Her renal graft drains into a continent neobladder which she catheterized via an umbilical stoma. She is immunosuppressed using tacrolimus and prednisone. Mycophenolate was discontinued in the first few months after transplantation. A biopsy was done in the first 2 months after transplantation when her creatinine, which was 1.4 mg/dL at best, had increased to 2–2.3 mg/dL. This showed subepithelial nodules in arterioles suggestive of CNI toxicity, but no evidence of rejection. The tacrolimus dose was decreased with improvement in renal function but only to serum creatinine concentrations of 1.7–1.9 mg/dL. A repeat biopsy a few weeks later showed mild interstitial fibrosis and tubular atrophy similar to the previous biopsy but no other specific abnormalities. Imaging of her graft did not show any evidence of obstruction. Since her transplant, she has had recurrent urinary tract infections and febrile pyelonephritis requiring several hospital admissions. She consistently has elevation of serum creatinine to 3–3.4 mg/dL concurrent with infections, and then improvement after treatment to 1.7–2 mg/dL. She presents after recently having had a positive pregnancy test performed by a medical facility; she later had vaginal bleeding and a follow-up test was negative. She is currently in a stable relationship with her long-term boyfriend; they use a condom for contraception. She and her boyfriend now want to discuss pregnancy, however. In addition to immunosuppressive medications, she is taking labetolol, sodium bicarbonate, and aspirin.

This patient represents a high-risk obstetric situation. She has significant renal graft dysfunction and would be at high risk for accelerated graft failure during pregnancy. Graft dysfunction would increase the risk of pregnancy-related complications such as pre-eclampsia and prematurity. Recurrent urinary tract infections would likely have additional adverse effects on the graft and pregnancy. She would be at higher risk for requiring a caesarean section which could risk the viability of her neobladder.

In kidney transplant recipients, the risk that pregnancy will adversely affect long-term graft function is low if baseline kidney function is well preserved. With pre-existing renal function impairment as defined by a serum creatinine >1.5 mg/dL, there is an increased risk of further deterioration of graft function during and after pregnancy. Graft loss within 2 years has been reported in as many as 14% of kidney recipients after pregnancy. This course is similar to what is seen in non-transplant recipients with CKD and is exacerbated by inadequate blood pressure control. Existing proteinuria tends to increase during pregnancy, then return to baseline levels after delivery. The number of reported pregnancies in other solid organ transplant recipients is small. Reported rates of early graft loss after pregnancy have varied from 3–9% in liver transplant recipients to 23% in lung recipients.

Neuropsychiatric problems

Mood disorders

Mood disorders, most notably depression, are common in patients awaiting organ transplantation. Despite an improved quality of life after transplantation, depression persists in a significant number of patients. In the heart transplant population, the incidence of depression has been shown to climb from 15% early after organ transplantation to as high as 25–30% by 3 years. Other solid organ transplant recipients have been less systematically studied, but similarly have elevated rates of mood disorders compared with the general population. Major depressive disorder and post-traumatic stress disorder are the most frequent diagnoses. Not surprisingly, mood disorders can negatively affect quality of life and perceived ability to work, thereby impairing rehabilitation. Rates of depression are higher in those with less socioeconomic support. The patient's expectations of outcome after transplantation appear, however, to also play a role. Expectations are higher in those with higher levels of education and this has, in addition, been associated with development of depression.

Most classes of antidepressants have been used in recipients of organ transplants. Unfortunately, the majority of experience is anecdotal or comes from small non-randomized studies. Although there is little support to recommend any specific antidepressant with regard to efficacy, side effects and/or drug interactions may dictate use of one drug over another. The largest experiences with the use of antidepressants have been reported in kidney and heart transplant recipients. Selective serotonin reuptake inhibitors (SSRIs) have been used most widely and appear to have a favorable efficacy and side-effect profile. SSRIs have an inhibitory effect on the enzymes of the cytochrome P450 system in the liver and can potentially raise levels of tacrolimus, cyclosporine, and the TOR inhibitors. However, the effect is variable and it is reasonable to increase the frequency of therapeutic drug monitoring when these agents are initiated. Dosage adjustment for renal and liver function impairment also warrants consideration. Table 5.8

Table 5.8 Use of antidepressants in the setting of transplantation and potential interaction with hepatic metabolism of calcineurin inhibitors via the 3A4 isoenzyme of the cytochrome P450 system

Drug class	Effect on cytochrome P450 3A4[a]	Dose adjustment for liver disease[b]	Dose adjustment for kidney disease[b]	Special considerations in transplant patients
Serotonin reuptake inhibitors	Inhibits enzyme:			Greatest experience and documented safety using this class of drugs; nefazodone appears to have highest risk of causing CNI toxicity, citalopram the least
Fluoxetine (Prozac)	++	Y	N	
Paroxetine (Paxil)	++	Y	Y	
Citalopram (Celexa)	+	Y	Y (severe)	
Escitalopram (Lexapro)	++	Y	Y	
Sertraline (Zoloft)	+	Y	Y	
Fluvoxamine	++	Y	N	
Nefazodone	++	Y	N	

Table 5.8 (*Continued*)

Drug class	Effect on cytochrome P450 3A4[a]	Dose adjustment for liver disease[b]	Dose adjustment for kidney disease[b]	Special considerations in transplant patients
Monoamine oxidase inhibitors[c]				Little experience in transplant recipients; numerous and serious potential drug and dietary interactions; most recommend avoiding this class of drugs
Phenelzine	–	Y	N	
Tranylcypromine	–	Y	N	
Selegiline	–	Y (severe)	N	
Tricyclic antidepressants[c]				May cause hepatotoxicity; can cause or exacerbate cardiac conduction abnormalities, orthostatic hypotension
Amitriptyline	–	Y	Y	
Imipramine	–	Y	Y	
Desipramine	–	Y	N	
Nortriptyline	–	Y	Y	
Stimulants[c]				May be contraindicated in the presence of significant cardiovascular disease or HTN; can lower seizure threshold; advantage of having more rapid onset of action for treatment severe vegetative depression
Methylphenidate	–	N/A	N	
Dexamfetamine	–	N	N	
Modafinil	+ induces	Y severe	N[c]	
Other				
St John's wort	++ induces	N/A	N/A	Can markedly decrease levels of CNI and cause allograft rejection; not recommended
Bupropion (Wellbutrin)[c] (norepinephrine–dopamine reuptake inhibitor)	–	Y severe	Y	May cause less weight gain than other antidepressants; use with extreme caution with advanced liver disease
Trazadone (5-HT receptor antagonist)	+ not clinically significant	N	N	Can cause sedation and orthostatic hypotension
Mirtazapine (Remeron) (α_2-receptor blocker, serotonin receptor antagonist)	+ not clinically significant[c]	Y	Y	Can cause agranulocytosis, sedation; may exacerbate hyperlipidemia and weight gain
Benzodiazepines (e.g., alprazolam, clonazepam, diazepam)	+ not clinically significant	Y	Y	May cause respiratory depression if significant lung disease; sedating; potential for habituation and abuse

[a]Effect on isoenzyme: more potent (++), less potent (+), or no effect (–).
[b]Y, yes, N, no; severe, in the presence of moderate to severe liver or kidney disease.
[c]Metabolized via other cytochrome P450 isoenzymes; there may be significant interactions with other psychoactive drugs, antiarrhythmics, HMG-CoA reductase inhibitors, antihypertensive, and antifungal drugs.
CNI, calcineurin inhibitor; HTN, hypertension; N/A, not available.

outlines the pharmacologic considerations of the use of the most widely used drugs in these patients.

Tricyclic antidepressants (TCAs) can be effective in this group of patients, but because they also can interact with the hepatic metabolism of CNIs, close drug monitoring and dosage adjustments may be required. As TCAs have well-documented cardiovascular toxicity, such as conduction delay, orthostatic hypotension, and anticholinergic effects, the use of these drugs as a first-line agent in cardiac transplant recipients is not recommended, and they should be reserved for treatment of severe depression unresponsive to other drugs. Benzodiazepines can be useful for short-term treatment of anxiety or insomnia. Use of short-acting agents can avoid problems with drug accumulation in the presence of renal or hepatic dysfunction. They do not have metabolic interactions with immunosuppressive drugs. There is little information on the use of monoamine oxidase inhibitors in solid organ transplant recipients. Their use is not recommended due to severity of complications caused by drug interactions and the need for dietary restrictions (and hypotensive effects). The pharmokinetics of lithium can be significantly effected by other drugs that transplant recipients are commonly taking including diuretics, ACEIs, and β blockers, as well as by changes in renal perfusion due to CNIs. In addition long-term lithium use can cause CKD. For these reasons its use in transplant recipients for the treatment of bipolar disorder is not recommended. St. John's wort is a herbal drug that has long been used as a treatment for depression. Recently, it has been shown to induce the metabolism of CNIs, thereby decreasing drug levels that could put the patient at risk for rejection, so its use should be avoided. Finally, electroconvulsive therapy (ECT) has been used in a small number of patients with severe depression unresponsive to medical therapy with some success. There is concern that cardiac transplant recipients in particular may be at higher risk for complications due to increased sympathetic discharge as a result of the procedure, such that patients undergoing ECT should be carefully selected.

Compliance

Poor compliance with medical therapy is a risk factor for morbidity and mortality after transplantation. Non-compliance with immunosuppressive medications can of course put the patient at risk for rejection of the organ, which can severely decrease longevity of the transplant. The term "non-compliance" in the setting of organ transplantation usually connotes lack of adherence to a prescribed immunosuppressive regimen, although it also can negatively impact the course of a patient if it involves other medications (e.g., for treatment of hypertension or diabetes mellitus), or lifestyle choices, such as smoking and dietary indiscretion. Serious non-compliance with immunosuppressants is estimated to occur in 20–50% of patients. Non-compliance with immunosuppressants can take various forms from partial compliance where patients may take a "drug holiday," to "white coat adherence" where a patient may start taking the drugs shortly before a follow-up visit after a period of non-adherence, or stop taking the drugs altogether and present with irreversible graft dysfunction. Those with life-saving organ transplants such as heart, lung, and liver, would in theory suffer more severe consequences as a result of non-compliance compared with kidney transplant recipients who can restart dialysis if their graft fails; however, there is no documentation that rates of non-compliance differ among these groups. It has been said that the most useful function of monitoring immunosuppressive drug levels in a long-term transplant recipient is to be able to document compliance with these medications, but this measure would be insensitive in picking up patients with intermittent non-adherence who restart their drugs shortly before a follow-up visit. Socioeconomic factors can play a significant role in non-adherence because most drugs used to prevent rejection are costly. Loss of insurance drug coverage can lead to the patient not being able to afford the medication and to complete discontinuation of the medication or taking it less than prescribed in order to make it last longer. Compliance with drug therapy and confirming that the patient is able to afford the drug should be confirmed regularly even in the long-term patient.

There are several other factors that are associated with poor compliance, including pre-transplant non-compliance, substance abuse, poor social support, and personality disorders. Mood disorders themselves are not associated with higher rates of non-compliance. Non-compliance with other medical recommendations, such as smoking cessation, is more likely to be associated with non-compliance with the prescribed immunosuppressive regimen. Side effects of the anti-rejection medication, either perceived or real, can lead to non-compliance. This is particularly true with the cosmetic side effects that can be seen with corticosteroids or cyclosporine. Rates of non-compliance are higher in the adolescent transplant recipient, which is often related to cosmetic side effects. In kidney transplant recipients, those who receive living donor transplants are reported to have a higher rate of non-compliance, often related to the belief in the less intensive need for immunosuppressive medication in this setting. Although there are no easy answers as to how to prevent non-adherence, proactively addressing concerns about side effects and repetitive education as to the importance of anti-rejection therapy, especially in individuals deemed at high risk, may help to minimize this complication.

Further reading

Abbott KC, Oglesby RJ, Agodoa LY. Hospitalized avascular necrosis after renal transplantation in the United States. *Kidney Int* 2002;**62**:2250–6.

Ablassmaier B, Klaua S, Jacobi CA, Muller JM. Laparoscopic gastric banding after heart transplantation. *Obesity Surgery* 2002;**12**:412–15.

Alexander JW, Goodman HR, Gersin K, et al. Gastric bypass in morbidly obese patients with chronic renal failure and kidney transplant. *Transplantation* 2004;**78**:469–74.

Aliabadi AS, Pohanka E, Seebacher G, et al. Development of proteinuria after switch to sirolimus-based immunosuppression in long-term cardiac transplant patients. *Am J Transplant* 2008;**8**:854–61.

Armstrong KA, Campbell SB, Hawley CM, et al. Obesity is associated with worsening cardiovascular risk factor profiles and proteinuria progression in renal transplant recipients. *Am J Transplant* 2005;**5**:2710–18.

Asberg A. Interactions between cyclosporin and lipid-lowering drugs. *Drugs* 2003;**63**:367–78.

Aull MJ, Buell JF, Trofe J, et al. Experience with 274 cardiac transplant recipients with posttransplant lymphoproliferative disorder: a report from the Israel Penn International Transplant Tumor Registry. *Transplantation* 2004;**78**:1676–82.

Barbaro D, Orsini P, Pallini S, et al. Obesity in transplant patients: case report showing interference of orlistat with absorption of cyclosporine and review of literature. *Endocrinol Pract* 2002;**8**:124–6.

Barry JM. Treating erectile dysfunction in renal transplant recipients. *Drugs* 2007;**67**:975–83.

Bilchick KC, Henrikson CA, Skojec D, et al. Treatment of hyperlipidemia in cardiac transplant recipients. *Am Heart J* 2004;**148**:200–210.

Bordea C, Wojnarowska F, Millard PR, et al. Skin cancers in renal-transplant recipients occur more frequently than previously recognized in a temperate climate. *Transplantation* 2004;**77**:574–79.

Burroughs TE, Swindle J, Takemoto S, et al. Diabetic complications associated with new-onset diabetes mellitus in renal transplant recipients. *Transplantation* 2007;**83**:1027–34.

Cassiman D, Roelants M, Vandenplas G, et al. Orlistat treatment is safe in overweight and obese liver transplant recipients: a prospective, open label trial. *Transplant Int* 2006;**19**:1000–5.

Christenson LJ, Geusau A, Ferrandiz C, et al. Specialty clinics for the dermatologic care of solid-organ transplant recipients. *Dermatol Surgery* 2004;**30**:598–603.

Clive DM. Renal Transplant-associated hyperuricemia and gout. *J Am Soc Nephrol* 2000;**11**:974–9.

Conley E, Muth B, Samaniego M, et al. Bisphosphonates and bone fractures in long-term kidney transplant recipients. *Transplantation* 2008;**86**:231–7.

Coscia LA, Consantinescu ST, Moritz MJ, et al. Report from the National Transplantation Pregnancy Registry (NTPR): Outcomes of pregnancy after transplantation. *Clin Transplants* 2007;29–42.

Crespo-Leiro MG, Alonso-Pulpon LA, Vazquez de Prada JA, et al. Malignancy after heart transplantation: incidence, prognosis and risk factors. *Am J Transplant* 2008;**8**:1031–9.

Crone CC, Gabriel GM. Treatment of anxiety and depression in transplant patients. *Clin Pharmokinet* 2004;**43**:36.

Dalle IJ, Maes BD, Geboes KP, et al. Crohn's-like changes in the colon due to mycophenolate? *Colorectal Dis* 2005;**7**:27–34.

Davies NM, Grinyo J, Heading R, et al. Gastrointestinal side effects of mycophenolic acid in renal transplant patients: a reappraisal. *Nephrol Dialysis Transplant* 2007;**22**:2440–8.

Durieux S, Mercadal L, Orcel P, et al. Bone mineral density and fracture prevalence in long-term kidney graft recipients. *Transplantation* 2002;**74**:496–500.

Egbuna O, Zand MS, Arbini A, et al. A cluster of parvovirus B19 infections in renal transplant recipients: A prospective case series and review of the literature. *Am J Transplant* 2006;**6**:225–31.

European Renal Association–European Dialysis and Transplant Association. Long-term management of the transplant recipient. *Nephrol Dialysis Transplant* 2002;**17** (suppl 4):3–67.

First MR, Combs CA, Weiskittel P, Miodovnik M Lack of effect of pregnancy on renal allograft survival or function. *Transplantation* 1995;**59**:472–6.

Fleischer J, McMahon DJ, Hembree W, et al. Serum testosterone levels after cardiac transplantation. *Transplantation* 2008;**85**:834–39.

Foresta C, Schipilliti M, Ciarleglio FA, et al. Male hypogonadism in cirrhosis and after liver transplantation. *J Endocrinol Invest* 2008;**31**:470–8.

Fusar-Poli P, Lazzaretti M, Ceruti M, et al. Depression after lung transplantation: Causes and treatment. *Lung* 2007;**185**:55–65.

Fusar-Poli P, Picchioni M, Martinelli V, et al. Anti-depressive therapies after heart transplantation. *J Heart Lung Transplant* 2006;**25**:785–93.

Glicklich D, Kapoian T, Mian H, et al. Effects of erythropoietin, angiotensin II, and angiotensin-converting enzyme inhibitor on erythroid precursors in patients with posttransplant erythrocytosis. *Transplantation* 1999;**68**: 62–6.

Hanevold CD, Ho PL, Talley L, Mitsnefes MM. Obesity and renal transplant outcome: a report of the North American Pediatric Renal Transplant Cooperative Study. *Pediatrics* 2005;**115**:352–6.

Hariharan S, Adams MB, Brennan DC, et al. Recurrent and de novo glomerular disease after renal transplantation. *Transplantation* 1999;**68**:635–41.

Howard AD. Long-term posttransplantation care: the expanding role of community nephrologists. *Am J Kidney Dis* 2006;**47**(4 suppl 2):S111–24.

Hunt J, Lerman M, Magee M, et al. Improvement of renal dysfunction by conversion from calcineurin inhibitors to sirolimus after heart transplantation. *J Heart Lung Transplantation* 2005;**24**:1863–7.

Jain AB, Reyes J, Marcos A, et al. Pregnancy after liver transplantation with tacrolimus immunosuppression: A single center's experience update at 13 years. *Transplantation* 2003;**76**:827–32.

Johnson DW, Isbel NM, Brown AM, et al. The effect of obesity on renal transplant outcomes, *Transplantation* 2002;**74**:675–81.

Kahn J, Rehak P, Schweiger M, et al. The impact of overweight on the development of diabetes after heart transplantation. *Clin Transplants* 2006;**20**:62–6.

Kasiske B, Cosio FG, Beto J, et al. Clinical practice guidelines for managing dyslipidemias in kidney transplant patients: a report from the Managing Dyslipidemias in Chronic Kidney Disease Work Group of the National Kidney Foundation Kidney Disease Outcomes Quality Initiative, *Am J Transplant* 2004;**4**(suppl 7):13–53.

Kasiske BL, Maclean JR, Snyder JJ. Acute myocardial infarction and kidney transplantation. *J Am Soc Nephrol* 2006;**17**:900–7.

Kasiske BL, Snyder JJ, Gilbertson DT, Wang C. Cancer after Kidney Transplantation in the United States. *Am J Transplant* 2004;**4**:905–13.

Kasiske BL, Vazquez MA, Harmon WE, et al. Recommendations for the outpatient surveillance of renal transplant recipients. American Society of Transplantation. *J Am Soc Nephrol* 2000;**11**:S1–86.

KDIGO clinical practice guideline for the care of kidney transplant recipients. *Am J Transplant* 2009 Nov;9 Suppl 3:S1–155.

Kobashigawa JA, Katznelson S, Laks H, et al. Effect of pravastatin on outcomes after cardiac transplantation. *N Engl J Med* 1995;**333**:621–7.

Lebbe C, Euvrard S, Barrou B, et al. Sirolimus conversion for patients with posttransplant Kaposi's sarcoma. *Am J Transplant* 2006;**6**:2164–8.

Leblond V, Sutton L, Dorent R, et al. Lymphoproliferative disorders after organ transplantation: a report of 24 cases observed in a single center. *J Clin Oncol* 1995;**13**: 961–8.

Lemahieu W, Maes B, Verbeke K, et al. Cytochrome P450 3A4 and P-glycoprotein activity and assimilation of tacrolimus in transplant patients with persistent diarrhea. *Am J Transplant* 2005;**5**:1383–91.

Lentine KL, Brennan DC. Statin use after renal transplantation: a systematic quality review of trial-based evidence. *Nephrol Dialysis Transplant* 2004;**19**:2378–86.

Lhotta K. Beyond hepatorenal syndrome: glomerulonephritis in patients with liver disease. *Semin Nephrol* 2002; **22**:302–8.

Lindelow B, Bergh C, Herlitz H, Waagstein F. Predictors and evolution of renal function during 9 years following heart transplant. *J Am Soc Nephrol* 2000;**11**: 951–7.

McCune TR, Thacker II LR, Peters TG, et al. Effects of tacrolimus on hyperlipidemia after successful renal transplantation. *Transplantation* 1998;**65**:87–92.

McKay DB, Josephson MA. Pregnancy in recipients of solid organs – Effects on mother and child. *N Engl J Med* 2006;**354**:1281–93.

Maes B, Haday K, de Moor B, et al. Severe diarrhea in renal transplant patients: Results of the DIDACT study. *Am J Transplant* 2006;**6**:1466–72.

Meier-Kriesche HU, Arndorfer JA, Kaplan B. The impact of body mass index on renal transplant outcomes: a significant independent risk factor for graft failure and patient death. *Transplantation* 2002;**73**:70–74.

Mihalov ML, Gattuso P, Abraham K, et al. Incidence of post-transplant malignancy among 674 solid-organ-transplant recipients at a single center. *Clin Transplant* 1996; **10**:248–55.

Nankivell BJ, Borrows RJ, Fung CL-S, O'Connell PJ, Allen RDM, Chapman JR. The natural history of chronic allograft nephropathy. *N Engl J Med* 2003;**349**: 2326–33.

Neal D, Tom B, Luan J, et al. Is there disparity between risk and incidence of cardiovascular disease after liver transplant? *Transplantation* 2004;**77**:93–9.

Nisbeth U, Lindh E, Ljunghall S, et al. Increased fracture rate in diabetes mellitus and females after renal transplantation. *Transplantation* 1999;**67**:1218–22.

Oertel SH, Verschuuren E, Reinke P, et al. Effect of anti-CD 20 antibody rituximab in patients with post-transplant lymphoproliferative disorder. *Am J Transplant* 2005;**5**: 2901–6.

Ojo AO, Held PJ, Port FK, et al. Chronic renal failure after transplantation of a nonrenal organ. *N Engl J Med* 2003; **349**:931–40.

Ong CS, Keough AM, Kossard S, et al. Skin cancer in Australian heart transplant recipients. *J Am Acad Dermatol* 1999;**40**:27–34.

Otley CC, Berg D, Ulrich C, et al. Reduction of immunosuppression for transplant-associated skin cancer: expert consensus survey. *Br J Dermatol* 2006;**154**:395–400.

Paya C, Fung J, Nalesnik M, et al. Epstein-Barr virus-induced posttransplant lymphoproliferative disorders. *Transplantation* 1999;**68**:1517–25.

Penn I. The effect of immunosuppression on pre-existing cancers. *Transplantation* 1993;**55**:742–7.

Ratz Bravo AE, Tchambaz L, Krahenbuhl-Melcher A, et al. Prevalence of potentially severe drug-drug interactions in ambulatory patients with dyslipidemia receiving HMG-CoA reductase inhibitor therapy. *Drug Safety* 2005;**28**: 263–75.

Rogers CC, Alloway RR, Alexander JW, et al. Pharmacokinetics of mycophenolic acid, tacrolimus and sirolimus after gastric bypass surgery in end-stage renal disease and transplant patients: a pilot study. *Clin Transplant* 2007;**22**:281–91.

Satchithananda DK, Parameshwar J, Sharples L, et al. The incidence of end-stage renal failure in 17 years of heart transplantation: A single center experience. *J Heart Lung Transplant* 2002;**21**:651–7.

Schaar CG, van der Pijl JW, van Hoek B, et al. Successful outcome with a 'quintuple approach' of posttransplant lymphoproliferative disorder. *Transplantation* 2001;**71**: 47–52.

Schwenger V, Morath C, Zeier M. Use of erythropoetin after solid organ transplantation. *Nephrol Dial Transplant* 2007;**22**(suppl 8):viii47–9.

Shah N, Al-Khoury S, Afzali B, et al. Posttransplantation anemia in adult renal allograft recipients: prevalence and predictors. *Transplantation* 2006;**81**:1112–18.

Shane I, Addesso V, Namerow PB, et al. Alendronate versus calcitriol for the prevention of bone loss after cardiac transplantation. *N Engl J Med* 2004;**350**: 767–76.

Sharif A, Moore RH, Baboolal K The use of oral glucose tolerance tests to risk stratify for new-onset diabetes after transplantation: an underdiagnosed phenomenon. *Transplantation* 2006;**82**:1667–72.

Sharma RK, Prasad N, Gupta A, Kapoor R. Treatment of erectile dysfunction with sildenafil citrate in renal allograft recipients: A randomized, double-blind, placebo-controlled, crossover trial. *Am J Kidney Dis* 2006;**48**: 128–33.

Sibanda N, Briggs JD, Davison JM, et al. Pregnancy after organ transplantation: A report from the UK Transplant Pregnancy Registry. *Transplantation* 2007;**83**: 1301–7.

Sifontis NM, Coscia LA, Constantinescu S, et al. Pregnancy outcomes in solid organ transplant recipients with exposure to mycophenolate mofetil or sirolimus. *Transplantation* 2006;**82**:1698–702.

Silverborn M, Jeppsson A, Martensson G, Nilsson F New-onset cardiovascular risk factors in lung transplant recipients. *J Heart Lung Transplant* 2005;**24**:1536–43.

Stallone G, Schena A, Infante B, et al. Sirolimus for Kaposi's sarcoma in renal-transplant recipients. *N Engl J Med* 2005;**352**:1317–23.

Stasko T, Brown MD, Carucci JA, et al. Guidelines for the management of squamous cell carcinoma in organ transplant recipients. *Dermatol Surg* 2004;**30**:642–50.

Stephany BR, Alao B, Budev M, et al. Hyperlipidemia is associated with accelerated chronic kidney disease progression after lung transplantation. *Am J Transplant* 2007;**7**:2553–60.

Sucato GS, Murray PJ. Gynecologic health care for the adolescent solid organ transplant recipient. *Pediatr Transplant* 2005;**9**:346–56.

Tsai DE, Douglas L, Andreadis C, et al. EBV PCR in the diagnosis and monitoring of posttransplant lymphoproliferative disorder: results of a two-arm prospective trial. *Am J Transplant* 2008;**8**:1016–24.

Vincenti F, Friman S, Scheurermann E, et al. Results of an international, randomized trial comparing glucose metabolism disorders and outcome with cyclosporine versus tacrolimus. *Am J Transplant* 2007;**7**:1506–14.

Wagoner LE, Taylor DO, Price GD, et al. Paternity by cardiac transplant recipients. *Transplantation* 1994;**57**: 1337–40.

Walsh SB, Altmann P, Pattison J, et al. Effect of pamidronate on bone loss after kidney transplantation: a randomized trial. *Am J Kidney Dis* 2009;**53**:856–65.

Weber SA, Naftel DC, Fricker FJ, et al. Lymphoproliferative disorders after paediatric heart transplantation: a multi-institutional study. *Lancet* 2006;**367**:233–9.

Webster AC, Craig JC, Simpson JM, et al. Identifying high risk groups and quantifying absolute risk of cancer after kidney transplantation: a cohort study of 15,183 recipients. *Am J Transplant* 2007;**7**:2140–51.

Wilkinson A, Davidson J, Dotta F, et al. Guidelines for the treatment and management of new-onset diabetes after transplantation. *Clin Transplant* 2005;**19**:291–8.

Zuber J, Anglicheau D, Elie C, et al. Sirolimus may reduce fertility in male renal transplant recipients. *Am J Transplant* 2008;**8**:1–9.

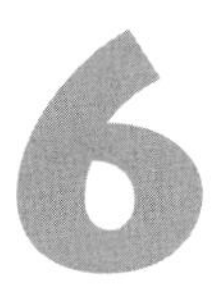

Pediatric transplantation

William Harmon

Children's Hospital Boston and Harvard Medical School, Boston, Massachusetts, USA

Although organ failure is far less common in children than in adults, pediatric organ transplantation has held an important position in the transplant community since its earliest days. Children make up a small fraction of all organ recipients. They represent about 2.3% of all active candidates and about 6.8% of all recipients. Children make up the majority of those receiving intestinal transplants. In contrast, virtually no children received pancreas transplants. Although the indications for transplantation, techniques, procedures, and immunosuppression for children are similar to those in adults, there are important differences in the approaches to treatment, e.g., the causes of end-stage organ failure in children are substantially different from those seen in adults. The lack of appreciation for the consequences of those etiologies could compromise graft and patient survival. Furthermore, the long-term goals of transplantation in children may be substantially different than those in adults, once again providing important guidance for the proper treatment and care of these patients, e.g., growth and development are clearly recognized as unique end-points for children, and immunosuppression plans and monitoring protocols are often modified based on this concern.

Furthermore, as current immunosuppression requires constant and unrelenting adherence to fixed schedules, it should not be surprising that older children and adolescents are at high risk for failure to follow the protocols and that they suffer the inevitable consequences. Thus, appropriate research efforts designed to minimize the number and frequency of administration of immunosuppressive medications, and to eliminate the medications with the worst side effects (particularly cosmetic side effects) become high-priority projects. Recent studies have shown outstanding outcomes in young children, suggesting that their immune responses are not a substantive barrier, and that they may become ideal candidates for long-term tolerance protocols. This is particularly relevant because children, who have the longest projected lifespan after organ transplantation, have the most to gain from long-term graft function and freedom from serious complications of chronic immunosuppression.

Considering the developmental phases of children, especially as they progress through adolescence, it is universally understood that they should have individually defined follow-up programs, designed to assure appropriate care of their grafts while providing them full rehabilitation status so that they can undertake all of the activities common to their peers. Recognizing the importance of pediatric organ transplant procedures as well as the substantial differences in their care, the National Institutes of Health, through the National Institute of Allergy and Infectious Diseases, has sponsored specific pediatric organ transplant research initiatives for over a decade. The first of these was the Collaborative Clinical Trials in Pediatric Transplantation (CCTPT), which supported several immunosuppression minimization studies in pediatric kidney transplantation.

Primer on Transplantation, 3rd edition.
Edited by Donald Hricik.

The CCTPT has been replaced by the more comprehensive Clinical Trials in Organ Transplantation in Children (CTOTC) which has recently established multicenter clinical trial consortia in pediatric kidney, heart, and lung transplantation. Importantly, these groups will be undertaking innovative trials designed to enhance immunosuppression for children while defining their unique immunologic responses, not only to the graft but also to infectious diseases. Each of these trials involves important mechanistic studies.

Pediatric organ transplantation is not a large clinical program in any single transplant center. Thus, pediatric transplant professionals, including physicians, surgeons, nurses, and investigators, have formed multicenter data registries designed to collect and analyze information concerning indications, outcomes, and complications of their procedures. Examples of these include the North American Pediatric Renal Trials and Collaborative Studies (NAPRTCS), Studies in Pediatric Liver Transplantation (SPLIT), the Registry of the International Society of Heart and Lung Transplant's (ISHLT) pediatric section, and the Pediatric Heart Transplant Study Group (PHTSG). Each of these registries has provided invaluable information about all aspects of organ transplantation in children and they have made these data available through periodic reports and websites. Importantly, their results have spawned subsequent prospective research trials. Nevertheless, the small numbers of pediatric transplant procedures results in an inevitable lack of precision of epidemiologic and outcome data in children compared with adults. Furthermore, clinical trials in children obviously require longer enrollment periods because of the inevitable paucity of appropriate candidates. Despite these handicaps, the determined efforts by the pediatric transplant community to cooperate in both data collection and multicenter clinical trials has resulted in a vibrant collaborative effort to describe and improve organ transplantation in children.

The fundamental indications for organ transplantation, the basic surgical procedures, the immune response to a solid organ transplant, and the complications of the immunosuppressive agents are similar or identical in children and adults. Insofar as these issues have been addressed by other chapters in this text, they are not repeated in this chapter. However, those issues that are clearly unique for pediatric recipients of organ transplants or which require substantial modification of typical protocols will be described in detail. Thus, this chapter is an important adjunct to the other resources provided in this primer, but it does not replace them. The data to support the information in this chapter come from multiple sources. However, the data about transplant rates, death on the waiting list, and outcomes come from the Scientific Registry of Transplant Recipients (SRTR) and represent transplantation in the USA.

Causes, demographics, and conservative treatment of children with end-stage organ disease

The etiologies of end-stage organ failure in children are generally substantially different than those in adults. Many children are born with congenital malformations that affect vital organs or have hereditary diseases that are expressed early in life. There are several consequences of these disorders. First, unlike adults whose acquired diseases are frequently degenerative and progressive, children with congenital organ malformations have fixed or unchanging disorders. Thus, the number of complicating conditions may be substantially reduced. On the other hand, abnormal organ function dating from the earliest period of life can seriously impair growth and development, resulting in additional handicaps. Furthermore, as many of these lesions, such as congenital heart disease or serious urologic malformations, require surgical reconstruction, many young patients with end-stage organ failure have had substantial surgical histories before requiring organ transplantation. And, although these specific malformations will not recur in a transplanted organ, any associated anatomic or physiologic abnormalities will require ongoing vigilance and repair. Furthermore, hereditary disorders, such as cystic fibrosis, autosomal recessive polycystic kidney disease, or cystinosis, may not be cured by an organ transplant. The ongoing physiologic abnormalities associated with these disorders may affect the new organ as well as other organ systems. Thus, those treating children with these types of disorders should have broad experience in dealing with their consequences.

End-stage renal disease

In general, adults develop end-stage renal disease (ESRD) from the complications of diabetes mellitus, hypertension, or simply growing older. As life expectancy lengthens, the potential for ESRD resulting from these disorders increases, probably explaining the marked increase in the number of patients receiving chronic dialysis in the USA. These types of disorders are rarely seen in children. Although children can suffer from hypertension, renal disease is typically the cause rather than the consequence of the hypertension. Although children certainly can develop diabetes mellitus at an early age, and despite the fact that the incidence of type 2 diabetes is expanding rapidly (particularly in the obese adolescent population), it is quite unusual for end-stage diabetic nephropathy to occur before the third decade of life. Congenital kidney and urologic abnormalities are major causes of the ESRD in children, but are rarely seen in adults. Furthermore, most hereditary disorders have an onset early in life and thus are generally expressed in the youngest patients.

One important exception to that general rule is autosomal dominant polycystic kidney disease. This disease, the most common lethal inherited disorder in white people, typically is not fully expressed until adulthood and is rarely appreciated in children, except as the earliest manifestations found in family members of affected patients. Comparisons of the causes of ESRD are shown in Table 6.1. For children, hereditary and congenital abnormalities, such as reflux nephropathy and renal dysplasia, account for slightly more than 50% of the cases of ESRD in children presenting for kidney transplantation. Focal sclerosis and various forms of glomerulonephritis account for about a quarter of the cases. Diabetes mellitus as a cause of ESRD in children is barely noticeable, and hypertension is not reported as a cause. In contrast, diabetes and hypertension account for slightly more than 70% of adults with ESRD. Urinary tract disorders and cystic kidney disease account for less than 5% and glomerulonephritis is the etiology in approximately the same percentage of adults as children with ESRD. Clearly, these differences in the causes of ESRD in children and adults require substantially different approaches to treatment and follow-up.

Table 6.1 Etiology of end-stage renal disease in children and adults

Etiology	Pediatric (%)	Adult (%)
Dysplasia/Hypoplasia	16.0	
Urinary tract disorders	24.0	2.0
Polycystic kidneys	5.7	2.4
Hereditary	5.0	
FSGS	11.7	
Glomerulonephritis	10.9	7.6
Pyelonephritis	1.8	
SLE and immune	1.9	
Tumor	0.5	
Infarct/Trauma	1.3	
Diabetes	0.1	43.8
Hypertension		27.1
Other	9.5	11.6
Unknown	6.1	5.0

Pediatric data abstracted from NAPRTCS. *Pediatr Transpl* 2007;**11**:366.
Adult data abstracted from USRDS Annual Report 2007.
FSGS, focal glomerulosclerosis; SLE, systemic lupus erythematosus.

Overall, there are slightly more boys than girls who develop ESRD, probably related to obstructive uropathy and other urinary tract disorders found early in life. In general, 60% of children receiving kidney transplants are boys. There is a slightly higher incidence of ESRD in African–American children compared with their prevalence in the overall population, approximately 17%. This fraction is substantially smaller than what is reported in adults. White children represent 61% and Hispanic children about 16% of pediatric kidney transplant recipients. Although children might have ESRD from birth, transplantation is frequently performed later in life as chronic kidney disease progresses into ESRD. Adolescents make up about 50% of pediatric kidney transplant recipients, with 6–10 year olds and 1–5 year olds representing 25% each. It is unusual for children aged <1 year to be treated with kidney transplantation. They are typically treated with conservative measures and dialysis until they are big enough to receive a kidney from an adult donor (see below). The incidence of ESRD in children, in contrast to what is reported in adults, has been relatively constant over the past 30 years. In general, there are about 500 pediatric kidney transplant candidates who are active on the deceased donor waiting list at any time and the number of living and deceased donor kidney transplants performed each year is in the range of 700–900.

Treatment with chronic dialysis is generally safe and effective in children with ESRD. Annual mortality rate of children treated with chronic dialysis is much lower than that reported in adults, probably 1% in contrast to the 15–20% reported for adults. Thus, the life-saving potential for kidney transplantation in children is not quite as acute as it is for adults. The one exception to this is in small infants for whom mortality rates of both dialysis and transplantation are much higher than in older children. Mortality risk, therefore, may make kidney transplantation more immediately necessary in infants who are not stable on dialysis. Nevertheless, virtually all programs agree that kidney transplantation is a much more appropriate and successful treatment than dialysis for ESRD in children.

There are indications that the outcome of preemptive kidney transplantation in children is superior to that in children who have undergone chronic dialysis. As children often receive living donor kidney transplants and as they have preference on the deceased donor list, there is no reason as such for them to have long periods of chronic dialysis before transplantation. Nevertheless, given the relative safety of dialysis and the substantial benefits of optimal preparation before transplantation, children with ESRD can be best prepared for kidney transplantation by undergoing necessary corrective surgery, such as urologic reconstruction, and necessary preparation such as completion of immunization schedules, and maximization of nutritional status, before the transplant procedure. In general, there are almost no emergency indications for pediatric kidney transplantation and a pediatric transplant program will collaborate with the dialysis team to provide optimal comprehensive care for children with ESRD. There are virtually no contraindications to kidney transplantation for children with ESRD, except perhaps for a very limited life expectancy, such as in children with metastatic Wilms' tumor or other organ failures.

Case: recurrent disease in kidney transplantation
A 12-year-old boy underwent living related donor kidney transplantation for focal segmental glomerulosclerosis (FSGS). The onset of FSGS occurred 3 years before that, with nephrotic syndrome that was not responsive to typical corticosteroid treatment. He was also treated with plasmapheresis, cyclophosphamide, and mycophenolate mofetil (MMF) at various times, all without any response. His renal function deteriorated over a 2-year span and he began chronic peritoneal dialysis 6 months before transplantation. As a result of sustained hypertension and proteinuria, measured at 5 g/day, he underwent bilateral native nephrectomies 3 months before transplantation. Both parents were ABO compatible and his mother volunteered to be the donor. He received three treatments of plasmapheresis and he was started on cyclosporine 5 days before transplantation. The transplant was technically successful and he started to make urine immediately. Within the first 24 hours, he made 6.5 L of urine and his serum creatinine fell from 7.5 mg/dL to 1.2 mg/dL in that time span. On the second postoperative day, his urine protein:creatinine ratio was 4.4, suggesting recurrence of FSGS.

Liver failure in children

The number of children awaiting liver transplantation has been relatively stable for the past several years. The number of pediatric liver candidates on the waiting list grew from 492 in 1997 to a peak of 703 in 2001, and has subsequently declined to 361 in 2006. This change in absolute numbers of candidates has been similar for both adults and children. A large number of children on the waiting list had been in an inactive status, likely representing early listing in order to be eligible for accumulation of waiting time credit. The change of allocation system in the USA in the early twenty-first century made urgency, rather than waiting time, the primary indication for liver transplantation. Subsequently, the number of children and adults awaiting liver transplantation has decreased, probably reflecting a more realistic estimate of the need for transplantation. Most commonly, diseases that inevitably progress to liver failure, rather than acute irreversible liver failure, account for the diagnoses of over 90% of the children listed for liver transplantation. Among these, cholestatic liver disease, principally biliary atresia, represents over 50% of the total population. Eighty percent of the children with biliary atresia are aged <5 years at the time of transplantation. Thus pediatric liver transplantation tends to be a procedure performed largely in infants and young children.

Attempts to prevent progression of biliary atresia with various surgical techniques, such as Kasai's procedure, are still recommended but are eventually unsuccessful in the majority of cases. If successful, however, the procedure does produce outcomes that are generally as good as liver transplantation. Metabolic liver diseases represent the next most common indication for liver transplantation, representing about 12% of recipients. In some cases, the children do not have overall liver failure but may lack specific functions, such as defects in the urea cycle. In these cases, morbidity results from acute and unexpected episodes of hyperammonemia which can sometimes be treated and prevented by appropriate diet and medications. In patients with Crigler–Najjar syndrome, hyperbilirubinemia can be treated with phototherapy and enteric administration of binding agents. As above, however, intermittent episodes of kernicterus can result and become irreversible despite supportive treatment. In other circumstances, an isolated liver dysfunction may result in other organ damage, such as occurs in primary oxalosis. In this setting, most programs will recommend simultaneous liver and kidney transplantation in order to prevent recurrent oxalate damage to kidneys and other organs. Wilson's disease can often be managed medically for long periods of time but will sometimes progress to chronic liver disease or acute fulminant liver failure. The indications and timing of liver transplantation in these unusual situations generally require judgment that is best developed through experience in specialized pediatric liver transplant programs. In some cases, liver function is not affected, but portal hypertension and its consequences can be the indication for transplantation, such as in autosomal recessive polycystic kidney disease or cystic fibrosis.

The next most common indication for liver transplantation in children is fulminant liver failure which most commonly occurs in either infancy or early adolescence. Unfortunately, the cause of the liver failure is often unknown, probably in more than half the cases. Another 15% are related to acetaminophen toxicity. The decision to proceed with liver transplantation in this setting of liver failure in children is very difficult, because some of these patients will recover spontaneously. Once again, the need for experience-based decision-making is paramount. Cirrhosis represents about 10% of the children receiving liver transplantation, most commonly resulting from autoimmune hepatitis. As with other forms of liver failure, a large fraction of these children have an undefined etiology. Liver tumors are very uncommon in children and represent less than 5% of children undergoing liver transplantation. Hepatoblastoma represents about 1% of all pediatric cancers but most of these patients are unsuitable for surgical resection because of the extensiveness of the tumor. Most of these patients undergo pretransplant chemotherapy and radiation to reduce the chance of recurrence. Often, this leads to primary treatment of the tumor and avoidance of transplantation. Those who require transplantation frequently have excellent outcomes. On the other hand, hepatocellular carcinoma often recurs after liver transplantation, obviously limiting its success. Clearly, active collaboration among oncologists, pediatric hepatologists, and the liver transplant team is essential to assure the best outcome for these patients. The typical diagnoses of adult liver transplant candidates, such as hepatitis C, alcoholic liver disease, and cirrhosis, are uncommon in children.

Case: a jaundiced patient

The parents of a 9-month-old infant just moved from Saint Lucia to the USA and bring their jaundiced infant son to the pediatric hospital. The child had been noted to be jaundiced soon after birth and was not responsive to phototherapy. He was taken to the UK, where the diagnosis of biliary atresia was made and he was treated with Kasai's procedure. His jaundice stabilized but did not resolve. He did not thrive well and was always noted to have ascites and to be jaundiced. Despite special diets, he now weighs only 5.2 kg, and some of that is clearly related to the ascites. He is deeply jaundiced, although his liver function tests are all normal. His serum bilirubin is 32 mg/dL, with 28 mg/dL noted to be direct. He has had no immunizations because he has been "too sick."

Evaluation of children for liver transplantation requires an experienced multidisciplinary approach that assesses both the indications for transplantation and the likelihood that a successful transplantation will improve the candidate's medical status. Contraindications to pediatric liver transplantation include extrahepatic malignancy, uncontrolled systemic or locally invasive infection, multisystem organ failure, irreversible neurologic injury, and other uncorrectable systemic disorders. The benefits of liver transplantation have to be weighed against the potential complications and early mortality, especially for disorders that have other modes of treatment, such as metabolic diseases. The management of children awaiting liver transplantation is essential for good outcomes and particular attention must be paid to the nutritional status of the recipients, particularly infants. There has been recent focus on mortality among children awaiting liver transplantation and there has been a proposal that no child should die awaiting organ transplantation. The mortality among pediatric liver transplant candidates is highly dependent on age: children older than 6 years of age have a mortality rate similar to that found in adults, but younger children have the highest death rates among all candidates. This rate is approximately 600–800 per 1000 patient-years at risk, and is three to four times greater than that observed in all other age groups. At total of 103 pediatric liver transplant candidates died in 2006 before transplantation. Recent attempts to preferentially allocate donors to high-risk pediatric recipients have been undertaken in an attempt to lower this rate. As with kidney transplantation, the number of liver transplantations performed in children each year has been quite stable, averaging 500–600 per year over the past decade.

Heart failure in children

About 25% of children considered or listed for heart transplantation are aged <1 year, with the remainder evenly split between cohorts aged 1–10 and those aged 11–17 years. There appears to be a slight predominance of boys, and the ethnicity generally reflects the overall population. The two major etiologies of heart failure in children are cardiomyopathy and congenital structural heart disease. The ratio of these two diagnoses is highly dependent on candidate age at listing: for infants aged <1 year, most have congenital structural heart disease – as high as 75% in previous years. However, as the surgical techniques for repairing congenital lesions have improved, the number of children listed for transplantation has decreased and the proportion listed because of cardiomyopathy has increased from 25% to 35%. Cardiomyopathy accounts for 50% of heart failure cases for children aged 1–10 years and for 75% for adolescents listed for heart transplantation. A small fraction, <5% in all age groups, is listed for other reasons, such as re-transplantation. Hypoplastic left heart syndrome has been the predominant diagnosis in infants undergoing heart transplantation. In infants, if heart transplantation is performed, it is generally done as a primary treatment, whereas, in older children and adolescents, it is performed after corrective surgery has been unsuccessful. More recently, the use of heart transplantation as primary therapy for infants has been decreasing, probably reflecting increased use of corrective, staged repairs. Cardiomyopathy subtypes are not evenly distributed: dilated cardiomyopathy represents about 75% of those listed for heart transplantation, with smaller fractions of restrictive cardiomyopathy (12%), myocarditis (8%), and hypertrophic cardiomyopathy (5%).

The number of children listed for heart transplantation has remained relatively stable over the last decade, during which here have been 400–500 children listed for heart transplantation at any time in the USA. More recently, the number of patients who have received transplants has increased slightly to 314 in 2006. The number of children who died while awaiting heart transplantation decreased to 59 in 2006, likely reflecting improvements in the treatment of chronic heart failure and adjustments in the allocation system that have provided better opportunities for children to receive heart transplants in a timely manner.

Support for pediatric heart transplant candidates by the use of extracorporeal devices is still uncommon but is increasing in frequency. Ventricular-assist devices (VADs) appropriate for young children and infants have been developed only recently. On the other hand, extracorporeal membrane oxygenation (ECMO) has been used more successfully in young children than in adults. In addition, the increased use of VADs and human homograft material for those who require surgery has resulted in higher rates of sensitization among pediatric heart transplant candidates. Unfortunately, the presence of anti-donor antibodies results in longer times on the waiting list, less likelihood of being appropriately matched for transplant, and poorer graft survival than that observed in unsensitized recipients. Techniques for reducing, preventing, and treating pre-sensitization are currently under investigation.

As with other transplant evaluations, pediatric heart transplant candidates must be assessed for clear indications for heart transplantation and to determine whether or not transplantation represents a viable option. Thorough evaluation of the candidate's pulmonary vascular resistance is an essential component of the overall evaluation process. As is the case with other pediatric organ transplant candidates, there are very few absolute contraindications to heart transplantation, and these include active and severe infection, active malignancy, immunodeficiency states that would be worsened by chronic immunosuppression, and severe and uncorrectable organ failure or dysfunction, particularly neurologic dysfunction.

Chronic lung disease in children

The number of pediatric lung transplants reached a peak in the late 1990s at slightly fewer than 100 transplants per year. The number has been stable since 2000 at about 60–70 per year. For infants aged <1 year, congenital heart disease and pulmonary vascular disease are the primary indications for lung transplantation. Certain congenital abnormalities such as surfactant protein B deficiency can also be treated with lung transplantation. In older children, aged 1–10 years, cystic fibrosis is the most common diagnosis, representing about a third of cases. Idiopathic pulmonary arterial hypertension is another important indication. About 75% of lung transplant candidates are adolescents and cystic fibrosis is the primary diagnosis for about two-thirds of them. There are over 30 000 patients with cystic fibrosis in the USA. Despite the identification of the gene responsible for cystic fibrosis, treatment currently remains symptomatic and supportive rather than curative. Nevertheless, these treatments have been very successful and mean survival time has improved over the past 30 years from the mid-teens to age >30 years. Most of the deaths are related to respiratory failure. As a result of the prolonged survival time, at least 80% of transplant candidates for lung transplantation who have cystic fibrosis are aged >18 years at the time of listing. The indications for listing and transplantation are somewhat subjective but typically include a decline in pulmonary function as measured by the forced expiratory volume in 1 second (FEV_1) of 30% or more.

Key points 6.1 Cystic fibrosis and pediatric lung transplantation

- Over 30 000 patients in the USA have cystic fibrosis (CF)
- CF accounts for approximately a third of lung transplantations performed in children between ages 1 and 10
- CF accounts for approximately two-thirds of lung transplantations performed in adolescents

Intestinal failure in children

Children make up the predominance of candidates awaiting intestinal transplantation, comprising about three-quarters of the list. The number of pediatric candidates on the intestine waiting list has increased almost threefold, to 140 in 2006. The primary diagnoses leading to intestinal failure and indication for transplantation include three major categories. The first is the anatomic loss of the intestine due to short bowel syndrome, most commonly related to jejunal–ileal atresia, midgut volvulus, and abdominal wall defects such as omphalocele. Also, neonates may suffer necrotizing enterocolitis, midgut volvulus, and vascular thrombosis. In general, infants with <35 cm of small bowel and an ileocecal valve are likely to remain dependent on total parenteral nutrition (TPN), eventually becoming transplant candidates. Infants requiring more than 50% of their caloric intake via intravenous routes are also likely to require intestinal and possibly liver transplantation. The second category of disorders includes neuropathic diseases such as Hirschsprung's disease or myopathic diseases such as chronic interstitial pseudo-obstruction syndrome. The third category consists of congenital diseases of the intestinal epithelium such as microvillous inclusion disease and epithelial dysplasia.

Most of these children can be treated and can thrive through the use of chronic TPN. Indeed, TPN may allow intestinal adaptation to occur if provided for a long enough period of time, and it is certainly possible for children to have normal growth and development while receiving TPN. Current survival rates for home TPN at 1 and 5 years are 90% and 75% respectively. The complications of chronic TPN include sepsis, liver failure, and loss of central venous access sites. Thus, the decision to progress to listing for intestinal transplantation may be similar to that for kidney transplantation, i.e., the alternative treatment is quite safe and effective, although it seriously impairs quality of life. The decision about intestinal transplantation is, however, complicated by the relatively poor outcome of the procedure, in contrast to that of kidney transplantation.

Pancreatic failure in children

The incidence of diabetes mellitus in children is increasing, similar to what is seen in adults. Other causes of pancreatic failure in children include hemolytic–uremic syndrome, cystic fibrosis, and chronic pancreatitis. The major complications of these latter forms of pancreatic failure are gastrointestinal dysfunction and diabetes mellitus. Both of these disorders can, however, be treated with exogenous medications such as oral pancreatic enzymes and insulin. As a result of the low morbidity and high efficacy of these treatments, replacement of pancreatic function by pancreas or islet transplantation is of questionable utility. Indeed, only a handful of children have received pancreas transplants, so few in fact that virtually no registries include those numbers. The balance of clinical improvement related to pancreas transplantation, the burden of chronic immunosuppression, and overall long-term success rates has generally resulted in decisions not to transplant children.

Donors for pediatric organ transplantation

Living donors

Children traditionally have been more likely to receive organ transplants from living donors than have adults. There are several reasons for this practice. Outcomes of living donor kidneys have had superior outcomes compared with deceased donor kidneys, with half-lives that may be up to twice as long as even ideal deceased donors. Parents generally are very willing to be donors for their own children. Transplant surgery has progressed to the point that an adult kidney may be transplanted into an infant as small as 6 kg, the size typically achieved by such children at

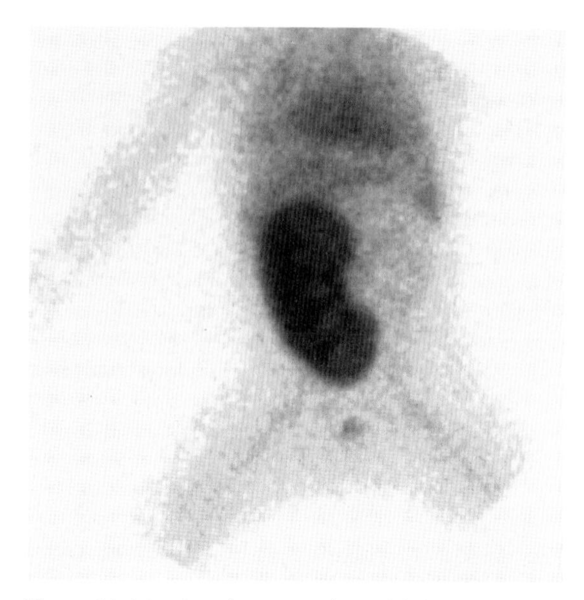

Figure 6.1 Mag-3 nuclear scan of an adult living-donor kidney into a 6.5 kg infant. The graft is well perfused but not concentrating tracer yet. Note the relative size of the graft compared to the recipient's liver and heart.

the first birthday (Figure 6.1 and see below). Indeed the longest projected half-lives are achieved when a living adult donor kidney is transplanted into an infant.

Evaluation and preparation of living donors for pediatric kidney transplantation should follow the same guidelines as for any other recipient. It is important to understand, however, that minors aged <18 years cannot be used as living donors. There is virtually universal agreement on this issue, as stipulated in the outcome of the Amsterdam Conference on the Care of Living Donors and on World Health Organization Guiding Principles on Human Cell, Tissue and Organ Transplantation that have been reiterated in the recent Istanbul Declaration. The principle underlying this prohibition against using minors as living donors is based on the ethical concept of volunteerism. Typically, minors are not considered capable of providing independent and truly voluntary permission.

The use of living donors for pediatric liver and lung transplantation has probably been more widely practiced than for adult recipients. Small lobes of donor liver or lung can be utilized as satisfactory organs for young children. The morbidity and mortality for such living donors is probably less than when living donors are used for adult recipients, although such statistics are very difficult to come by. Evaluation of potential donors for pediatric liver or lung transplantation should follow the usual protocols and standards. The outcome of these types of living liver or lung transplant procedures may not, however, be uniformly superior to deceased donor transplants as is the case with kidney transplantation. Therefore, the proper use of living donors for pediatric liver and lung transplant candidates remains controversial.

Deceased donors

Pediatric candidates remain a small fraction of all potential organ transplant recipients. In some cases, size matching of organs between donor and recipient is quite important, particularly in heart and lung transplantations. However, as noted above, adult kidneys can be used for even small infants if proper techniques are used (see Figure 6.1). Also, adult livers can be "split" with the smaller component or lobe going to be pediatric recipient and the remainder of the liver going to another recipient, typically an adult. Similar techniques can be utilized for deceased donor lungs. However, here are technical complications related to these reduction or splitting techniques, and recipients of such organs typically have more complications, and lower graft survival rates and half-lives. In addition, adult recipients of split livers may also have complications relating to the procedures performed on the donor graft.

The Organ Procurement and Transplant Network (OPTN), which is responsible for allocation of organs for transplantation in USA, has generally provided preference for pediatric recipients in all of its allocation rules. This was first evident in the initial allocation policy for deceased donor kidneys. Pediatric candidates aged <15 years were provided preference for organs that were recovered from donors aged <10 years. Unfortunately, this allocation policy, although probably shortening the time that pediatric candidates were required to spend waiting for a transplant, preferentially provided some young recipients with high-risk donor kidneys. Specifically, graft thrombosis became an important cause of early graft failure, affecting up to 5% of pediatric deceased donor transplants. A retrospective analysis of risk factors for graft thrombosis identified young donors and young recipients independently to be at high risk. Thus, a policy that specifically assigned high-risk donors to high-risk recipients could have been predicted to result in suboptimal outcomes. Indeed, infants receiving deceased donor transplants during that era had the worst outcomes of any age group.

A change in allocation policy that provided additional "points" to pediatric candidates was substituted. This policy provided these points only after a certain waiting time, varying between 6 and 18 months depending on the candidate's age. This prescribed waiting time was provided in order to allow pediatric candidates sufficient time to receive offers from well-matched donors. Unfortunately, the number of points necessary to reach the top of the waiting list varied among regions and eras. In addition, the waiting time provided to candidates to permit sufficient opportunity for well-matched donors almost invariably did not result in transplants as planned. More recently, therefore, the OPTN once again changed its allocation policy to provide preference for pediatric recipients. The most recent change permits pediatric candidates to be placed at the top of the waiting list for donors aged <35 years as soon as they are listed. This new policy has resulted in a marked decrease in waiting time for pediatric kidney candidates; many of them now receive grafts within 6 months of listing. Unfortunately, another unintended consequence has occurred. It appears as if this strong preference has shifted the ratio of living donor and deceased donor grafts for children. before this allocation policy, up to 60% of donors for pediatric kidney transplants were living donors. For the first 1–2 years after this allocation change, that ratio has reversed. The pediatric community is currently reviewing these results but early analysis suggests that the ease of obtaining deceased donors and the rapidity with which these grafts can be transplanted have to be balanced against the expected shorter half-life of deceased donor transplants compared with living donor grafts.

The OPTN has also provided preference for pediatric candidates awaiting liver, heart, and lung transplantation with varying policies, e.g., children have a separate urgency score, known as pediatric end-stage liver disease (PELD), rather than the model used for adult liver allocation, known as model for end-stage liver disease (MELD). In general, PELD provides better assessment of mortality risk for children awaiting liver transplant than MELD. However, recent analysis demonstrated that the MELD score is numerically higher for adolescents than the PELD one, and thus it has been substituted. In addition, OPTN has provided specific status 1 criteria for pediatric liver recipients which provides some preference for the sickest candidates. As candidates for combined liver–intestinal transplantation may have higher mortality while awaiting transplant, there are efforts to further refine liver allocation to provide additional benefit for them. The number of both candidates and size-specific donors is small, and wider sharing of these donors beyond typical OPO borders might alleviate some prolonged waiting episodes, and perhaps mortality, for infants and young children awaiting liver transplantation.

Similarly, despite the potential complications in adult recipients of split livers, policies that may require consideration of splitting donor livers more frequently could reduce pediatric candidate mortality. These latter two policies are currently under consideration by the OPTN. As a result of the stringent need for matching size of donor and recipient for heart transplants, small pediatric recipients may have a severe handicap because of the lack of size-matched donors in their local area. Also, adolescents will be in competition with adults of about the same size. Thus the OPTN has been focused on broader sharing of pediatric donor hearts because an appropriately sized donor for a small recipient may be a greater distance than is typically true for adult transplantation. Sharing even at a national level is being considered. Furthermore, children are now being given preference for organs recovered from pediatric donors in an effort to shorten waiting time. The allocation of lungs for transplant is based on a new system that assesses both the urgency of the recipient and the probability of good outcome. As children aged <12 years have a different mix of the etiologies for chronic lung failure, they are allocated donor lungs in a manner different from older children and adults. There are considerations of providing preference for pediatric lung candidates to receive young donor lungs, comparable to the kidney, liver, and heart allocation systems.

Death on the waiting list

Unfortunately, some candidates die while awaiting organ transplantation. The mortality on the waiting list may be higher for young pediatric candidates than for older children and adults. The number of children awaiting all types of deceased donor organ transplants over the past decade is shown in Figure 6.2. This figure shows the number of active transplants on the last day of each calendar year and is a relatively accurate indicator of the balance of additional new candidates and candidates who have either received grafts or died. As noted, the number of listed pediatric candidates has actually decreased over the last 5 years, probably because of more appropriate listing criteria for liver and lung transplantation. As a result of the success of chronic dialysis, death on the waiting list for kidney transplantation tends to be lower than for other organs. In contrast, waiting list deaths for liver transplant candidates are more common. The development of the PELD and MELD systems was designed to allocate organs to

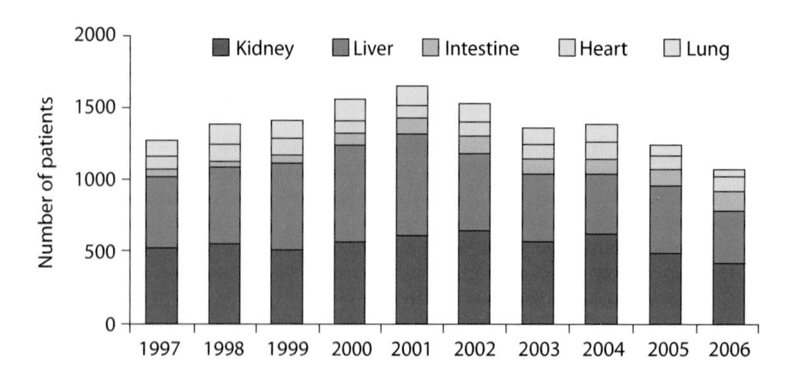

Figure 6.2 Number of pediatric transplant candidates on the deceased donor waiting list on the last calendar day of each year, by type of graft. (Reprinted from Magee JC, Krishnan SM, Benfield MR, et al. Pediatric transplantation in the United States, 1997–2006. *Am J Transplant* 2008;8:935–45.)

those most urgently in need of them. However, because of their declining health condition, the mortality risk rises substantially. Currently, children older than 6 years have a mortality risk the same or slightly lower than that of older children and adults, approximately 50 deaths per 1000 patient-years at risk. However, the risk for infants aged <1 year is 10- to 20-fold higher, between 500 and 1000 deaths per 1000 patient-years at risk. In 2006, 103 pediatric candidates for liver transplantation died before they could receive a graft.

The number of heart transplant candidates who died before they could receive a graft has declined slightly over the past decade, to 59 deaths in 2006, equivalent to 89 deaths per 1000 patient-years. In that same year, 54 pediatric candidates received lung transplants but 16 died while waiting. There has been great variation in the mortality rate while awaiting intestinal transplant, likely due to small numbers of candidates awaiting combined liver–intestinal transplantation. For candidates listed initially for intestinal-alone transplantation across all age ranges, the death rate was 379 per 1000 patient-years in 2006. As a result of all of these death rates, the OPTN set a strategic goal of eliminating death on the waiting list for pediatric organ transplant candidates. Obviously, accomplishment of that goal would require improvement in artificial life support for children with organ failure, substantial preference for children compared with adults on the waiting list, wider sharing of appropriate organs from size-matched young donors, and perhaps innovative surgical techniques. Although elusive and ambitious hopefully this goal is achievable.

Key points 6.2 Death on organ transplant waiting lists among children

In 2006:

- 103 liver transplant candidates
- 59 heart transplant candidates
- 16 lung transplant candidates

Strategic goal of the Organ Procurement Transplant Network: eliminate all deaths among children on organ transplant waiting lists!

Pediatric organ donors

Although the accidental death rate among children is lower than in adults, it does rise during adolescence. Furthermore, as children frequently have few complicating medical disorders, they are more likely to be appropriate organ donor candidates if they have terminal disorders. The number and percentage of pediatric organ donors have decreased somewhat over the past 10 years. The distribution of generations has, however remained constant, with about 60% of donors ranging between the ages of 11 and 17 years. And, while the number of adult donors is substantially greater than that of pediatric donors, the percentage of organs transplanted versus the organs recovered from deceased donors is dramatically greater. Within the pediatric age range the vast majority of organs recovered from pediatric donors are transplanted. What may be even more striking is the balance between pediatric organ donors and pediatric transplant recipients. As shown in Figure 6.3, less than 10% of kidneys recovered from pediatric donors were transplanted into pediatric recipients early in this decade. This ratio may be changing with the new pediatric kidney allocation system. Nevertheless, the number of pediatric donor kidneys that were transplanted into adults was more than five times the number of adult donor kidneys that were transplanted into children. The same patterns are similar for pediatric heart, lung, and liver donors. Only in pediatric intestinal transplants are the majority of organs recovered from pediatric donors transplanted into pediatric recipients.

Given the present shortage of deceased organ donors and in view of the decreased number of pediatric organ donors, there has been a broad range of efforts to increase organ donations including donation after cardiac death (DCD). DCD has been increasing among all donor age groups from just a handful in the late 1990s to 647 in 2006. Children comprise about 12% of DCD donors and about 8% of pediatric donors were from DCD. As organ donation is generally unusual in a pediatric hospital, the introduction of DCD protocols may require more time and effort to be developed and enforced. Pediatric intensive care units have well-developed end-of-life and withdrawal-of-support practices in place, and these were developed before the DCD

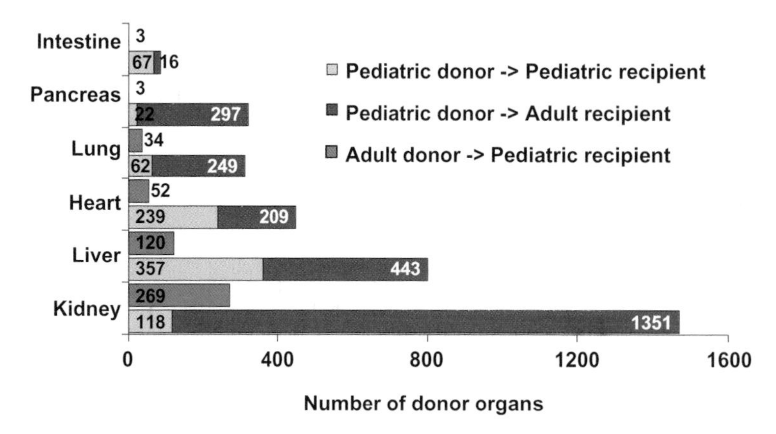

Figure 6.3 Number of deceased donor grafts recovered from pediatric and adult donors and transplanted into pediatric and adult recipients by organ type, 2003. More pediatric donor organs are transplanted into adults than adult organs into children. (Adapted from Magee JC, Bucuvalas JC, Farmer DG, et al. Pediatric transplantation. *Am J Transplant* 2004;4(suppl 9):54.)

protocols became practical. Based on recent policies advanced by the Joint Commission (JCAHO) and the OPTN, there is new emphasis on developing DCD protocols.

Key points 6.3 Pediatric organ donors

- Higher conversion rates than adult donors, usually because of absent comorbidities
- Currently comprise 12% of DCD donors
- Organs from very young donors associated with more thrombosis and other technical problems
- The large majority of kidneys, hearts, lungs, and livers procured from children are transplanted into adult recipients

Wait list management

As pediatric organ transplant programs are generally small and perform fewer than 50–100 transplantations per year, the complexity and difficulties of managing a large list of transplant candidates is generally not as common as in adult programs. Nevertheless, the need to assure that the candidate listing data are correct and up to date is equally important for pediatric candidates. Of similar importance is the need to assure that the candidate's transplant status is stable and unaffected by intercurrent illness or severity of disease.

Peritransplant procedures

Successful organ transplantation requires careful preparation of the candidate before transplantation, a team effort in the immediate postoperative setting, and careful maintenance of the graft after the patient is discharged from the hospital. Each of the organ systems has unique components of this effort.

Pediatric kidney transplantation

Histocompatibility matching used to play a large role in allocation of deceased donor kidneys and in choosing a living donor. Although better donor matching does result in longer graft half-lives, this influence has been lessened because of overall improvement in immunosuppression. However, kidney transplants still require blood-type matching and negative cross-matches between donors and recipients. Both of these requirements have been modified lately based on more sensitive cross-match techniques, and desensitization procedures in a few circumstances. As chronic hemodialysis or peritoneal dialysis provides a lifesaving option, pediatric kidney transplantation does not have to be undertaken as an emergency procedure under any circumstances. Indeed, the presence of chronic dialysis permits preparation of the candidate so that the transplantation can be undertaken under the best possible circumstances rather than under the most risky or difficult circumstances. As noted above, approximately 25% of children receive kidney transplants pre-emptively, i.e., without prior dialysis treatment. Other children may undergo periods of chronic dialysis in order to stabilize their nutrition, to perform necessary corrective surgery before transplantation, or because suitable donors have not been identified. In addition, particularly for children with acquired diseases such as FSGS or lupus nephritis, a period of chronic dialysis permits the underlying disease to "burn out" and for the child to have previously used medications such as steroids or cytotoxic agents tapered and discontinued. Sometimes, renal function deteriorates suddenly and dialysis is necessary before transplantation can be undertaken.

There are several indications for native nephrectomies, either before transplantation or during the transplantation procedure. Children who have urologic malformations and obstructive uropathy may develop a urinary-concentrating defect and have large amounts of urine output. If this continues after transplantation, appropriate hydration, particularly if the recipient is an infant, may be compromised. If children have ongoing proteinuria, particularly those infants who have congenital nephrotic syndrome with extraordinary protein losses, these conditions will also compromise postoperative care. Pyelonephritis in kidneys of children with serious urogenital malformations may also complicate post-transplant care. Sometimes, chronic kidney disease in children can cause serious hypertension. When hypertension either is difficult to control or requires substantial antihypertensive medications, consideration of pretransplant nephrectomy may be appropriate. Thus, polyuria, proteinuria, ongoing hypertension, and infection may be indications for elective pretransplant native nephrectomy. In some programs, this is performed before the transplantation procedure and, in others, during it. In the particular circumstance of children with severe proteinuria, however, the native nephrectomies are preferentially performed before the transplantation in order to allow sufficient time for the candidate's nutritional status to be improved. One other special circumstance for which pre-transplant nephrectomy should be considered is the transplantation of an adult kidney into an infant recipient. In that situation, there is ongoing concern about sufficiency of blood flow to the transplanted kidney (see Figure 6.1). Perfusion of native kidneys may add a complicating factor to this concern for adequate blood flow and may suggest that they be removed before implantation of the new graft.

Generally, children >30 kg can receive the same surgical implantation techniques as adults. Smaller children and infants will require an individualized approach, for which the key issue is the appropriate matching of blood vessel size and anticipation of circulatory volume requirements. For young children and infants, <10 kg, the transplant incision is generally a midline laparotomy with anastomosis of the donor kidney onto the aorta and inferior vena cava. For slightly older children, there is reasonable variability based on the relative size of the donor organ and the recipient, and any pretransplant surgery performed on the recipient. Thus, the anastomosis may be to the great vessels or to the femoral or iliac vessels, depending on the relative size of the donor and recipient vessels. In addition, some children have vascular abnormalities that require special techniques. In some situations, en bloc implantation of organs recovered from infant donors may be used, as shown in Figure 6.4. The implantation of the transplant ureter into the recipient's bladder is typically performed in a manner designed to prevent vesicoureteral reflux. Perioperative management of the pediatric recipient also requires attention to specific or unique details. Intraoperatively, there is substantial emphasis on prevention of complications from underlying systemic disease and maintenance of optimal perfusion of the transplanted kidney. In general, particularly when there is a substantial size mismatch between the donor graft and the recipient, there is a need to

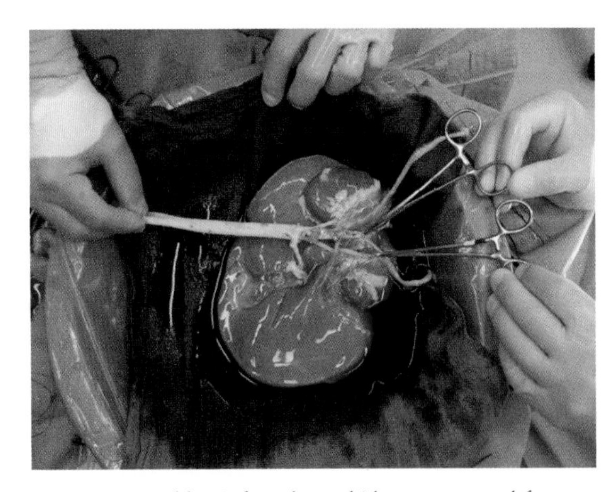

Figure 6.4 En bloc infant donor kidneys recovered for transplantation into infant requiring combined liver–kidney transplantation. Note long segment of vena cava recovered to replace a thrombosed segment in recipient.

expand the circulatory volume to allow for adequate perfusion of the adult donor allograft. In extreme circumstances, the recipient's cardiac output doubles after perfusion of the graft is achieved, and up to 50% of the cardiac output is directed toward perfusion of the transplanted kidney. In general, central venous pressure is kept high, in the range of 8–12 cmH_2O with a mean arterial pressure >70 mmHg. Sometimes, an infusion of dopamine is required. Postoperatively, the child is often cared for in an intensive care unit or at least requires intensive care nurse monitoring. Typically, the urine output for the first 48 h is replaced on an equal basis and may reach extraordinary levels. In this setting, careful management of fluid and electrolyte status by experienced staff is essential. Hyperglycemia, hyponatremia, hypocalcemia, acidosis, and hypokalemia are all possible without appropriate management. After 48 h, fluid intakes are gradually tapered to more usual levels. In the circumstance of adult kidneys being transplanted into young children or infants, the recipients must continue to receive greater than usual amounts of fluid for many months or years, to avoid underperfusion of the graft.

Children who have delayed graft function may need to undergo hemodialysis or peritoneal dialysis until the renal dysfunction resolves. Of course, this complicates postoperative care substantially. If transplant biopsy is required to assess for acute rejection or to determine the status of the graft, it can be performed in the usual percutaneous manner, generally under ultrasound guidance, even if the graft is intraperitoneal. In this latter circumstance, however, bleeding is more common because of lack of appropriate tamponade, so appropriate vigilance is necessary.

Case: infant kidney transplant

A 6-month-old infant is referred to the pediatric hospital for treatment of congenital nephrotic syndrome. An older brother with the same disorder had died at 3 months of age from sepsis and peritonitis. He has an 11-year-old sister who appears healthy. His mother's pregnancy was complicated by polyhydramnios and an amniocentesis had demonstrated elevated levels of α-fetoprotein. Soon after birth, severe proteinuria was noted. He was treated with periodic infusions of salt-poor albumin, but had many complications. He became dehydrated at 3 months of age and infarcted the tips of two toes on his left foot. He developed an episode of *E. coli* peritonitis just before referral and was treated with intravenous antibiotics, albumin infusions, and intravenous immune globulin. On presentation, he was markedly malnourished with depleted muscle mass, with marked anasarca. He weighs 5.9 kg. His hematocrit is 24%, blood urea nitrogen (BUN) 12 mg/dL, serum creatinine 0.1 mg/dL, and serum albumin 0.9 g/dL. Both parents wish to be worked up as possible kidney donors as well as his sister and two uncles.

Pediatric liver transplantation

Blood type compatibility is generally observed for liver transplantation, with possible exceptions for the youngest recipients. Histocompatibility matching is typically not performed and cross-matching is performed only after the procedure. As noted above, allocation of deceased donor livers for transplantation is based on a medical urgency, indicating that grafts are allocated to recipients most likely to die without a transplant. Thus, it is highly likely that these candidates will be quite unstable at the time of transplantation. To the credit of the transplant teams, postoperative mortality does not seem to be related to the severely compromised condition of these candidates at the time of transplantation. For pediatric recipients, particularly infants, careful attention must be paid to assuring adequate nutritional support before transplantation. Recovery of deceased donor livers follows typical protocols, but particular care must be provided to the graft vessels and supplemental splenic or carotid arteries should be recovered. Living donor liver recovery also has been previously described and the approach depends upon the lobe to be removed. Laparoscopic left lateral lobe recovery has been reported, but open procedures are more common. The actual procedure is dependent on the source of the graft, with some variations related to whole versus reduced-sized grafts. Up to 50% of children receive technical variant grafts, including living donor liver grafts and reduced-sized grafts. These partial liver transplants tend to have complicated vascular and biliary anastomoses, creating postoperative problems with graft perfusion and biliary outflow. In addition, those with a cut edge tend to have biliary leaks and postoperative infections. Improvements in surgical techniques and preoperative management have reduced the need for lengthy hospitalization following liver transplantation. Typically patients requiring intense monitoring and abdominal ultrasonography is performed to assess perfusion of the graft on a periodic basis. As with kidney transplantation, fluid management is undertaken to assure adequacy of graft perfusion. Frequently anticoagulants in the form of aspirin, heparin dextrans, or prostacyclin are provided to prevent graft thrombosis. Careful assessment for postoperative complications, including bleeding and bile leaks as well as for infection and electrolyte abnormalities, is essential.

Pediatric heart transplantation

Blood-type-compatible donors are typically used for heart transplantation. However, very young candidates, aged <2 years, may receive blood-type-incompatible grafts if their anti-A and anti-B antibody levels are low. Typically, allocation of hearts for transplantation is not based on histocompatibility matching, although knowledge of donor antigens may be valuable to predict positive cross-matches. Although these cross-matches cannot typically be performed before transplantation, they certainly complicate the postoperative management and success, so knowledge about potentially positive cross-matches, based on specificity of pre-formed antibodies, may be valuable. As noted above, many infants and young children have high levels of anti-HLA antibodies, likely related to extracorporeal perfusion or the use of homografts before transplantation. As this level of sensitization limits transplant options for these patients, new protocols designed to "de-sensitize" them are being explored.

As with liver transplantation, allocation of hearts for transplantation is based on urgency criteria, but, in addition, there are stronger restrictions with respect to size mismatches. Therefore, children, particularly young children, may wait and suffer many complications related to chronic heart failure before the transplantation. Importantly, until very recently, there were no appropriate VADs available for small children. Heart transplant surgical techniques have been described previously. These techniques may be complicated by prior surgery for correction of congenital heart disease, leading to more complex surgery requirements for the transplant. In addition, abnormal placement of the great arteries and other structures might require innovative approaches to ensure that the donor heart functions properly. In general, postoperative management is similar to that provided to other children undergoing cardiopulmonary bypass. Systolic function often recovers rapidly but diastolic dysfunction may persist for weeks. Particular attention must be paid to pulmonary vascular resistance which can cause right heart failure. In addition, cardiac arrhythmias are more common in this setting. Maintenance of an appropriate heart rate is important for maintaining cardiac output and can be regulated by atrial pacing or chronotropic agents. Surveillance for acute rejection is typically performed by routine intracardiac biopsy. Many programs perform biopsies on a weekly basis in the early postoperative period.

Pediatric lung transplantation

Matching on the basis of blood type and histocompatibility typing for lung transplant is similar to what is done for heart transplant. In general, there is no time for performing pretransplant cross-matches but attention to recipient antibodies to donor HLA antigens might provide predictive value. Typically, bilateral sequential lung transplants rather than single lung transplant is the procedure of choice in children because of the concern for growth of the implanted lungs. Postoperatively, attention is paid to graft dysfunction related to reperfusion injury. All patients undergo bronchoscopy and perfusion lung scan soon after transplantation. Infection is the most common longer-term complication. The lung is the only transplanted solid organ exposed constantly to outside contamination. Maintenance of appropriate fluid and electrolyte balance is necessary in order to avoid pulmonary edema. If living donors are used, typically there are two donors, each of whom supply a single lobe. The results of the living donor transplants seem to be about as good as those for deceased donor transplants.

Pediatric intestinal transplantation

In general, identical blood group matching is preferred for intestinal transplantation, although the clinical condition of the recipient would dictate the possible use of ABO-incompatible blood types. Critically ill liver–intestine or multivisceral recipients may possibly receive ABO-incompatible grafts, but this practice is generally avoided in isolated intestine transplants. The non-identical blood type transplants may be associated with hemolytic reactions because of the large lymphoid load included with the allograft. In general, cytotoxic cross-matches should be negative before implementation because of a detrimental effect of positive cross-matches on outcome. This is particularly true for isolated intestinal transplants. In the setting of a combined liver–intestine transplant, however, cross-matching may not be necessary. Size matching is important for successful intestinal transplantation and, indeed, donors smaller than the recipient may be necessary because of a smaller abdominal cavity. Unfortunately, organs from intestinal donors seem more susceptible to necrotizing enterocolitis. As the intestine is so sensitive to perfusion injury, meticulous care of the donor before transplantation to avoid cardiac arrest or circulatory collapse is important. The recipient operation may be complicated by vascular abnormalities occurring before transplantation. In all these cases, concern for maintenance of adequate graft perfusion is uppermost. As surveillance for rejection requires appropriate biopsy material, and as allograft mucosal biopsy remains the only method to confirm clinically suspected acute rejection, appropriate access to a site for biopsy is necessary.

Post-transplant monitoring

Pediatric recipients of organ transplants are typically followed very closely by members of the transplant team in the immediate post-transplant period. Many programs have established protocols for the frequency of surveillance and its components. The American Society of Transplantation developed a clinical practice guideline for follow-up of the kidney transplantation and this contained proposed guidelines for the follow-up of pediatric kidney transplant recipients. In general, the pediatric community felt that more frequent and more intense follow-up was necessary for children, based on their unique complications, the possibility of more frequent early acute rejection episodes, the potential for infection related to a more naïve immune response to pathogens before transplantation, and the potential for non-adherence to prescribed immunosuppression protocols. Typically, these transplant recipients are assessed for graft function and complications of both the transplant and the immunosuppressive medications being used. Pediatric programs usually taper the initial immunosuppression slowly to lower maintenance levels during the first post-transplant year.

Some programs, typically heart and intestinal transplant programs, perform surveillance graft biopsies in order to be vigilant for acute rejection. Kidney transplant programs, based on excellent outcomes from multicenter clinical trials, have started to perform surveillance kidney biopsies also, but more frequently to assess for nephrotoxicity than for acute rejection. In general, although patients are frequently referred back to their primary care physicians or subspecialists closer to home, pediatric transplant recipients continue to be monitored at their transplant centers on a periodic basis. Appropriate adjustment of immunosuppressive medication as the patient grows becomes increasingly important with lengthening time after transplantation. Of equal importance is the assessment of adherence to the transplant follow-up protocols. Unfortunately, there have been multiple reports of children, particularly adolescents, who have lost their grafts from presumed non-adherence to immunosuppression regimens. Without good methods of assessing adherence, however, it is very difficult to determine whether these reports are accurate. In the same vein, proposals for behavior modification that may lessen the incidence of non-adherence are compromised by lack of accuracy of assessment of their efficacy. Nevertheless, increasing attention is being paid to this problem by pediatric care teams because of its detrimental effects on long-term outcomes. Perhaps the combination of behavioral techniques to improved adherence as well as the development of immunosuppressive agents or protocols that require less vigilance on the individual patient's part may prove to be successful in the future.

Immunosuppression for pediatric transplantation

In general, children receive the same immunosuppressive medications after organ transplantation as adults. However, most of these medications have not been tested in controlled clinical trials and few of them have specific pediatric indications. This situation is changing, however, because the Food and Drug Administration (FDA) provides some benefit to pharmaceutical companies that seek and achieve pediatric indications. Furthermore, the establishment of multicenter clinical trial groups permits specific testing of some of these medications in children. Dosing of medications for children is usually indexed against some measure of body mass, either weight or body surface area. Furthermore, infants and young children cannot swallow pills and they frequently metabolize medications at substantially different rates from adults. Thus, they frequently require special formulations and schedules.

Virtually all organ transplant recipients receive multidrug regimens, typically double or triple therapy. In addition, many receive induction therapy with lymphocytotoxic or modifying antibodies. Many of the protocols are center specific and based on experience rather than controlled trials. Recently, some trials sponsored by the CCTPT have evaluated certain combinations. In most cases, the immunosuppression is maximized soon after the transplantation, and then is very slowly tapered to lower maintenance levels over several months to years. In general, kidney transplant recipients receive substantial immunosuppression in order to prevent acute rejections because every acute rejection leaves the transplanted kidney damaged and shortens the ultimate graft survival. Most commonly, these patients receive triple immunosuppression, including corticosteroids, and at least half receive treatment with an induction antibody. Heart transplant recipients also receive substantial immunosuppression but much more frequently receive steroid-free protocols because of their long-term detrimental cardiovascular complications. They often receive high doses of calcineurin inhibitors (CNIs) early after transplantation and that may account for the high incidence of nephrotoxicity in these patients.

Liver transplant recipients infrequently receive induction antibody treatment and often have steroid-free immunosuppression protocols. The overwhelming majority of liver transplant recipients have a CNI-based immunosuppression protocol, most often tacrolimus. Typically, tapering of immunosuppression is more aggressive in these recipients; they do have higher frequencies of acute rejection but the regenerative capabilities of the liver probably account for the fact that the rejection episodes have less deleterious effects on long-term outcome. Some liver transplant recipients are reduced to monotherapy for maintenance. There is less information about intestinal and lung transplant recipients because of the low number of procedures performed each year. However, intestinal transplant recipients frequently receive very high levels of immunosuppression, particularly early on because of the frequency and severity of acute rejection. Similarly, lung transplant recipients may also have high rates of rejection. Unfortunately both of these types of transplants have substantial morbidity related to post-transplant infections, thereby complicating the decision about immunosuppressive techniques even more.

Induction antibodies

Retrospective data from the NAPRTCS registry have consistently shown a beneficial effect of prophylactic induction antibody use in pediatric kidney transplant recipients. Several studies have demonstrated an 8–10% improvement in 5-year graft survival for both living and deceased donor kidney transplant recipients who received induction antibody compared with those who did not. However, a large randomized controlled trial of the monoclonal antibody OKT3 showed no beneficial effect other than a delay of the first acute rejection episode. Similarly, retrospective analyses of interleukin-2 (IL-2) receptor-blocking antibodies have shown that they are well tolerated and may delay or prevent acute rejections. Nevertheless, well-controlled trials of their efficacy on long-term graft survival are lacking, so the use of these antibodies for pediatric organ transplant recipients is based mostly on center bias and experience. Currently, there are two polyclonal antibodies available, ATGAM and Thymoglobulin. The latter is much more commonly used. Typically it is provided, particularly in the setting of delayed graft function, for 10–14 days after transplantation. A recent report suggests daily monitoring of CD3+ lymphocyte subsets as a guide to therapy: the daily dose is given only when the CD3+ lymphocyte count exceeds a certain level, such as 20 cells/mm^3.

There is an increasing trend for the use of Thymoglobulin after pediatric kidney and heart transplantation, and it is proving to be both safe and probably effective in preventing acute rejection in the early post-transplantation period. Orthoclone OKT3 is a mouse monoclonal antibody directed against the T3 antigen on most circulating lymphocytes. Although it apparently depletes lymphocytes from the peripheral circulation, it is not truly a "lytic" antibody because mouse antibodies do not bind human complement. As noted above, a controlled trial of Orthoclone OKT3 in pediatric kidney transplant recipients demonstrated delay of the first acute rejection episode but no effect on long-term graft survival or the incidence of acute rejections. Currently, Orthoclone OKT3 is not used for induction treatment in virtually any pediatric organ transplant recipients but it is sometimes used for treatment of acute rejection episodes, particularly in intestinal transplant recipients.

A newer monoclonal antibody, alemtuzumab (Campath-1H) causes profound lymphocyte depletion for at least 3–6 months. Recent innovative protocols utilizing alemtuzumab induction for pediatric kidney and liver transplants have demonstrated that it is generally safe and quite effective in preventing early acute rejection episodes and allowing minimization protocols for these recipients. Larger studies will be necessary before alemtuzumab is more widely utilized. There are two non-depleting antibodies that block the IL-2 receptor on mature lymphocytes, daclizumab and basiliximab. Both of these antibodies have been utilized for induction treatment in children and there is broad experience with their safety. In general, they are used only during the immediate post-transplant period. However, some innovative protocols suggest that longer-term use may be safe and possibly allow pediatric recipients to avoid other toxic immunosuppressants, specifically corticosteroids. Experimentation with chronic use of these antibodies has started, but unfortunately daclizumab production has now ceased, making further study unlikely.

Maintenance immunosuppressive drugs

There are currently six classes of immunosuppressive medications that are used for chronic prophylactic treatment for pediatric transplant recipients. Each class is discussed below.

Corticosteroids

Corticosteroids have been used for many decades and were felt to be necessary for graft survival for kidney transplantation until recently. Typically, corticosteroids are given in high doses immediately after the transplantation and then tapered to low daily or alternate-day schedules. Lower doses and less frequent dosing have been associated with fewer chronic side effects. These side effects are particularly difficult for pediatric recipients, and include hypertension, hyperglycemia, cosmetic changes, specifically cushingoid appearance and weight gain, psychological changes, osteoporosis, growth retardation, hypercholesterolemia, etc. The growth retardation effects are particularly noticeable after kidney transplantation. As noted, alternate-day dosing can ameliorate many of these effects but steroid withdrawal or avoidance is the most preferable. Until very recently all attempts to withdraw steroids from pediatric kidney transplant recipients were unsuccessful. However, in at least four recent trials, two of which were randomized and controlled, steroids have been completely eliminated after pediatric kidney transplantation, so it is likely that the appropriate use of other medications will permit steroid-free transplantation for a large number of pediatric kidney transplant recipients. As noted above, liver and heart transplant recipients frequently avoid or withdraw steroids altogether.

Azathioprine and mycophenolate mofetil

Azathioprine and MMF are anti-proliferative agents that have been used frequently in pediatric transplant recipients. More recently, enteric-coated mycophenolic acid (Myfortic), has been introduced as an alternative, but there is less pediatric experience with its use. Myfortic dosing studies in children have demonstrated slightly higher area values for under the curve (AUC) than in adults with comparable doses, but the clinical significance of this is not known. Azathioprine was the first approved medication shown to prevent rejection and it has had wide applicability. However, for the past decade, it has been principally replaced by MMF. In general, both of these medications can cause granulocytopenia and MMF has been associated with gastrointestinal complications, particularly in younger children. Although several studies have assessed the pharmacokinetics and safety of MMF, there are no clear guidelines to concentration-controlled dosing. MMF has been used in combination with all other immunosuppressants except azathioprine and there are no contraindications to these combinations. MMF dosing has been evaluated in children and the dosing is typically prescribed based on the body surface area, with recommended doses ranging between 600 and 1200 mg/m^2 per day in two to three divided doses. When diarrhea occurs, the more frequent dosing with lower dose amounts has been tried, but often azathioprine is substituted instead, in doses of 1–2 mg/kg per day. More precise dosing of MMF or azathioprine can be achieved by compounding liquid preparations from the pill forms that are supplied.

Calcineurin inhibitors

CNIs have been the mainstay of organ transplantation for the past 20–30 years. Cyclosporine was the first of this class of medications that was introduced and its use led to marked improvements in virtually all types of organ transplant outcomes. Early use of cyclosporine in children was, however, somewhat complicated by a lack of clinical trials and understanding of its pharmacokinetics. Young children, in particular, were found to metabolize cyclosporine more quickly than adults, and this led to under-dosing. The proper dosing was corrected only after institution of protocols using two to three times a day dosing and indexing based on body surface area. Typical starting doses for children aged <6 years are 500 mg/m^2 per day, administered three times a day, whereas older children receive 15 mg/kg per day, administered twice daily. Doses are adjusted to attain protocol-specific target blood levels.

The complications of cyclosporine in children are similar to those in adults and include nephrotoxicity, hypertension, and hyperlipidemia. However, hypertrichosis, gingival hyperplasia, and facial dysmorphism are particularly disturbing to children, especially adolescents, so long-term use has been compromised. Tacrolimus was first approved for liver transplantation but subsequently has been used extensively for kidney, intestine, heart, and lung transplantation. It is particularly attractive for pediatric use because it lacks the cosmetic side effects of cyclosporine, although it shares most of the other complications. Early use of tacrolimus in children was marred by a very high incidence of post-transplant lymphoproliferative disease (PTLD) and other serious side effects such as hyperglycemia. However, these complications may have been related to doses that were excessive. Subsequent protocols, utilizing lower doses, have had fewer side effects. In general, oral dosing of tacrolimus begins at 0.1 mg/kg twice daily, but are adjusted to achieve target trough blood levels. Typical levels are 5–20 ng/L, with more recent maintenance levels closer to the lower level, in order to avoid nephrotoxicity. Both cyclosporine and tacrolimus come in liquid preparations, which makes pediatric dosing more convenient. Unfortunately, the taste of both is unpleasant.

TOR inhibitors

Target of rapamycin (TOR) inhibitors include sirolimus and everolimus, although the latter is not available in the USA at this time. These new drugs have unique mechanisms of action, which means that they can be combined with virtually all other immunosuppressants, although caution should be observed in the combination of a CNI and a TOR inhibitor for children. These medications have long durations of action, resulting in a once-a-day dosing for adults. Children appear to have quicker metabolism, however, and they often need to be administered twice a day. Sirolimus is available as pills or liquid and its dose can therefore be tailored easily for children. Typical target levels are between 7 and 15 ng/mL, but these seem to be center specific. Major complications of the TOR inhibitors include hyperlipidemia, thrombocytopenia, impaired wound healing, and proteinuria.

Co-stimulation blockade

Co-stimulation blockade is the general term used to describe a novel immunosuppression strategy. Most immunosuppressants have been designed to eliminate or block the action of lymphocytes which typically mediate organ transplant rejection. This new approach, on the other hand, is designed to enhance natural regulatory mechanism or block activation stimuli. Antigen recognition alone is not sufficient for full T-cell activation. T cells require two distinct signals for full activation. The first signal is provided by the engagement of the T-cell receptor (TCR) with the MHC plus peptide complex on antigen-presenting cells (APCs) and the second "co-stimulatory" signal is provided by engagement of one or more T-cell surface receptors with their specific ligand on APCs. Signaling through the TCR alone without a co-stimulatory signal can lead to a prolonged state of T-cell anergy.

The best characterized and perhaps most important co-stimulatory signal is that provided by interaction of CD28 on T cells with either B7-1 or B7-2 on APCs.

The CD28/CTLA-4–B7-1/B7-2 T-cell co-stimulatory pathway is a unique and complex pathway that regulates T-cell activation. After activation, T cells express another CD28 family member, CTLA-4, that has a higher affinity for B7-1 and B7-2, and functions to provide a "negative" signal resulting in physiologic termination of T-cell responses. Ligation of CD28 by B7-1 or B7-2 is blocked by CTLA4Ig, a recombinant fusion protein that contains the extracellular domain of CTLA-4 fused to an IgG heavy chain tail. There have been several candidate molecules tested in preclinical and pilot human trials. There is only one molecule, belatacept, in final clinical testing and likely to become widely available in the near future. Belatacept is slightly modified variant of CTL-4–Ig and its initial trials in human renal transplant recipients has been encouraging. As belatacept is administered parenterally once a month, there is promise that its chronic use may lead to improved adherence among recipients, which might be particularly appropriate for adolescents.

Immunosuppression combinations and minimization protocols

As noted above, most protocols for pediatric organ transplant recipients consist of two or three drugs. The most common regimen for kidney transplantation is prednisone–MMF–tacrolimus. Liver and heart transplant programs are more likely to use steroid-sparing regimens and typically two-drug protocols. The combination of prednisone–CNI–rapamycin is particularly potent in preventing acute rejection, but is also associated with an unacceptably high incidence of PTLD in susceptible pediatric recipients, specifically those who are seronegative for Epstein–Barr virus (EBV) at the time of transplantation and receive an organ from an EBV-seropositive donor. Recently, minimization protocols involving tacrolimus alone or the combination MMF–sirolimus have been proposed in small pilot trials and offer some promise.

Outcomes of pediatric organ transplantation

Pediatric kidney transplantation

Young children used to have the worst outcomes after kidney transplantation, but recent reports show that children aged <10 years now have the best long-term outcomes of all age groups of children and adults (Figure 6.5), with 5-year living donor graft survival rates at 85–89%. Unfortunately, these excellent outcomes are not shared by adolescent recipients whose graft survival rates are worse than any other

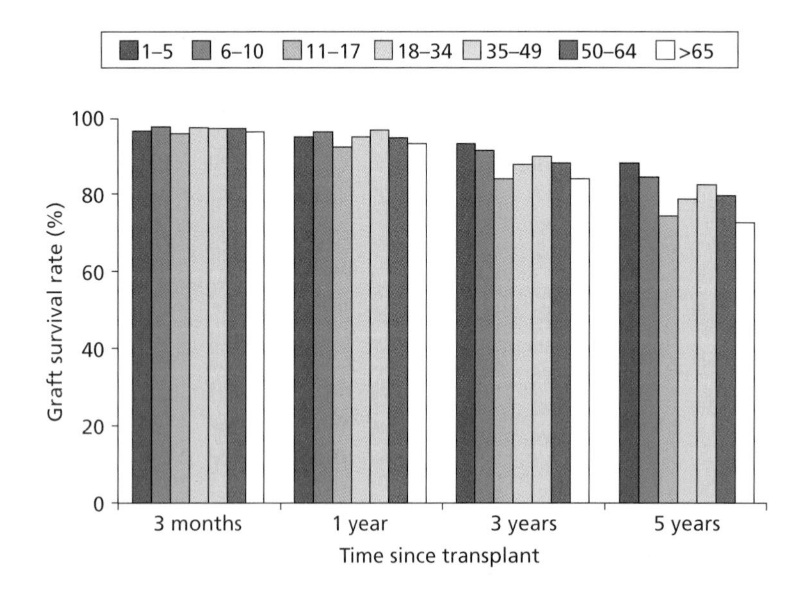

Figure 6.5 Living donor kidney transplant graft survival rates in various age group cohorts. Recipients aged <10 years have the best 5-year graft survival rates of all age groups whereas adolescents are worse than all except elderly recipients. (Reprinted from Magee JC, Krishnan SM, Benfield MR, et al. Pediatric transplantation in the United States, 1997–2006. *Am J Transplant* 2008;8:935–45.)

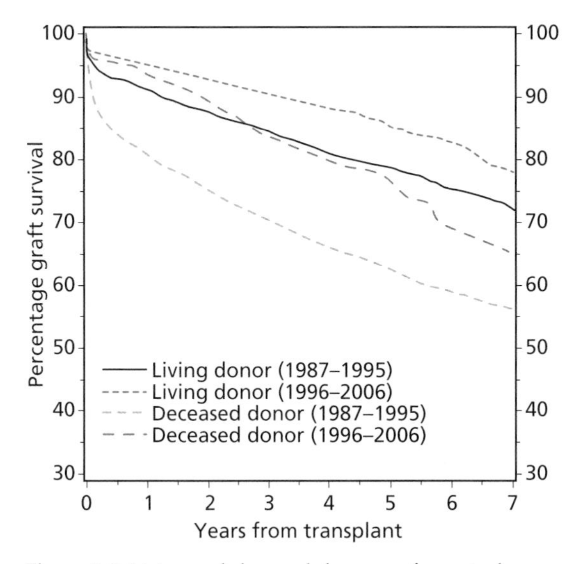

Figure 6.6 Living and deceased donor graft survival rates from two eras. Note the overall improvement in graft survival. Living donor grafts have better long-term survival than deceased donor grafts in both eras. (Adapted from Smith JM, Stablein DM, Munoz R, Hebert D, McDonald RA. Contributions of the Transplant Registry: The 2006 Annual Report of the North American Pediatric Renal Trials and Collaborative Studies (NAPRTCS). *Pediatr Transplant* 2007;**11**:366–73.)

age groups except very elderly people, with 5-year graft survival rates for living donor transplants of about 74%. Although graft survival after deceased donor kidney transplantation has improved significantly over the past decade, the results of living donor kidney transplants remain significantly better than deceased donor (Figure 6.6), between 10% and 15% better at 5 years, depending on recipient age. The major causes of graft failure are, in order, chronic allograft nephropathy, vascular thrombosis, recurrent disease, and acute rejection. Acute rejection rates have fallen substantially in kidney transplantation and only about 15–20% of pediatric kidney transplant recipients have an acute rejection episode in the first year. Mortality rates after kidney transplantation are very low, probably because of excellent early graft survival and alternative treatments if the graft does fail. Current 5-year patient survival rate is about 95%, with slightly higher survival after living donor compared with deceased donor transplants and also higher for older children and adolescents compared with infants. The major causes of death are, in order, infection, cardiovascular causes, and malignancy.

Pediatric liver transplantations

Mortality rates after liver transplantation in children have improved substantially over the past decade, especially for infants, whose 1-year patient survival rates are now about equal to all other age groups (Figure 6.7). Overall 3-year patient survival rate is about 84% in children. The best 5-year patient survival rates are seen in the 6–10 year olds, at 89%. Graft survival for living donor recipients are better than for deceased donor recipients for all age groups: 3-year graft survival rates for living versus deceased donor recipients were 83% versus 80% for <1 year olds and 79% versus 76% for 1–5 year olds. Overall long-term graft survival rates from the SPLIT registry are shown in Figure 6.8. Risk factors for poor outcome include size and malnutrition at the time of transplant, re-transplantation, malignancy, and fulminant hepatic failure. Very young children have lower acute rejection rates, as with other organ transplants, but have somewhat lower graft and patient survival, probably related to technical and donor issues. In general, technical variant grafts (split livers, reduced-size donors) do not have outcomes as good as whole-liver grafts.

One study showed that living donor grafts for infants did better than split deceased donor grafts. The major cause of death after liver transplantation is infection. Bacterial infections are the most common cause for many of the early years, but fungal and viral sources, principally EBV and cytomegalovirus (CMV), are also important. Graft failure is another important cause of mortality. Although up to 50% of pediatric liver recipients have acute rejection episodes in the first 6 months, virtually all are reversed and few cause graft failure or death. Chronic rejection occurs in up to 25% by 10 years, but late graft loss is much less common in liver transplant recipients than in other organ transplants. About 10% of liver transplant recipients develop PTLD. Ten years after transplantation, about three-quarters of pediatric liver transplant recipients have mild-to-severe chronic kidney disease.

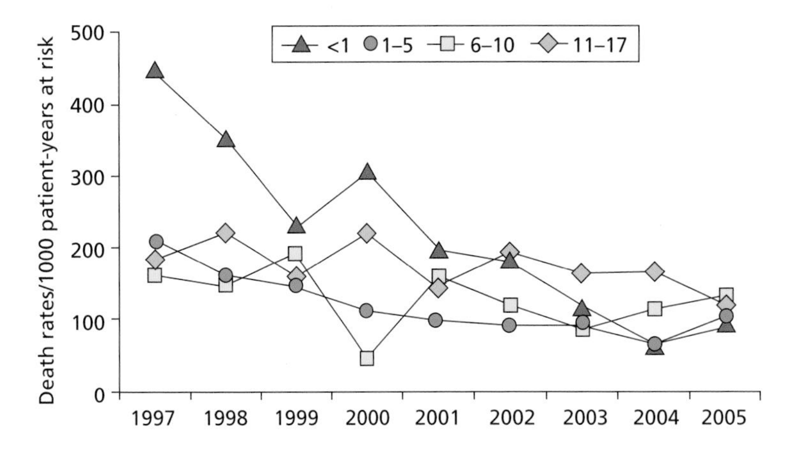

Figure 6.7 Death rates for various pediatric age groups during the first year after deceased donor liver transplantation. Very young candidates now have the same risk as older children. (Reprinted from Magee JC, Krishnan SM, Benfield MR, et al. Pediatric transplantation in the United States, 1997–2006. *Am J Transplant* 2008;8:935–45.)

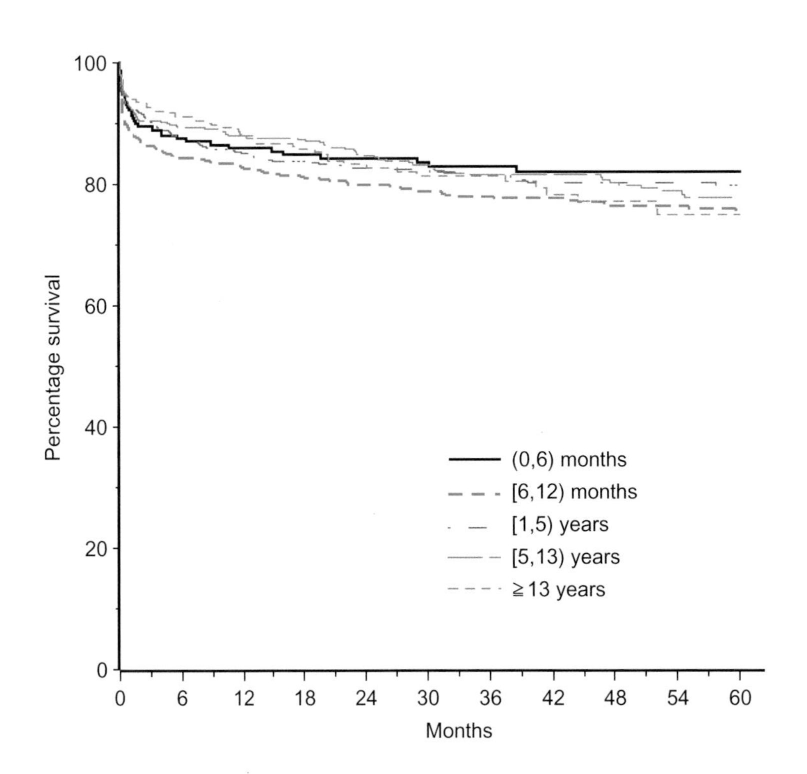

Figure 6.8 Graft survival rates for various pediatric age groups after liver transplantation by age. (From SPLIT Annual Report, with permission [unpublished].)

Pediatric heart transplantation

Overall patient survival rates after heart transplantation in children, according to the Pediatric Heart Transplant Study Group, are 85%, 75% and 64%, respectively, at 1, 5 and 10 years post-transplantation. As with organ transplants in children, outcomes of pediatric heart transplants have improved over the past decade and now are similar or better than those in adults. Graft and patient survival rates are related to recipient age. Infants have a 1-year patient survival rate of 81% compared with 91% for adolescents

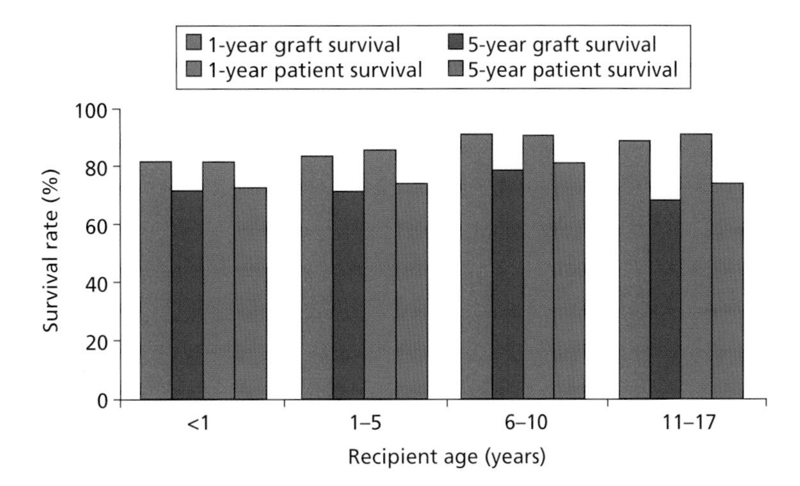

Figure 6.9 One- and five-year patient and graft survival after heart transplantation by age group cohort. Note poor long-term outcomes in adolescents. (Reprinted from Magee JC, Krishnan SM, Benfield MR, et al. Pediatric transplantation in the United States, 1997–2006. *Am J Transplant* 2008;8:935–45.)

(Figure 6.9). However, 6–10 year olds have the best 5-year survival rate – 81%. Adolescents have disappointingly low long-term graft survival rates, similar to kidney transplants. Infants tend to have lower survival rates overall, as do those who required cardiac assist devices or respirators pretransplantation. Congenital heart disease as an indication for heart transplantation was thought to be a risk factor for poor outcome, but recent data show that these children do as well as children without congenital heart disease. Nevertheless, children with previous Fontan procedures, especially those with protein-losing enteropathies, are probably at risk for post-transplant complications and worse outcomes. With increasing graft survival rates, attention has turned to long-term morbidity. Recent studies have shown progressive decline in renal function late after heart transplantation in children. There is a 10-year actuarial risk of 12% for chronic kidney disease and 4% for ESRD. Importantly, those who develop renal disease have a ninefold risk of death compared with those who do not.

Case: a second heart transplant

A 17-year-old girl received a heart transplant in 1996 because of presumed viral myocarditis. Her transplant worked well initially, but she had three acute rejection episodes in the first postoperative year. All three episodes were treated with methylprednisolone pulse therapy, and the last one was also treated with intravenous antilymphocyte globulin when the response to steroids was thought to be incomplete. After that, her surveillance biopsies did not show acute rejection, but apparently did show some "chronic changes." She was treated with cyclosporine, azathioprine, and low-dose steroids for several years. In the past 2 years, however, her cardiac echoes have shown a "stiff" heart and she was hospitalized three times for treatment of pulmonary edema. During the most recent hospitalization, her serum creatinine was noted to be 3.5 mg/dL, and a review of her chart revealed that her renal function had been deteriorating slowly over the past 5 years. A 24-hour urine collection contained 2.5 g protein. She is now developing ascites and is hospitalized for fluid control.

Pediatric lung transplantation

Survival after lung transplantation tends to be poorer than with other types of organ transplants. Figure 6.10 shows that 3-year graft survival rates for <1, 1–5, 6–10, and 11–17 year olds are 64%, 70%, 81%, and 57%, respectively. Unfortunately, graft survival continues to deteriorate subsequently and the 5-year graft survival rate for adolescents is 24%. The major cause of death immediately post-transplantation is infection, particularly pneumonia. By 1 year post-transplantation, bronchiolitis obliterans causes most graft failures. Risk factors for early graft loss include prolonged ischemia time, mechanical ventilation pre-transplantation, and early graft dysfunction. Risk factors for bronchiolitis obliterans include the incidence of acute rejection and prolonged ischemia time. Young children may be at decreased risk for

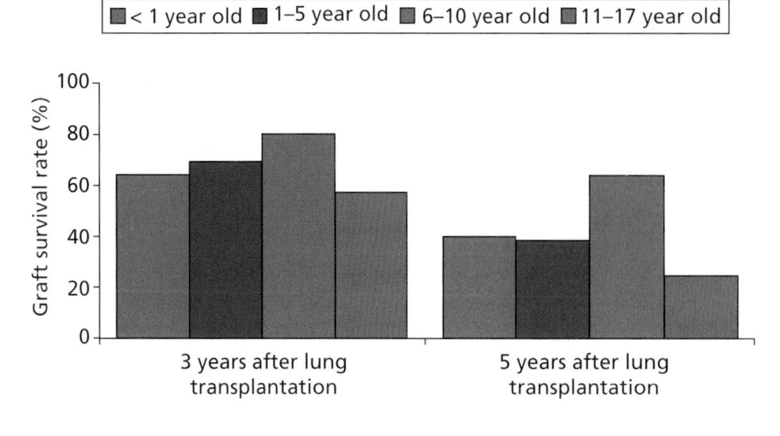

Figure 6.10 Three- and five-year lung transplant graft survival by recipient age group cohort. (Reprinted from Magee JC, Krishnan SM, Benfield MR, et al. Pediatric transplantation in the United States, 1997–2006. *Am J Transplant* 2008;8:935–45.)

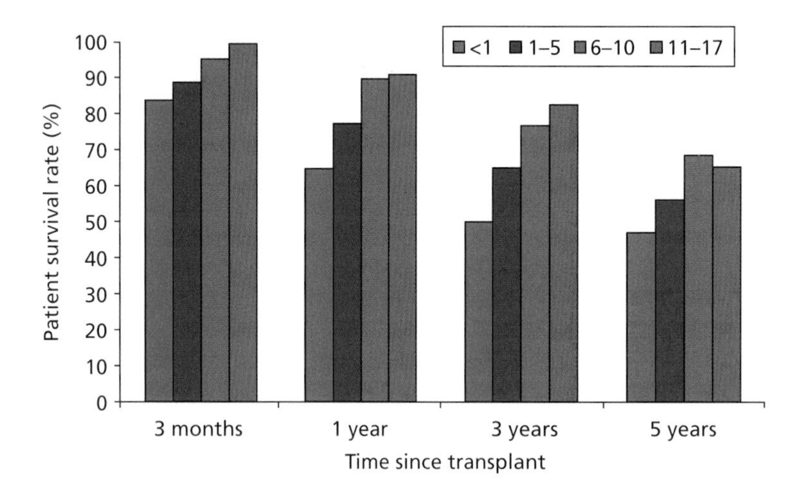

Figure 6.11 Short- and long-term patient survival after intestinal transplantation in pediatric age group cohorts. (Reprinted from Magee JC, Krishnan SM, Benfield MR, et al. Pediatric transplantation in the United States, 1997–2006. *Am J Transplant* 2008;8:935–45.)

bronchiolitis obliterans, possibly related to a lower incidence of acute rejections.

Case: cystic fibrosis

A 19-year-old girl has been followed at a pediatric hospital for her entire life because of cystic fibrosis. She has had multiple hospitalizations for pulmonary infections. During this time, her liver function has been normal, but she has developed low-level hyperglycemia, with fasting blood sugars in the 150–200 mg/dL range. Despite appropriate medications and dietary supplements, she appears to be malnourished and she currently weighs only 41 kg. Over the past year, her pulmonary function has been deteriorating more rapidly and her most recent FEV_1 is 40% less than it was last year. Although she finished her first year of college, she is now too weak to return for her sophomore year. She approaches the lung transplant program for information about lung transplantation.

Pediatric intestinal transplantation

Graft survival after intestinal transplantation tends to be poor. Five-year graft survival rates for <1, 1–5, 6–10, and 11–17 year olds are 39%, 54%, 45%, and 48%, respectively. As a result of alternative treatments, specifically TPN, patient survival is 5–25% higher at 5 years (Figure 6.11). Unlike other organ transplants, adolescents have better long-term survival. Acute rejection has been very common after intestinal transplantation, with some reports as high as 70–90%. More recent data suggest lower levels, perhaps 40–50%. Acute rejection is reported as the major cause of graft loss and the cause of about 10% of the deaths. Infections are common, probably related to the intensity of immunosuppression; CMV and EBV infection are common and have recently been modulated by the introduction of specific monitoring, prophylaxis, and immunosuppression adjustments.

Key points 6.4 Post-transplant lymphoproliferative disease (PTLD) in pediatric transplantation

Higher incidence than in adults, in part because Epstein–Barr virus mismatches (seropositive donor to seronegative recipient) are more common

Incidence varies with the transplanted organs, in descending order:
- Lung and intestinal transplants
- Liver and heart transplants
- Kidney transplants

Pediatric organ transplant complications

In general, children have the same complications and side effects of transplantation and chronic immunosuppression as adults, but two deserve special mention: PTLD and growth retardation.

PTLD is a serious complication of organ transplantation, and can be fatal, particularly if it progresses to lymphoma. PTLD is generally related to EBV infection and, although it can occur as a recurrent infection, it is much more common if the infection occurs anew during immunosuppression. For organ transplant recipients, the virus is often transmitted with the graft, especially when an organ from a seropositive donor is transplanted into a seronegative recipient. CMV infection has been associated with an increased risk of developing PTLD, as have several different types of immunosuppression. There is likely no single agent responsible for the severity of the infection, but the more intense the regimen, especially if lymphocytotoxic antibodies are used, the more likely the development of PTLD. The true incidence of disease is difficult to assess because there are substantial differences in reporting. In general, the incidence of PTLD after pediatric kidney transplantation is probably 5% or less, after liver or heart transplant 5–10% , and higher for lung and intestinal transplantation. There are indications that the incidence of PTLD might be decreasing, perhaps because of preventive measures. Some programs recommend prophylaxis with valganciclovir, perhaps to prevent concomitant CMV infection. Many programs now prospectively monitor blood by polymerase chain reaction (PCR) for EBV and adjust the immunosuppression when there is evidence of viremia.

Children with chronic organ dysfunction frequently exhibit growth retardation and developmental delays, likely related to metabolic disorders and malnutrition. This is particularly true for children with ESRD and the use of recombinant human growth hormone has been particularly useful in treating this disorder. If normal organ function can be established after transplantation and satisfactory nutrition established, satisfactory growth rates can be restored. The use of chronic corticosteroids will inhibit normal growth, however, so many programs are now avoiding or withdrawing chronic immunosuppression with steroids for this reason. If steroids must be given, alternate-day dosing has been shown to provide equivalent protection against rejection and much better growth potential. Growth hormone is not approved for use following organ transplantation and some reports have linked its use to increased rates of rejections.

Further reading

North American Pediatric Renal Trials and Collaborative Studies. *Annual Report*. Available at: www.naprtcs.org. accessed 22 September 2010.

Aurora P, Boucek MM, Christie J, et al. Registry of the International Society for Heart and Lung Transplantation: tenth official pediatric lung and heart/lung transplantation report – 2007. *J Heart Lung Transplant* 2007;**26**: 1223–8.

Bar-Dayan A, Bar-Nathan N, Shaharabani E, et al. Kidney transplantation from pediatric donors: size-match-based allocation. *Pediatr Transplant* 2008;**12**:469–73.

Bartosh SM, Ryckman FC, Shaddy R, Michaels MG, Platt JL, Sweet SC. A national conference to determine research priorities in pediatric solid organ transplantation. *Pediatr Transplant* 2008;**12**:153–66.

Benden C, Boehler A, Faro A. Pediatric lung transplantation: literature review 2006–2007. *Pediatr Transplant* 2008;**12**: 266–73.

Boucek MM, Aurora P, Edwards L, et al. Registry of the International Society for Heart and Lung Transplantation: Tenth Official Pediatric Heart Transplantation Report – 2007. *J Heart Lung Transplant* 2007;**26**:796.

Canter CE, Kirklin J, eds. *Pediatric Heart Transplant*, Vol **2**. ISHLT monograph series. Philadelphia: Elsevier, 2007.

Canter CE, Shaddy RE, Bernstein D, et al. Indications for heart transplantation in pediatric heart disease. *Circulation* 2007;**115**:658.

Chen JM, Davies RR, Mital SR, et al. Trends and outcomes in transplantation for complex congenital heart disease: 1984–2004. *Ann Thorac Surg* 2004;**78**:1352.

Ching YA, Gura K, Modi B, Jaksic T. Pediatric intestinal failure: nutrition, pharmacologic, and surgical approaches. *Nutr Clin Pract* 2007;**22**:653–63.

Dehghani SM, Derakhshan A, Taghavi SA, Gholami S, Jalaeian H, Malek-Hosseini SA. Prevalence and risk factors of renal dysfunction after liver transplant: a single-center experience. *Exp Clin Transplant* 2008;**6**:25–9.

Dharnidharka VR, Araya CE. Post-transplant lymphoproliferative disease. *Pediatr Nephrol* 2009;**24**:731–6.

Duffy JP, Farmer DG, Busuttil RW. A quarter century of liver transplantation at UCLA. *Clin Transpl* 2007:165–70.

Fine RN, Webber SA, Olthoff KM, Kelly DA, Harmon WE, eds. *Pediatric Solid Organ Transplantation.* Oxford: Blackwell, 2007.

Fine RN. Management of growth retardation in pediatric recipients of renal allografts. *Nature Clin Pract Nephrol* 2007;**3**:318–24.

Gupta J, Amaral S, Mahle WT. Renal transplantation after previous pediatric heart transplantation. *J Heart Lung Transplant* 2008;**27**:217–21.

Herlenius G, Fagerlind M, Krantz M, et al. Chronic kidney disease – a common and serious complication after intestinal transplantation. *Transplantation* 2008;**86**: 108–13.

KDIGO Clinical Practice Guideline for the Care of the Kidney Transplant Recipients. *Am J Transplant* 2009;**9** (supp 3).

Lacaille F, Vass N, Sauvat F, et al. Long-term outcome, growth and digestive function in children 2 to 18 years after intestinal transplantation. *Gut* 2008;**57**:455–61.

Mazor R, Baden HP. Trends in pediatric organ donation after cardiac death. *Pediatrics* 2007;**120**:e960–6.

Merion RM, ed. SRTR Report on the State of Transplantation. *Am J Transplant* 2008;**8**:909–1026.

Mian SI, Dutta S, Le B, Esquivel CO, Davis K, Castillo RO. Factors affecting survival to intestinal transplantation in the very young pediatric patient. *Transplantation* 2008; **85**:1287–9.

Mohanka R, Basu A, Shapiro R, Kayler LK. Single versus en bloc kidney transplantation from pediatric donors less than or equal to 15 kg. *Transplantation* 2008;**86**:264–8.

Moonnumakal SP, Fan LL. Bronchiolitis obliterans in children. *Curr Opin Pediatr* 2008;**20**:272–8.

Pironi L, Forbes A, Joly F, et al. Survival of patients identified as candidates for intestinal transplantation: a 3-year prospective follow-up. *Gastroenterology* 2008;**135**:61–71.

Puliyanda DP, Toyoda M, Traum AZ, et al. Outcome of management strategies for BK virus replication in pediatric renal transplant recipients. *Pediatr Transplant* 2008;**12**: 180–6.

Smith JM, Stablein DM, Munoz R, Hebert D, McDonald RA. Contributions of the Transplant Registry: The 2006 Annual Report of the North American Pediatric Renal Trials and Collaborative Studies (NAPRTCS). *Pediatric Transpl* 2007;**11**:366–73.

Souilamas R. Lung transplantation in cystic fibrosis pediatric population myth or reality. *J Cyst Fibros* 2008;**7**: 460.

Studies of Pediatric Liver Transplantation (SPLIT). A summary of the 2003 Annual Report. *Clin Transpl* 2003: 119–30.

Sweet SC, Aurora P, Benden C, et al. Lung transplantation and survival in children with cystic fibrosis: solid statistics – flawed interpretation. *Pediatr Transplant* 2008;**12**: 129–36.

Yashar S, Wu SS, Binder SW, Cotliar J. Acute graft-versus-host disease after pediatric solid organ transplant. *J Drugs Dermatol* 2008;**7**:467–9.

7 Kidney and pancreas transplantation

Joshua J Augustine, Kenneth A Bodziak, Aparna Padiyar, James A Schulak, and Donald E Hricik
University Hospitals Case Medical Center and Case Western Reserve University, Cleveland, Ohio, USA

In 2004, the international transplant community celebrated the fiftieth anniversary of the first successful kidney transplantation performed between identical twin brothers by Dr Joseph Murray and colleagues at the Peter Bent Brigham Hospital in Boston. Since that time, remarkable strides have been made to increase the success of kidney transplantation and to prolong the lives of patients with end-stage renal disease (ESRD). General advances in medical science, including improvements in surgical techniques and the development of effective antimicrobial agents, have undoubtedly played a role in this success story. However, the current success of kidney transplantation has been related more directly to an improved understanding of the mechanisms resulting in allograft rejection and the development of immunosuppressive drugs capable of preventing or reversing these processes. The introduction of cyclosporine in the early 1980s was associated with dramatic improvements in kidney transplant outcomes, a proliferation of transplant centers, and the serious development of extrarenal organ transplantation. The introduction of newer and more potent immunosuppressants since the mid-1990s has been associated with further improvements in traditional short-term benchmarks of success in kidney transplantation, as discussed below.

Pancreas transplantation is appropriately discussed in parallel with kidney transplantation because the diabetic patients who are candidates for this procedure almost always have chronic kidney disease (CKD) resulting from diabetic nephropathy. In the USA, most whole organ pancreas transplantations are performed as simultaneous pancreas–kidney (SPK) transplantations using organs from a common deceased donor. Pancreas after a previous kidney transplantation (PAK) is another approach. Pancreas transplantataion alone (PTA), performed before the need for kidney transplantation, is the least common modality. Islet cell transplantation is being performed increasingly but arguably remains experimental. This chapter will focus on the evaluation and selection of kidney transplant recipients and donors, their surgical and medical management, and their long-term outcomes and complications. Where appropriate, pancreas and islet cell transplantation are considered separately.

Patient and allograft outcomes

The number of patients wait-listed for a deceased donor kidney transplant has grown steadily over the past two decades. During the same time period, the number of deceased donor grafts available has grown only modestly. According to the Organ Procurement and Transplantation Network (OPTN) data 8097 deceased donor renal transplants were performed in the USA in 2006, a marginal increase from 7730 a decade ago. As discussed below, the largest proportion of the increase in deceased donors over the past few years can be attributed to the increased use of expanded criteria (ECD) and donor after cardiac

Primer on Transplantation, 3rd edition.
Edited by Donald Hricik.

death (DCD) donors. The demand for organs, with 24077 new kidney waiting list registrations in 2006 alone, far exceeds the increase in donors. For the wait-listed patient between the ages of 35 and 64 years, this shortage translated to a median wait time of 3.2 years in 2001. Since that time, it has been difficult to calculate median waiting times because of substantial regional variations in waitlist times. Eleven percent of candidates can expect to wait more than 5 years. The average age of wait-listed patients is rising, and currently over 15% of candidates on the waitlist are aged >65 years. Not surprisingly, there has been a progressive increase in the number of patients dying while waiting for a kidney transplant. White people have significantly shorter wait times (mean 1255 days) than African–American (1782 days), Hispanic, (1617 days) or Asian individuals (1787 days). The longest wait times are for patients with blood types B and O (1967 and 1764 days, respectively), with shorter wait times for patients with blood type A (1084 days) or AB (596 days). The number of living donor transplants performed in the USA rose from 3886 in 1996 to 4905 in 2006. Since 2001 the number of living donors has exceeded the number of deceased donors (Figure 7.1), though the rate of increase in living donors has actually decreased in recent years.

It is now well recognized that kidney transplantation offers a survival advantage and improved quality of life for eligible patients with ESRD when compared with dialysis-based renal replacement therapy. Compared with wait-listed patients who are maintained on dialysis, projected years of life are greater with transplantation, irrespective of age and the presence or absence of diabetes mellitus (Table 7.1). As discussed below, this survival advantage holds true even for recipients of kidneys from marginal or expanded criteria donors (ECDs). The traditional short-term benchmarks of success in kidney transplantation, i.e., 1-year allograft survival rate and the incidence of acute rejection in the first year post-transplantation, have improved steadily over the past five decades (Figure 7.2). As noted above, the most significant breakpoints occurred in association with the development of cyclosporine in the early 1980s and with the introduction of tacrolimus and mycophenolate mofetil (MMF) in the mid-1990s. Currently, irrespective of donor source, most transplant centers achieve 1-year graft survival rates of >90% and a 1-year incidence of acute rejection of <20%. As discussed below, recipients of living donor renal allografts experience both short- and long-term outcomes that are superior to those of patients who received deceased donor grafts.

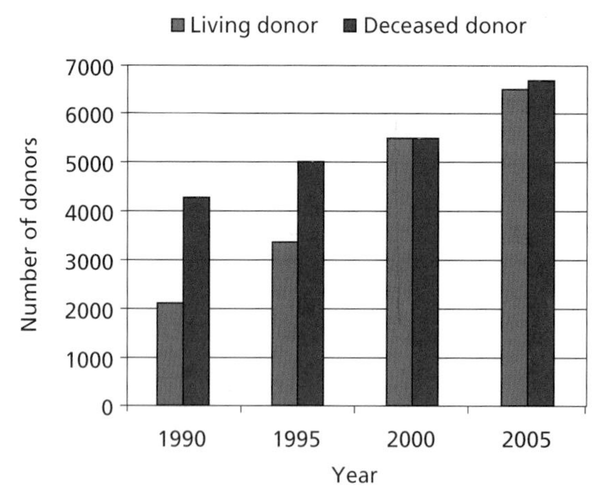

Figure 7.1 Numbers of living and deceased donors in the USA from 1990 TO 2005. (From www.OPTN.org.)

Table 7.1 Projected years of life based on retrospective analysis of patients receiving deceased donor kidney transplants versus waitlisted patients

Age and diabetic status	Projected years of life	
	With a kidney transplant (n = 46164)	Without a transplant (n = 23275)
20–39 years, no diabetes	31	20
20–39 years with diabetes	25	8
40–59 years, no diabetes	19	12
40–59 years with diabetes	22	8
60–74 years, no diabetes	12	7
60–74 years with diabetes	8	5

Adapted from Wolfe RA Ashby VB, Milford EL, et al. Comparison of mortality in all patients on dialysis, patients on dialysis awaiting transplantation, and recipients of a first cadaveric transplant. *N Engl J Med* 1999;**341**:1725–30.

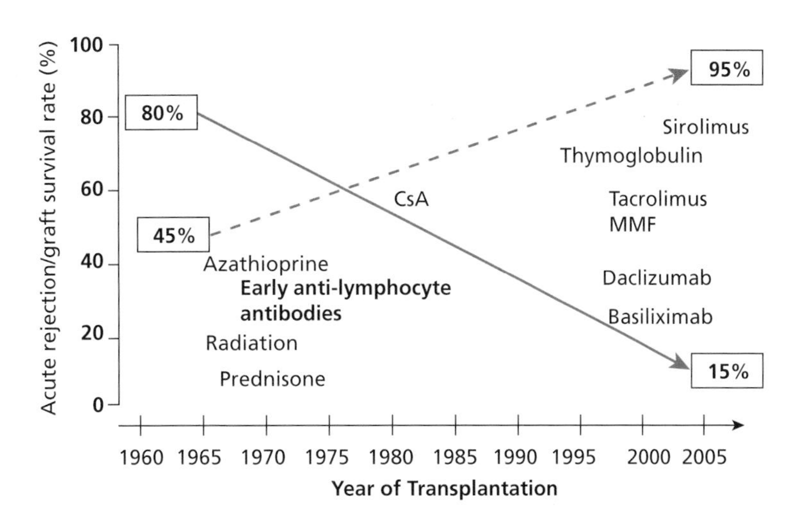

Figure 7.2 Changes in 1-year graft survival rates (dashed line) and in the incidence of acute rejection during the first transplant year (solid line) in deceased donor kidney transplant recipients during the past 50 years. CsA, cyclosporine; MMF, mycophenolate mofetil.

Improvements in the short-term outcomes of kidney transplant recipients have not been paralleled by robust improvements in long-term outcomes. There are a number of potential explanations for this disparity. The most common causes of long-term graft loss are "chronic allograft nephropathy" and death with a functioning graft. Immunosuppressive medications are expensive and non-compliance with medications based on inability to pay for the drugs tends to increase with time after transplantation. Although the calcineurin inhibitors (cyclosporine and tacrolimus) have served as the cornerstones for modern immunosuppression protocols, their nephrotoxic effects probably contribute to long-term allograft loss in a substantial minority of kidney transplant recipients and certainly do so in recipients of extrarenal organs. The epidemic of BK polyoma nephropathy was not anticipated 20 years ago and certainly has contributed to poor long-term outcomes after kidney transplantation in some patients. Although acute rejection is not common in the modern era, there is evidence to suggest that even a single episode of acute rejection has an even greater impact on long-term graft survival than was true in an earlier era. The importance of high titers of pre-existing anti-donor antibodies as a risk factor for hyperacute rejection has long been recognized. However, it has only recently been recognized that low titers of such antibodies detected either before or new after transplantation may contribute to allograft rejection even many years after transplantation. Finally, it is also possible that death with a functioning graft is related directly to the toxicities of the very immunosuppressants that have yielded such impressive short-term outcomes. The available maintenance drugs variably contribute to the risks of cardiovascular disease, infection, and malignancy – the main causes of late mortality in transplant recipients.

Key points 7.1 Common causes of late mortality after kidney transplantation

Cardiovascular disease

Infection

Malignancy

A discrepancy between supply and demand has also characterized pancreas transplantation in the past decade. The number of pancreata recovered increased by 53% between 1997 and 2006. However, the number of people waiting for pancreas transplants during that time period doubled to approximately 4000 during the same time period, resulting in increased waiting times for all types of pancreas candidates. The median waiting time for a PAK transplant increased from about 220 days in the late 1990s to 562 days in 2004. The median waiting time for an SPK rose from 380 days in 1997 to 451 days in 2005.

On the other hand, there have been recent downward trends in the number of SPK, PAK, and total pancreas transplant registrations. The total number of new pancreas waiting list registrations grew from 1740 in 1997 to a high of 2796 in 2000, and then fell to 2548 in 2006. Only PTA registrations showed a consistent increase from 1997 to 2006, growing from 187 to 404.

The most recent data from the Scientific Registry for Transplant Recipients (SRTR) indicates that patient survival rates are similar for PAK, SPK, and PTA recipients at 1 year (ranging from 95% to 97%), 3 years (ranging from 91% to 92%), and 5 years (ranging from 84% to 88%). However, the 10-year patient survival rate was lowest for PAK recipients at 64%, and similar for SPK and PTA recipients, with rates of 70% and 71%, respectively. Among pancreas recipients, those with SPK transplants experienced the best pancreas graft survival rates (86% at 1 year and 54% at 10 years). Pancreas graft survival rates for PAK and PTA recipients were similar to each other, with 1-year rates of 79% and 80%, respectively, and 10-year rates of 29% and 27%, respectively (Figure 7.3). Both registry analyses and single center experiences suggest that patient survival for SPK recipients is superior to that of patients with type 1 diabetes receiving deceased donor kidneys alone and possibly superior to that of patients with diabetes receiving HLA-mismatched living donor kidneys. However, in the absence of randomized trials, such analyses should be viewed with caution because of likely bias in the selection of healthier candidates for the combined transplants. As a result of early technical complications including thrombosis of the pancreas (in 5–10% of cases), 1-year pancreas graft survival is lower than 1-year kidney graft survival in SPK recipients. However, some studies suggest that, in SPK recipients in whom both organs are functioning at 1 year, the subsequent half-life of the pancreas allografts exceeds the half-life of the renal allografts. In SPK recipients, the incidence of acute rejection in the renal allograft is higher than that observed in comparable patients receiving kidney transplants alone. This is an intriguing observation that differs from the experience with other combined organ transplants (e.g., liver–kidney, heart–kidney) in which the non-renal organ appears to exert an immunoprotective effect manifested by relatively low rates of renal allograft rejection.

The major proven benefits of a technically successful pancreas transplantation are insulin independence and normal or near-normal control of blood glucose concentrations. Whether a pancreas transplantation prevents or retards the progression of microvascular complications of diabetes mellitus has been more difficult to prove, in part because many patients receive their pancreas allografts when these complications are already far advanced. Evidence suggesting improvements in diabetic retinopathy, enteropathy, or peripheral and autonomic neuropathy after pancreas transplantation is mixed at best, and there is little evidence for improvement in macrovascular disease. Nevertheless, anecdotal reports of improvements in all of these complications, together with the observation that glycemic control generally retards the development of diabetic complications in the general population, underscore the need for additional long-term studies and continue to provide motivation for whole organ pancreas transplantation among both patients and transplant professionals.

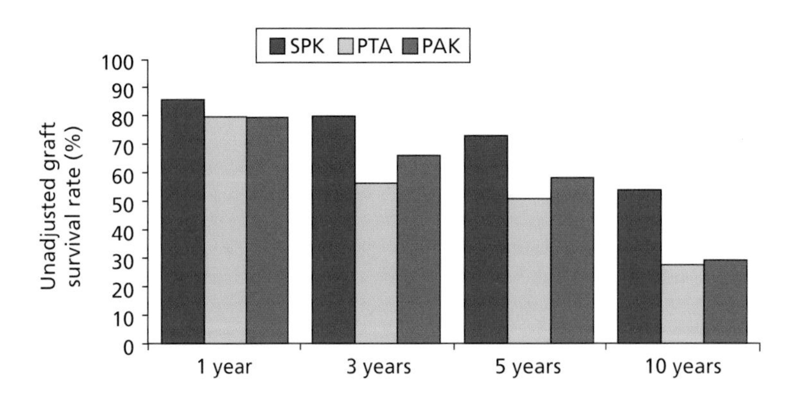

Figure 7.3 Pancreas graft survival by transplant type. SPK, simultaneous pancreas and kidney; PTA, pancreas transplant alone; PAK, pancreas after kidney transplantation. (From www.OPTN.org.)

Key points 7.2 Important facts regarding simultaneous pancreas kidney transplantation (SPK)

Most pancreas transplants are performed simultaneously with a kidney transplant from the same deceased donor

After SPK transplantation, short-term pancreas graft survival is lower than kidney transplant survival owing to early technical problems including thrombosis

Acute renal allograft rejection occurs more commonly after SPK transplantation than in diabetic patients receiving a kidney transplant alone

Non-randomized studies suggest that patient survival after SPK transplantation is superior to that of diabetic patients receiving a kidney transplant alone

Key points 7.3 Timing of kidney transplantation

Listing for deceased donor transplantation generally allowed only when glomerular filtration is <=20 mL/min

Long-term graft survival is optimized in patients who are transplanted pre-emptively (before the need for dialysis)

Pre-emptive transplantation for asymptomatic patients is generally performed when the glomerular filtration rate is <15 mL/min but can be performed with higher levels in patients with symptomatic uremia

Recipient selection and evaluation

Evaluation of kidney transplant recipients

In view of the survival advantage offered by kidney transplantation, all patients with advanced CKD should be considered as potential transplant recipients until deemed not suitable, or unless a pre-existing absolute contraindication is identified, as discussed below. In fact, referral of the patient for evaluation should be considered in advance of starting dialysis, because several studies have suggested a decreased risk for graft failure and death when transplantation is performed *pre-emptively*. Patients are generally not listed for deceased donor transplantation until the glomerular filtration rate (GFR) has fallen to <=20 mL/min. When pre-emptive transplantation is possible (most often in the setting of living donor transplantation), transplantation is generally performed when the GFR is <15 mL/min unless the patient is symptomatically uremic with higher values. Whenever possible, evaluation of the potential kidney transplant recipient should begin before the GFR falls to a level mandating initiation of dialysis.

Medical evaluation

Evaluation starts with a detailed medical history and physical examination. Standard laboratory testing varies from one center to another but generally includes ABO blood typing, a complete blood count, comprehensive metabolic panel, coagulation screen, and urinalysis. Additional studies include an EKG, chest radiograph, colonoscopy for patients aged >50 years, pap smears for women of reproductive age, mammography in women aged >40 years, a PPD (purified protein derivative) skin test, prostate-specific antigen for men aged >50 years, a urine drug screen, and serologic studies to determine prior exposure to human immunodeficiency virus (HIV), hepatitis B and C, cytomegalovirus (CMV), Epstein–Barr virus (EBV), varicella-zoster, and syphilis. Further evaluation is determined on a case-by-case basis and may include urodynamic evaluation, cystoscopy, and non-invasive imaging of the aortofemoral vasculature. These latter studies are protocol driven in some centers, or may be precipitated by findings elicited from the history or physical examination in others. At any step during the process, an absolute or relative contraindication may be identified and result in either a delay in listing the patient, or declaration that the patient is permanently ineligible for transplantation.

Contraindications to transplantation

Absolute contraindications to kidney transplantation are listed in Table 7.2 and generally include conditions that represent an ongoing threat to life, or conditions that are associated with high short-term mortality rates. There are many relative contraindications discussed below.

Cardiovascular disease Cardiovascular disease is the major cause of death among dialysis patients, and remains the major cause of mortality after transplantation, albeit at a much lower incidence. Risk factors for cardiovascular disease among patients with ESRD include increased age, hypertension, diabetes mellitus, dyslipidemia, smoking history, family history of premature cardiovascular disease, and prolonged

Table 7.2 Absolute contraindications to kidney transplantation

Chronic medical disease with life expectancy <2 years:
severe cardiomyopathy or irremediable ischemic heart disease
severe chronic obstructive pulmonary disease
hepatic cirrhosis
diffuse, pronounced vascular disease
Active malignancy, other than basal cell skin cancer
Active sepsis or other life-threatening infectious disease
Active substance abuse
Active peptic ulcer disease
Psychiatric illness impeding upon patient's compliance

duration of dialysis (>2 years). Pretransplantation evaluation for cardiovascular disease has become a subject of increasing controversy. Nuclear and echocardiographic stress testing predict myocardial infarction and cardiac death after transplantation, particularly in patients with diabetes. However, the sensitivity of non-invasive testing may be reduced in the ESRD population, and some have advocated cardiac angiography in higher-risk transplant candidates. That being said, there is little evidence supporting the benefit of intervention in otherwise asymptomatic patients in the absence of left main coronary artery disease, at least in the general population. In the Coronary Artery Revascularization Prophylaxis trial, 510 patients undergoing major vascular surgery were randomized to revascularization versus medical management. No survival benefit was demonstrated in either group, prompting guidelines from the American College of Physicians against revascularization in asymptomatic patients before non-cardiac surgery. For transplant candidates, preoperative cardiac stenting can be particularly problematic when antiplatelet agents such as clopidogrel are required for an extensive period, increasing the risk of bleeding or delaying transplant surgery. With these caveats in mind, most centers continue to perform screening studies in patients deemed to be at high risk based on age >50 years, presence of diabetes mellitus, or multiple conventional risk factors. Screening of such patients consists minimally of an EKG, echocardiogram, and a stress test with myocardial perfusion imaging. Coronary angiography should be considered when stress tests are positive or in any patient with symptomatic heart disease. Revascularization is generally recommended before transplantation in patients with critical coronary lesions. Inoperable coronary disease and/or advanced heart failure is a contraindication to transplantation.

As there is an increased prevalence of carotid artery disease among patients with ESRD, duplex imaging of the carotids should be considered in patients with asymptomatic carotid bruits and in those with a prior history of stroke or transient ischemic attack. Patients with adult polycystic kidney disease have an increased incidence of cerebral aneurysms. Screening with magnetic resonance (MR) angiography should be considered for such patients if they have a family history of cerebral aneurysms or unexplained stroke, or if they suffer from unexplained headaches.

Peripheral vascular disease occurs in 2.0–3.2% of renal transplant candidates. Traditional risk factors include diabetes mellitus, cigarette smoking, hypertension, dyslipidemia, older age, and male gender. For patients who manifest either clinical symptoms or physical findings consistent with aortoiliac disease, angiography and surgical intervention may be required before proceeding with transplantation.

Malignancy Immunosuppression may promote growth of existing malignant cells, so that all potential kidney transplant recipients should be screened for common cancers. In a review of more than 900 renal transplant recipients from the pre-cyclosporine era, Penn noted a 53% recurrence rate for all tumors when patients were transplanted within 0–24 months following their cancer treatment course, a 34% rate of recurrence when treatment finished 25–60 months before transplantation, and a 13% rate when treatment was completed >60 months pretransplantation. These observations led to the general concept that pre-existing cancer mandates treatment, complete remission, and a period of waiting before proceeding with transplantation. However, the recommended period of waiting varies depending on the type of tumor, its size, and the presence or absence of metastases before achievement of remission. No waiting may be necessary when a tumor is small and completely resected surgically (e.g., some renal cell or prostate cancers). For most solid tumors, a waiting period of 3–5 years is generally recommended.

Infection Active infection should be viewed as a contraindication to transplantation until the infection has been adequately treated. Transplantation of HIV-positive patients was not considered before the introduction of highly active anti-retroviral therapy (HAART). With the advent of HAART, acceptable graft and patient survival rates are now being achieved among selected patients. In the USA, transplantation of HIV-positive patients has been aided by an ongoing collaborative multicenter study sponsored by the National Institute of Allergy and Infectious Disease. Hepatitis C infection is common among hemodialysis patients with a reported prevalence 7.8% in the USA in 2002. As routine liver function tests are normal in most hepatitis C virus (HCV)-positive dialysis patients, many transplant centers recommend a liver biopsy before kidney transplantation in order to rule out chronic active hepatitis or cirrhosis. Antiviral therapy with interferon and/or ribavirin may be tried in an attempt to eradicate the virus before transplantation. Overall, HCV-positive transplant recipients enjoy better long-term survival rates than their dialysis counterparts, so that, in the absence of severe hepatitis or cirrhosis, a positive test for hepatitis C in itself is not a contraindication to transplantation. Patients testing positive for hepatitis B surface antigen (HBsAg) should undergo additional evaluation including tests for evidence of active viral replication and possibly a liver biopsy to rule out chronic active hepatitis. If either is present, kidney transplantation is contraindicated because of an increased risk of death from liver failure with initiation of immunosuppression. In the absence of evidence for active viral replication, the HBsAg-positive patient may proceed with transplantation, although liver function tests should be monitored regularly thereafter.

Patients with negative serologic tests for CMV or EBV should be informed of the potential risk for acquiring these viruses from seropositive donors. Varicella immunization should be performed before transplantation in patients who are seronegative for this virus. Patients with a positive PPD skin test and a normal chest radiograph are generally treated with isoniazid, although the timing of treatment (i.e. pre- or post-transplant) varies and depends on the likelihood and expected timing of transplantation.

Case

A 53-year-old man with ESRD from hypertension is being evaluated as a potential kidney transplant recipient. His pretransplant evaluation is unremarkable except for a past history of intravenous drug abuse that was discontinued 12 years ago. In addition, serologic studies indicated the presence of hepatitis C antibody. Polymerase chain reaction (PCR) studies confirm a positive, albeit low, viral load. A liver biopsy is performed and shows mild hepatitis without evidence for chronic active hepatitis or cirrhosis. Liver ultrasonography shows no evidence of hepatocellular carcinoma. The man is advised that his risk for severe liver disease after kidney transplantation will not be appreciably different than expected if he remains on dialysis. The patient opts to proceed with transplantation and is added to the center's waiting list.

Other relative contraindications As discussed in Chapter 5, the influence of obesity on post-transplant outcomes remains controversial, but most studies suggest an adverse effect on death-censored graft survival. In addition, obesity increases the risk of perioperative complications, including impaired wound healing and wound infection. The upper threshold of acceptable body mass index (BMI) varies from 35 kg/m^2 to 40 kg/m^2 across centers, and patients above those thresholds are encouraged to lose weight before proceeding with transplantation. Most centers have abandoned upper age limits for kidney transplantation and individualize decisions about transplantation of patients aged >65 years based on their overall health status. Use of tobacco products is, of course, frowned upon, but centers differ in opinions about smoking as a contraindication to kidney transplantation. Although smoking is considered an absolute contraindication in some centers, others consider smoking a contraindication only in patients with proven vascular disease.

A number of renal diseases are known to recur in transplanted kidneys (Table 7.3). The risk of recurrence should always be discussed with the potential recipient. However, the possibility of recurrent disease should only rarely preclude kidney transplantation. Exceptions to this rule include primary oxalosis for which prior or simultaneous liver transplantation may be required to prevent recurrence, and focal and segmental glomerulosclerosis in a patient who has lost a previous allograft from recurrence of this

Table 7.3 Approximate risk of recurrent disease after kidney transplantation

Recurrent disease	Risk (%)
Primary oxalosis	80–100
Membranoproliferative glomerulonephritis type 2 (dense deposit disease)	80–100
Diabetic nephropathy	80–100
Idiopathic hemolytic–uremic syndrome	50–75
IgA nephropathy	40–50
Focal and segmental glomerulosclerosis	30–50
Membranoproliferative glomerulonephritis type 1	30–50
Membranous nephropathy	10–30
Wegener's granulomatosis	20
Systemic lupus erythematosus	10
Fabry's disease	5

disease. For certain systemic immune disorders associated with ESRD (e.g., systemic lupus erythematosus, Goodpasture's disease, or Wegener's granulomatosis), it is generally agreed that recurrence in the transplanted kidney can be minimized by postponing transplantation until the systemic disease is in remission. It is less clear whether the risk of recurrence is higher when transplantation is performed in the face of persistent serologic activity (e.g., positive anti-DNA antibodies in lupus or positive anti-neutrophil cytoplasmic antibodies in Wegener's granulomatosis) in patients with clinically quiescent disease.

Wait-list management

The imbalance between supply and demand for kidney allografts has resulted in growth in the size of the waiting list, longer waiting times, and increased death rates among wait-listed patients. Particularly because prolonged exposure to dialysis is associated with a number of morbidities, most transplant centers have developed protocols for re-evaluation of wait-listed candidates on at least an annual basis. The protocol varies between centers but usually includes an interim medical history, and an update on viral serologies and cancer screening. Many centers repeat cardiovascular screening for high-risk patients on an annual basis. Patients with new, reversible contraindications to transplantation should be placed on "status 7" or "hold" status until the problem is rectified. Those with irreversible contraindications should be removed from the list.

Evaluation of pancreas transplant recipients

Patients referred for pancreas transplantation should fulfill the general eligibility criteria for kidney transplantation. However, many centers impose stricter limits on age (often excluding patients aged >55 years) and BMI (excluding patients with BMI >30 kg/m^2). Most centers perform pancreas transplantation only on patients with type 1 diabetes mellitus, defined by undetectable blood C-peptide levels. However, a number of studies have shown that pancreas transplantation can be successful in selected patients with type 2 diabetes mellitus, so that the presence of type 2 diabetes is no longer considered an absolute contraindication at some centers. As patients with diabetes, potential pancreas recipients are considered to be at high risk for cardiovascular disease so that, irrespective of age, most centers aggressively perform cardiovascular screening at the time of the initial evaluation and at least annually for waitlisted patients. For PAK or PTA candidates, renal function should be stable (GFR >40 mL/min for PAK on calcineurin inhibitor, >60 mL/min for PTA). Otherwise, an SPK should be considered.

Donor selection and evaluation

Deceased kidney donation

Donor factors affecting outcome

The outcomes of deceased donor allografts are influenced by the quality and function of the graft at the time of harvest. The age of the deceased donor has a significant impact on long-term graft survival. The 5-year graft survival rate is 72% when the deceased donor is aged between 18 and 34 years, and 61% when between 50 and 64 years. Prolonged cold ischemia time and HLA mismatching have a relatively smaller impact. The difference in graft survival between zero-mismatched kidneys and 6-antigen-mismatched kidneys is only 10% at 5 years post-transplantation. Similarly, graft survival in transplants with a cold ischemia time of <11 h versus those with a cold ischemia time of 32–41 h differs by only 6%. Through the use of variables including age, cold ischemia time, donor race, cause of death, history of hypertension or diabetes, and HLA match, computer models can provide relatively precise projections of graft half-life.

Organ evaluation and procurement

Once accepted to a waiting list, patients in the USA are registered with the United Network for Organ Sharing (UNOS), where a centralized computer network links all organ procurement organizations (OPOs) and transplant centers. OPOs are non-profit, federally funded organizations that are assigned to distinct geographic areas within the USA. They provide an integral link between donor and recipient, and are responsible for the retrieval, transportation, and preservation of organs nationwide. Inclusion and exclusion criteria for deceased donation, as well as medical evaluation and management of the deceased donor, are discussed in detail in Chapter 3. As noted in that chapter, infection with HIV is an absolute contraindication to deceased donation. In addition, the Center for Disease Control has generated criteria for behavior considered to represent a high risk for transmission of HIV, irrespective of the results of HIV testing (Table 7.4). Organs should not be accepted from donors meeting these criteria unless the transplant center deems that the benefits of transplantation outweigh the small risk of transmitting HIV. Under those circumstances, the center is obliged to notify the potential recipient about the high risk behavior.

In addition to providing help in obtaining consent, OPOs are responsible for obtaining the donor medical history, blood type, tissue type, size of the organ, and distance between donor and recipient. All of these factors are entered into a national database. A list of potential recipients is generated, ranked based on blood and tissue match and distance from the recipient. The computer will search nationally for a recipient who matches the donor at all identified HLA loci. Historically, almost 15% of transplanted kidneys have been allocated on the basis of a "perfect" match or zero mismatches. However, recent changes in UNOS bylaws now limit exportation of zero-mismatched kidneys to highly sensitized patients. With that exception, the kidney is usually allocated to a patient in the local area of the OPO according to an algorithm that takes into account waiting time, HLA-DR matching, panel reactive antibody (PRA) status, pediatric status, and geographic factors using the UNOS "points" system. It is important to note that, over the years, UNOS has modified the number of points assigned to each of these variables in an effort to improve the equity of allocation. Ethnicity, gender, religion, and financial status currently are not part of the point system. The transplant center caring for the top-ranked patient determines if the organ is suitable. If not, the next listed individual's transplant center is contacted, and so on.

Table 7.4 Center for Disease Control guidelines for high-risk behavior that must be considered in all potential kidney transplant donors

1. Men who have had sex with other men in the preceding 5 years
2. People who report non-medical intravenous, intramuscular, or subcutaneous injection of drugs during the preceding 5 years
3. People with hemophilia or related clotting disorders who have received human derived clotting factor concentrates
4. Men and women who have engaged in sex in exchange for money or drugs in the preceding 5 years
5. People who had had sex in the previous 12 months with any person described in items 1–4 above or with a person known or suspected to have HIV infection
6. Persons who have been exposed in the preceding 12 months to known or suspected HIV-infected blood through percutaneous inoculation or through contact with an open wound, non-intact skin, or mucous membranes
7. Inmates of correctional systems

Special considerations for pancreas donors

Most of the inclusion and exclusion criteria applying to potential donors for kidney transplantation are relevant to pancreas transplantation as well. However, donors with a history of diabetes mellitus are generally excluded. Elevations of pancreatic enzymes occur commonly in the hemodynamically unstable donor, may reflect ischemic injury to the organ, and often preclude acceptance of the pancreas for transplantation. Finally, transplant surgeons generally prefer younger, non-obese individuals for pancreas donation, so that potential donors aged >55 years and those with BMIs >35 kg/m^2 are often excluded. In some cases, a preliminarily accepted pancreas may be rejected during the harvesting procedure when visual inspection of the pancreas reveals evidence of fat necrosis or other injury.

New trends in deceased donor transplantation

Expanded criteria donors The ECD program was specifically developed to increase the pool of deceased donors, taking advantage of kidneys that previously were discarded. ECD kidneys are defined by donor characteristics associated with a 70% greater risk of kidney graft failure, at any point in time following transplantation, when compared with a reference group of "standard criteria" donors (SCDs) (Table 7.5). In the first 18 months after implementation of the ECD kidney allocation policy, there was an 18% increase in ECD kidney recovery and a 15% increase in ECD kidney transplantations. The ECD donor population currently constitutes about 20% of the donor pool. Inpatient costs are about 10% greater for ECD compared with SCD recipients, largely reflecting higher rates of delayed graft function and the accompanying need for dialysis and extended length of hospital stay.

Wait-listed patients must provide informed consent before consideration for an ECD kidney. Patients should understand that consenting for an ECD kidney does not influence waiting time for an SCD kidney. However, the increasing age of the donor population makes ECD kidneys more likely to be available. Thus, the main reason to consider ECD grafts is to decrease waiting time for transplantation. This may be particularly appealing for patients with shortened life expectancies on dialysis (e.g., patients with diabetes, older patients) or for any patient anticipating extended waiting times for standard kidneys (e.g., highly sensitized patients). An ECD kidney that is thought to be non-transplantable as a single allograft may provide sufficient renal function when both donor kidneys are transplanted together into one recipient. Almost always, dual transplants of this kind involve elderly donors and recipients. Reported outcomes have been at least equivalent to those of single ECD kidneys.

Table 7.5 Defining characteristics of expanded criteria donors for deceased donor kidney transplantation

Age >60 years
or
Age >50 with at least two of the following 3:
History of hypertension
Cerebrovascular accident as the cause of death
Terminal serum creatinine concentration >1.5 mg/dL

Donation after cardiac death Transplantation of kidneys from non-heart-beating donors (i.e., DCDs) has increased markedly over the last decade. A comparison of all DCD to brain-dead donor kidney transplants in the USA between January 1993 and June 2000 found elevated rates of delayed graft function after DCD transplantation, but equivalent graft and patient survival rates at 1, 6, and 10 years. Currently in the USA, fewer then half of OPOs perform the majority of DCD kidney transplantations. Many centers remain reluctant to transplant DCD kidneys for a variety of reasons. However, UNOS recently mandated that all OPOs develop protocols for harvesting organs from DCDs. It has been estimated that increasing the utilization of DCD grafts represents an opportunity to increase the supply of kidneys, by as much as 25%.

Allocation according to net survival benefit Although there have been trends toward older recipients receiving older organs, the current allocation system does not mandate who should receive a given organ based on its quality. There is concern that significant graft years may be lost by transplantation of younger donor kidneys into older recipients with potentially shorter lifespans. Such concern has led to the idea of a utility-based "net lifetime survival benefit" allocation system, similar to that seen for lung and heart transplants. In proposed models, the incremental survival benefit (i.e., the difference between estimated transplant lifespan with a given kidney minus predicted waiting list lifespan without a transplant) is determined from statistical modeling of donor and recipient factors. The model assumes that transplantation increases the overall life expectancy compared with remaining on the waiting list for most candidates. New allocation policies based on net survival benefit are currently being scrutinized by UNOS.

Living kidney donation

Donor trends

The number of living donor kidney transplants has increased over time, and in the USA the number of live donor transplants surpassed that of deceased donors for the first time in the year 2000, when over 5000 transplantations from each donor source were performed. However, since 2005 this trend has reversed. As the waiting list has grown, an increased demand for donor kidneys has fueled an increase in living donation. Short- and long-term outcomes in kidney transplantation have been consistently superior with living versus deceased donors (Figure 7.4), further increasing the demand for living kidney donation. In addition to the obvious advantage of avoiding long wait-list times, recipients of living donor transplants have longer graft half-lives and patient survival than recipients of deceased donor grafts. One-year and 5-year graft survival rates for living versus deceased donor grafts is 95% versus 89%, and 80% versus 67%, respectively. Patient survival rates at 1 and 5 years for living donor recipients is 98% and 90%. By comparison, for deceased donor recipients, 1- and 5-year patient survival rates are 95% and 82%, respectively. Living donors must go through a rigorous evaluation program to ascertain their eligibility for donation, and tend to be healthier than age-matched individuals in the general population. Also, living donor allografts avoid the cold ischemia time and subsequent ischemia–reperfusion injury typical of deceased donor transplantation. In contrast, most deceased donors have comorbid conditions around the time of death.

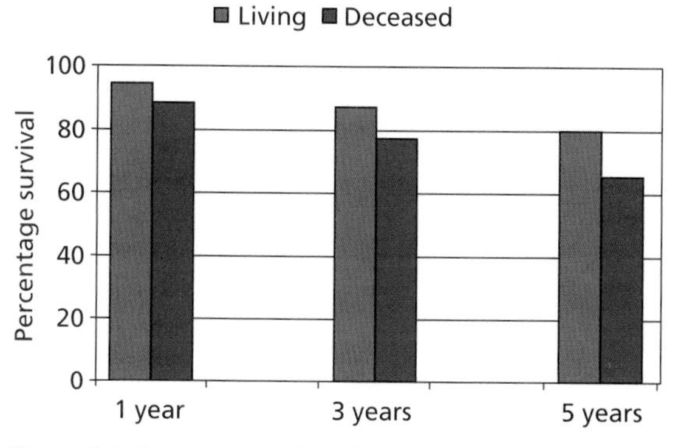

Figure 7.4 Comparison of graft survival rates in living versus deceased donor kidney transplant recipients from 1997 to 2004. (From www.OPTN.org.)

Laparoscopic donor nephrectomy has become a standard of practice for live donor nephrectomy at most centers, and decreased morbidity associated with the laparoscopic technique has also contributed to the increase in living donor transplants. The laparoscopic approach has been associated with less post-operative pain, less blood loss, quicker convalescence, and quicker return to work compared with open nephrectomy. Laparoscopic nephrectomy is a longer, more technically challenging procedure, and for this reason concern has been raised that the donor kidney may be at risk for more ischemic injury before implantation. However, long-term renal function in recipients appears to be comparable when the laparoscopic and open donor techniques have been compared.

The number of unrelated living donor transplants has also increased in the past 20 years and represents the greatest percentage increase among donor types. In the 1980s to 1990s, less then 10% of living donor kidneys came from unrelated donors and, at that time, were primarily from recipient spouses. Recently, unrelated donors have more commonly included friends, workmates, members of places of worship, and even strangers. In the era of modern immunosuppressive therapy, living unrelated donor kidneys have had a survival rate similar to that of living related kidneys, and allograft survival with unrelated donors remains superior to that with deceased donors.

Occasionally, transplant centers will receive requests from those who want to donate a kidney anonymously, with no specific target recipient. A series of ethical considerations and practice guidelines for so-called non-directed donation has been published. Most experts agree that non-directed donors should not be solicited but may be considered for donation after initiating contact with a transplant center. Most also agree that centers should choose a recipient in a similar manner to a deceased donor recipient, through the UNOS points system. Additional attention may be given to matching of donor and recipient age and body size, while avoiding any medically irrelevant biases that may exist from the donor or the transplant center itself.

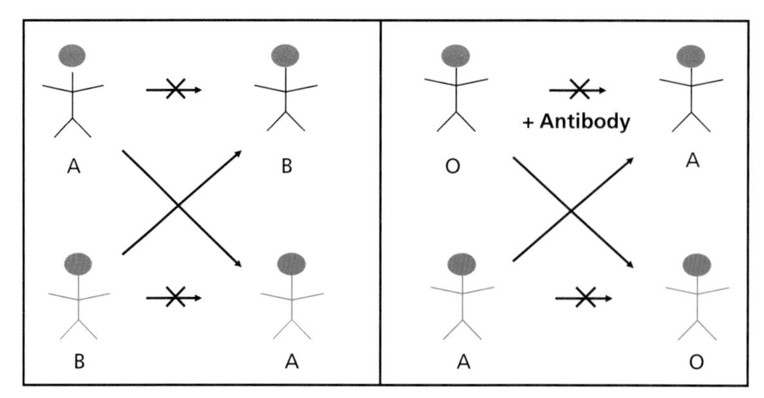

Figure 7.5 Examples of the potential utility of a paired donor exchange program. In the left panel, two ABO-incompatible donor recipient pairs exchange to facilitate two ABO-compatible transplants. In the right panel, transplantation is precluded in the upper pair by a positive cross-match and in the lower pair by ABO incompatibility. If the recipient in the upper panel has a negative cross-match to the donor in the lower panel, exchange between the couples facilitates two successful kidney transplants.

Many potential non-directed donors do not pursue further work-up after initial contact with transplant centers, particularly after learning about the extent of the donor work-up required. However, if such prospective donors do continue to request evaluation, psychological evaluation is a key component of the work-up. A significant percentage of such donors have been found to be unsuitable, not only on physical grounds, but also on psychological or motivational grounds. Centers must be wary of a desire from such donors to relieve a psychological burden or to look for secondary gain either from the media or through a relationship with the recipient or others. Ultimately, only a small percentage of applicants progress to non-directed donation, and donors who are deemed suitable typically exhibit a rational desire to improve the well-being of others and have a pre-existing pattern of benevolent and charitable behavior.

Non-directed donation may also be used to benefit a loved one or friend through a policy of donor exchange. A live-donor exchange involves a living donor–recipient pair who are incompatible due to either blood-type mismatch or a positive antibody cross-match. The donor agrees to donate to a second compatible recipient in exchange for a donation from a second donor to the primary recipient. Recipients with type O blood may be disadvantaged by this system because donors with type O typically donate regardless of recipient blood type. Therefore recipients with type O who participate in a living donor exchange must rely on a type O donor who elicits a positive cross-match in the primary recipient (Figure 7.5). One-year patient and graft survival rates were excellent in a recent series of living donor or exchange recipients that included patients who were highly sensitized.

Some UNOS regions have also developed a live-donor/deceased donor exchange program. In such a system, an incompatible living donor agrees to donate to a transplant candidate on the waiting list. Selection is based on points akin to selection of a deceased-donor recipient. In exchange, the incompatible recipient becomes a candidate for the next ABO-identical or O-type deceased donor kidney. One criticism of this policy is that it may deplete O-type donors from the deceased donor pool, and further disadvantage type O recipients on the waiting list.

Another recent approach aimed at increasing the number of living donor kidney transplants involves the use of antibody desensitization protocols. Such protocols have used plasmapheresis and intravenous immunoglobulin (IVIG)-based therapies to decrease the concentration of circulating antibodies against HLA, allowing transplantation despite an initially positive cross-match. High dosage of IVIG alone (2 mg/kg) given monthly until a cytotoxic cross-match becomes negative has been used with some success in highly sensitized patients. Other groups have found greater success using plasmapheresis, IVIG at lower dosages, ± treatment with an anti-CD20 antibody (rituximab). Success appears to depend on the antibody titer before therapy. Most studies show high rejection rates of 30–50% despite recipient conversion to a negative cross-match, and aggressive and costly desensitization treatment is frequently continued after transplantation. Even with successful conversion to a negative antibody cross-match, alloantibodies tend to persist and may potentially contribute to chronic rejection post-transplantation. Similar protocols have been used to allow transplantation in the presence ABO blood type incompatibility. One center used pre- and post-transplant plasmapheresis with either splenectomy or rituximab in 40 ABO-incompatible recipients. Recipients with an ABO titer of <1 : 8 proceeded with transplantation. Rejection rates were high at 3 months (30%) but the 1-year graft survival rate was excellent at 95%, likely due to aggressive post-transplant monitoring and treatment with ongoing plasmapheresis, steroids, and/or rituximab after either rejection or a rise in ABO titers.

Most agree that donor exchange programs are superior to desensitization protocols in that the cost of therapy is significantly reduced and rejection rates are substantially lower. However, broadly sensitized patients and patients with blood type O may not find success with donor exchange programs and may benefit from desensitization protocols. Further analyses of such protocols are required, because both treatment regimens and outcomes remain variable between transplant centers.

Donor evaluation

The medical evaluation of the living kidney donor consists of basic tests to confirm adequate renal function in the absence of kidney disease, as well as excellent overall health in the donor. Most centers demand that a donor be of legal adult age (18 years) and able to provide informed consent. The upper limit of age for the donor varies among institutions and may not be as important as the donor's overall health status. However, the realization that renal function declines with age may make an older donor less desirable.

A history and physical examination are key components of the donor evaluation. Any history of major illness, including cardiovascular, pulmonary, or liver disease is noted, and donor candidates with significant comorbidities are typically excluded. Active malignancy and infection are usually also contraindications. Screening for syphilis and tuberculosis is performed, and donors are screened for viral infections such as hepatitis B, hepatitis C, and HIV, and excluded if active infection is present. Titers of antibodies against CMV and EBV are also measured to assess the risk of transmission of these viruses to the recipient.

Renal functional impairment and/or proteinuria is a contraindication for kidney donation. Some centers rely on 24-hour urine collections for both creatinine clearance and proteinuria. Others use more accurate assessments of GFR based on clearances of various isotopes, most commonly iothalamate. A GFR of 80 mL/min per 1.73 m^2 is the typical lower cut-off value for donation. Albumin:creatinine ratios are effective and accurate in ruling out abnormal albumin excretion, and total protein:creatinine ratios will also capture non-glomerular protein excretion.

Urinalysis is used to rule out pyuria or hematuria. Hematuria typically requires evaluation of the urogenital tract to look for mucosal abnormalities or kidney stones. A history of multiple kidney stones is generally a contraindication for donation. Occasionally patients with a history of a remote solitary kidney stone or with small microcalcification found on renal imaging will undergo a metabolic work-up for kidney stones. If such a work-up is unrevealing or can be corrected over time with medical therapy, donation is allowed at many centers.

If the potential donor has hematuria and no source of bleeding is found with renal imaging and cystoscopy, one must also consider glomerular hematuria, which may be associated with defects in the glomerular basement membrane. Potentially deleterious kidney diseases such as Alport's syndrome or IgA nephropathy must be considered in such patients. Even thin basement membrane disease, a condition once thought benign, has recently been associated with deteriorating kidney function over time. Risk of familial kidney diseases in a living related donor must be considered when the recipient has kidney failure due to polycystic disease, Alport's syndrome, or nephrotic syndrome. Polycystic kidney disease in the donor can be ruled out with renal ultrasonography, which serves as a highly sensitive screening test if the donor is aged >30 years.

Blood pressure measurement is a key component of the donor work-up, and patients with hypertension are generally excluded. There is no clear evidence that hypertension predisposes to kidney failure in patients with a solitary kidney, but there is an association with higher blood pressure and progression to kidney failure in the general population. A cut-off of ≥140/90 mmHg in the office and/or the need for blood pressure medication is generally used as an exclusion criteria. However, a significant percentage of patients with mild elevations in blood pressure in the office will have normal readings using ambulatory blood pressure monitoring, and such home monitoring can be a valuable tool in evaluating the potential donor. Some centers have expanded living donor criteria to include subjects with mild hypertension, although most agree that this is probably not wise in African-American individuals.

Donor candidates are usually screened for diabetes mellitus. One challenge commonly encountered is a younger donor candidate with no evidence of diabetes mellitus, but with an extensive family history of the disease, sometimes including the recipient candidate. A glucose tolerance test may be performed in a donor with a family history of disease, and donors with glucose intolerance should be excluded. Donors with an extensive family history of diabetes mellitus, particularly if they have other risk factors such as obesity, may be excluded as well. A history of gestational diabetes in women is also a relative contraindication, because approximately a third will go on to develop type 2 diabetes mellitus.

Other tests such as a chest radiograph and EKG are standard in the donor evaluation. Donors should undergo age-appropriate screening for malignancy, such as mammograms and pap smears in women, prostate evaluation in men, and colonoscopy in age-appropriate adults. Specific findings on history and physical examination may prompt further studies, such as cardiac stress testing or pulmonary function studies. A history of clotting or deep venous thrombosis is a relative contraindication for donation, because surgery itself creates a risk for recurrent thrombotic events. Pregnancy is a contraindication for donation, but future planned pregnancy is not, as many case series of normal successful pregnancies have been reported after kidney donation. Two recent studies suggest a slightly increased risk of pre-eclampsia in women who have previously donated a kidney. Finally, the donor medical evaluation includes a study that details the anatomy of both kidneys and their vascular supply. Angiography was once the norm, but less invasive modalities such as CT, MR, or digital subtraction angiography have largely supplanted conventional angiograms. These imaging studies are critical to rule out any anatomic abnormality that may exclude a donor. Identification of multiple renal arteries may make vascular implantation more challenging or lead to the harvesting of the right kidney despite the increased technical challenge of right nephrectomy.

A careful psychosocial evaluation is necessary to ensure that the donor is free from psychiatric illness and appropriately motivated. A donor seeking secondary gain through either financial reimbursement or improvement in social status should be excluded. It is also critical that the donor be highly motivated and willing to undergo some degree of risk to benefit the recipient. Donors should be screened in the absence of family members or the recipient. They should not feel overt pressure or undue anxiety about proceeding, and must be allowed to stop the evaluation process at any time. Finally, donors must be counseled on the fact that recipient outcomes may not always be optimal. Under recent UNOS mandates, each transplant center is obliged to identify a living donor advocate whose purpose is to objectively assess and counsel potential donors based on the above principles.

Case

A 29-year-old woman was being evaluated as a potential donor to her 61-year-old father who has ESRD from diabetic nephropathy. Her older brother and two paternal uncles have type 2 diabetes mellitus. She has a history of gestational diabetes during an otherwise uncomplicated pregnancy 2 years earlier. An oral glucose tolerance test was performed. Fasting blood glucose was normal but postprandial glucose was elevated, indicating impaired glucose tolerance. In view of concerns that the she was at high risk for developing overt diabetes mellitus in the future, she was advised against kidney donation.

Living kidney donor outcomes

Donor mortality after surgery is extremely low, but not absent. Mortality rates of 3 in 10 000 and complication rates of around 1% have been reported.

Long-term outcomes have been examined in living donors via retrospective analyses. Life expectancy in living donors exceeds that of the general population, due in part to the selection of healthy candidates for kidney donation. A recent survey from the University of Minnesota contacted donors 20 years after donation. Of 773 donors, information was gathered on 464 (60%), and serum creatinine was measured in 74 (9.5%). Mean serum creatinine was 1.2 ± 0.04 mg/dL (range 0.7–2.5 mg/dL). Proteinuria was seen in approximately 10% of donors, and hypertension was common, occurring in more than a third of those surveyed. However, the great majority with proteinuria had either trace or 1+ protein on a dipstick, with no impairment in renal function, and hypertensive rates were no different from aged-matched rates from the general population.

Long-term data are lacking on kidney donors who may be at higher risk, including obese donors. Obesity has increased in the general population and a higher percentage of modern-era kidney donors are obese. Donor nephrectomy in obese donors appears to be safe, with no increased risk of major complications or hospital length of stay after laparoscopic nephrectomy in one series. Obese donors in this study also had no increased proteinuria or renal dysfunction in the first year after donation. There is concern, however, that obese donors may be at greater risk for renal functional deterioration over time. Obesity is an independent risk factor for the development of proteinuria in the general population, and after non-transplant nephrectomy in one series. In kidney donors, higher BMI correlates with risk of developing hypertension, and hypertension correlates with a risk of developing proteinuria after donation.

Controversies in living donor transplantation

Soliciting for organ donation On a small scale, organ solicitation has likely gone on for years through local venues such as newspapers and places of worship. More recently, widespread solicitation has been made available through media sources such as the internet. New websites have been set up by third parties allowing wait-listed patients to advertise for organs and to communicate online with potential donors. Some worry that an unfair allocation of organs may result from such widespread solicitation. Recipients may not always be forthright in self-portrayals, and certain descriptions may be used to stimulate an emotional response from prospective donors. Whether portrayals are accurate or not, responses to such solicitation may lead to the bypassing of recipients with longer waiting times or better immunologic matching. Although some recipients may capitalize on such solicitation, others may not have the resources or the charisma to gain similar benefit.

Arguments supporting widespread organ solicitation describe a potential increase in the overall donor pool by increasing awareness of the unmet need for organ donation. With the current shortage of available donors relative to numbers on the waiting list, desperate patients will naturally pursue such means. Organ solicitation is not illegal, provided that it does not involve financial compensation. However, in an attempt to maintain fair allocation, some have recommended that anyone responding to such solicitation be offered the chance to donate in a non-directed fashion.

Financial compensation for organs Another concern about widespread donor solicitation is the potential for financial compensation and trafficking of organs. As a direct emotional link is often absent in this type of organ exchange, financial recompense may be used to fill the void. In the USA, the National Organ Transplant Act (NOTA) of 1984 contains a specific title prohibiting the sale of organs, although it does allow for reimbursement for donor travel and lodging expenses. Some argue that this law should be amended, and that a regulated system of reimbursement for organ donation in the USA is needed to combat the long and growing waiting list for deceased donor kidneys. A regulated system could eliminate kidney brokers, and may be superior to the black market trade in kidneys that exists in other countries and even in the USA.

One suggestion would allow for government-sponsored life insurance and life-long medical coverage for living donors, reimbursement for lost wages and travel expenses, and a modest cash compensation for "inconvenience, anxiety, and/or pain." Government-based compensation would eliminate the potential injustice of kidneys being purchased exclusively by wealthy recipients. A recent public poll found that a majority was in favor of some compensation for expenses, including medical costs and insurance coverage for living donors. Lifelong health insurance has been considered an appropriate award for living donors; however, many believe that any cash compensation would attract an indigent population willing to donate for the money alone. Donors desperate to repay debt may be clouded in their judgment and may not give true informed consent.

Systematic reimbursement for organ donation has been described in other nations, and some studies have suggested the process as an effective way to reduce or even eliminate patients on the waiting list. Impoverished young men have been the primary targets for donation under one such system and, despite reimbursement, compensation for kidney donation has not resolved debt. In addition, although altruistic donors are lauded as heroes in the USA, paid donors in other countries have been ostracized. The vast majority of Iranian paid donors attempt to hide their history of donation, and describe organ donation as a form of "prostitution."

Some argue that kidney sales would actually diminish the number of altruistic donations from family and friends. This has been observed in Iran, where living unrelated donation for reimbursement has dominated over altruistic living donation. Surveys from paid donors have revealed that the great majority would not donate again if given the chance, with percentages roughly inverse to those from surveys from altruistic donors in the west. Nevertheless, the debate over donor compensation continues in the USA, where concerns for donor welfare and exploitation have been weighed against the goal of improving survival by increasing the number of living donor transplants and diminishing recipient waiting time.

Surgical techniques and complications

Kidney graft procurement

Deceased donor kidney graft procurement

Multiorgan retrieval from heart-beating, brain-dead donors is the most common scenario for deceased organ donation. A median sternotomy and midline laparotomy (see Figure 7.6a) allow for isolation of the great vessels in the chest, at the diaphragm, and at the iliac bifurcation. This exposure also permits rapid cannulation of the distal aorta in case of donor instability. Further dissection defines anatomic variations, assesses organ quality, and prepares the field for cold flush with preservation solution after aortic clamping. Elements essential for good organ preservation at the time of aortic clamping include previous intravenous bolus of heparin, rapid arrest of the donor metabolism by decreasing donor body temperature (aortic cold flush and ice slush packing of the peritoneal cavity), and complete removal of intragraft blood by flushing with preservative solution.

Grafts are removed in a standard order: first the heart, then the lung(s), liver. and pancreas, and finally the kidneys. When used, the intestine is removed with the liver and pancreas before the kidneys. The kidneys can be removed en bloc, attached to the aorta and vena cava (see Figure 7.6b), and then separated on

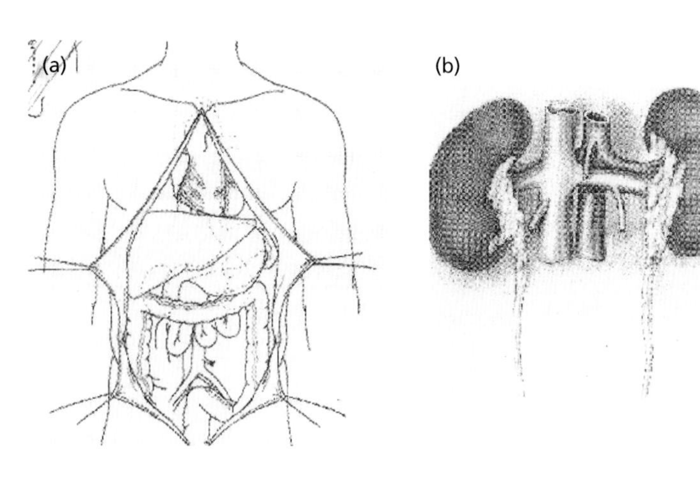

Figure 7.6 The multiorgan donor procurement operation. (a) Exposure is facilitated by a median sternotomy and midline laparotomy. (b) En bloc kidney removal. Note the piece of aorta and vena cava with attached renal vessels. The ureters are removed, retaining as much length as possible.

the back table. Alternatively, they can be separated *in situ* and then removed. Perinephric fat should be cleared to allow inspection for neoplastic lesions, and superficial cysts or masses should be opened and biopsied. Renal biopsy may be performed to evaluate histology in grafts deemed to be marginal on the basis of clinical parameters.

Organ retrieval from non-heart-beating donors follows the declaration of death using standard criteria after withdrawal of life support. The latter should be performed either in the operating room or in close proximity to the operating room in order to decrease warm ischemia time. Rapid organ cooling is accomplished by prompt laparotomy, placement of an aortic cannula for cold flushing of the organs, and installation of ice slush in the peritoneal cavity.

Live donor procurement

The goal in performing live donor nephrectomy, regardless of technique, is to safely procure the kidney while exposing the patient to the lowest chance for morbidity. Before renal artery occlusion, systemic anticoagulation is achieved by the administration of heparin. Generous administration of intravenous fluids during the procedure assures good diuresis. After removal, the kidney is immediately flushed with cold preservation solution and packed in ice until preimplantation preparation is performed.

Open and mini-incision nephrectomy Traditionally, open nephrectomy has been performed through a large flank incision (16–22 cm) that sacrifices the tip of the twelfth rib, and extends to the border of the rectus muscle. Smaller, less painful incisions are now preferred and often result in postoperative recovery times similar to those following laparoscopic nephrectomy. The kidney is dissected out of Gerota's fascia and the renal artery and vein are divided after transfixion sutures or staples are employed proximally. The site of ureter transaction is chosen to maximize length.

Laparoscopic nephrectomy Laparoscopic donor nephrectomy, first reported in 1995, was initially reserved for left kidneys with standard anatomy, and was associated with an increased risk for delayed graft function compared with open donors. More recently, successful recovery of right or left kidneys has been performed and transplant outcomes are comparable to kidneys procured using the open technique. Previous abdominal surgery may preclude the laparoscopic technique.

Appropriate positioning of the patient is essential. Pneumoperitoneum is accomplished through the placement of a 12-mm trocar using the open technique. Two other 5-mm trocars are placed under direct vision. This approach requires the use of both a 10-mm and a 5-mm laparoscopic camera at different times during the dissection. Inflation pressures are kept around 10–12 mmHg, and intravenous fluids are administered generously, to minimize renal dysfunction. The hand-assisted approach starts with a midline periumbilical incision (6–8 cm in length) to place the hand port and to establish pneumoperitoneum. Graft dissection is performed as described for the open technique; once it is completed a brief period of deflation is recommended to improve graft blood flow and to establish a brisk diuresis. The preferred technique is to gain control of the renal artery and vein by the use of staplers. Use of a single-three row stapler followed by section with scissors affords greater blood vessel length. The kidney is removed through the hand port. With the non-hand-assisted laparoscopic procedure, organ dissection is performed through the three ports with delay of the larger incision (midline or lower quadrant transverse) until the kidney is ready for removal. Similar periods of hospital recovery and return to normal activities have been observed with the laparoscopic approach when compared with the mini-incision approach.

Key points 7.4 Important facts regarding laparoscopic donor nephrectomy (compared with traditional open nephrectomy)

Higher cost, mostly related to longer operative time

Shorter length of hospital stay

Shorter period of rehabilitation

Higher rate of delayed graft function in the recipients, but no discernible effect on long-term outcomes

Organ preservation

Although kidneys may be preserved for up to 72 h, particularly when preserved by pulsatile perfusion, most surgeons perform kidney transplantation in less than 24 h to minimize the risk of delayed graft function. University of Wisconsin solution (UW, Viaspan) or HTK solution (Custodiol) may be used. Although they differ significantly in their components, both are high in oncotic pressure and achieve similar periods of successful cold preservation. Preservation of kidney graft function for >24 h is best achieved by the use of a pulsatile preservation pump. This technique is associated with a decrease in the incidence of graft dysfunction and it may be used as a tool for assessing graft quality by observing the trends in perfusion pressure and perfusate flow and vascular resistance.

Kidney graft implantation

Adult transplantation

The extraperitoneal approach, using the iliac vessels for blood supply, has been the mainstay for single kidney transplantation since its inception (Figure 7.7). Arterial inflow to the graft is usually achieved by end-to-side anastomosis of the renal artery to the host common or external iliac artery. Alternatively, an end-to-end anastomosis to the hypogastric artery can be used. The recipient's saphenous vein can be used as a conduit to extend the renal artery if it is too short. Rarely, excision and replacement of the iliac artery with a prosthetic conduit can provide a location for anastomosis in patients with severe iliac artery atherosclerosis. Use of the proximal common iliac vessels or even the distal aorta and vena cava is occasionally necessary, especially in patients undergoing re-transplantation, or in patients with implantation of dual kidneys. Venous reconstruction is usually achieved by an end-to-side anastomosis between the renal vein and the external iliac vein. Venous length is rarely an issue when the left kidney is used. When necessary, the right renal vein can be lengthened by creating a venous conduit from the attached vena cava or by attachment of a hand-sewn segment of donor iliac vein.

The technique for ureteral implantation depends on the anatomy of the patient and the preferences of the surgeon. The anterior (Gregoir–Lich) ureteroneocystostomy is straightforward and therefore, more commonly used than the posterior (Ledbetter) approach. Use of a double J stents is a matter of surgical preference. In cases of a short ureter or small bladder, the use of the recipient ureter either as a pyeloureterostomy or ureter-to-ureter anastomosis can be used. Uncommonly, bladder augmentation, construction of an ileo-conduit, or a cutaneous ureterostomy may be necessary.

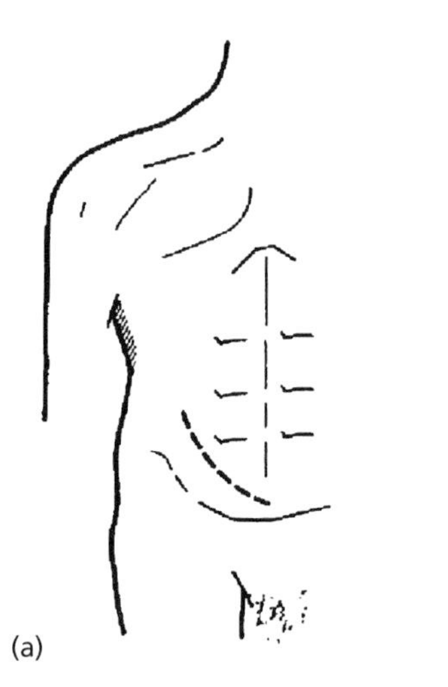

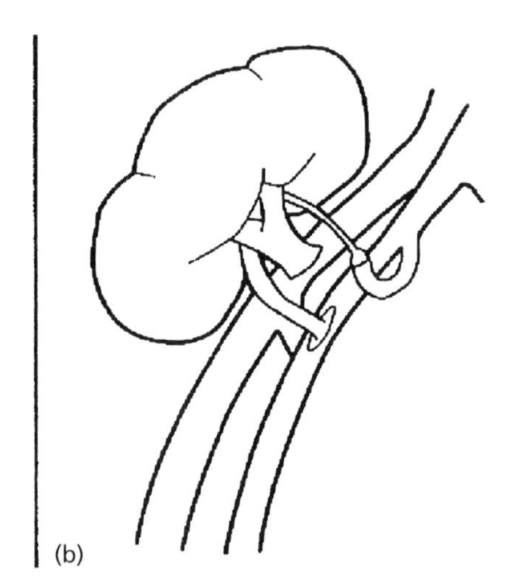

Figure 7.7 The recipient operation for kidney transplantation. (a) A lower abdominal incision is performed in an extraperitoneal approach. (b) The final anatomy of a revascularized renal allograft. Note the use of the internal iliac artery as a separate inflow for the polar renal artery.

Implantation of both kidneys from a deceased donor into a single recipient is an alternative strategy when donors exhibit marginal kidney function or histology. Transplantation of both kidneys can be performed on one side of the pelvis, if adequate recipient arterial supply exists. This approach avoids two incisions and leaves the contralateral iliac vessels intact, should future re-transplantation be needed.

Pediatric kidney transplantation

Transplantation using pediatric donors Kidneys from infant donors (<20 kg) have small renal vasculature that increases the risk of technical failure. In addition, transplantation of one small kidney may not provide adequate nephron mass for a large adult recipient. Such kidneys may be kept en bloc and transplanted into a single recipient, using the donor aorta and vena cava for the implantation. Some surgeons advocate suture pexy of the grafts in a position that preserves vascular inflow and outflow. The use of absorbable mesh for this purpose has been reported.

Transplantation into pediatric recipients Use of adult kidney grafts for pediatric recipients is standard procedure. In very small infants the graft is implanted intraperitoneally on the right side through a midline incision, using the recipient aorta and vena cava for revascularization. In children weighing >10 kg, the retroperitoneal approach can be used. Again, preference is for the right side. Care should be exercised at the time of reperfusion because a large kidney can take up to 30% of the total blood volume of a child. Graft hypoperfusion and subsequent risk of delayed graft function may be decreased by keeping the central venous pressure at ≥15 mmHg, particularly at the time of reperfusion. Bladder reconstruction before or at the time of transplantation may be necessary in children with very small bladders.

Kidney re-transplantation

A second transplantation is usually accomplished by placement of the kidney on the contralateral, unused side. Third and further re-transplants require both dissection in a reoperative field and removal of the previously failed graft in order to accommodate the new kidney. Immunosuppression, prior infections, fluid collections, and the occurrence of other surgical complications make the degree of scarring unpredictable. In rare occasions, an intraperitoneal approach is required with placement of the vascular reconstruction at the aorta and vena cava level.

Kidney transplantation in combination or after other abdominal organs

Simultaneous deceased donor kidney and pancreas transplantation is routine, and is usually accomplished through a midline, intraperitoneal approach. Most surgeons place the kidney graft on the left side and the pancreas graft on the right side of the pelvis using the iliac vessels as previously described. Portal venous drainage of the pancreas moves the graft to the mid abdomen, away from the pelvis, affording greater options for kidney placement (Figure 7.8). Compared with systemic venous drainage into the iliac venous system, portal drainage mimics normal physiologic drainage of the pancreas into the portal system. Although there has been some debate regarding the immune and metabolic advantages of systemic versus portal venous drainage, there is no clear consensus about clinically meaningful differences, and the approach has been left to surgeon discretion. With the portal drainage approach, the use of an additional

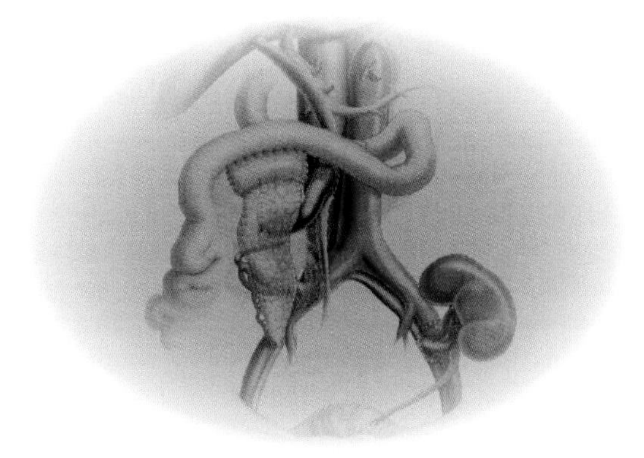

Figure 7.8 Simultaneous kidney and pancreas transplantation. Typically, the kidney graft is implanted on the left side of the pelvis. The pancreas graft is usually implanted on the right side using the iliac vessels or, as in this case, using the iliac artery for the arterial reconstruction and the portal vein for the venous implantation. Note the conduit to the portal vein. The exocrine pancreas is enterically drained using an anastomosis of the donor duodenal cuff with the recipient's small intestine.

conduit to the portal vein is usually necessary (Figure 7.8). Currently, drainage of the exocrine pancreas is accomplished most often by anastomosis of the donor duodenal stump to the small intestine of the recipient. However, some surgeons still prefer the older technique in which the duodenal stump is anastomosed to the recipient bladder. Kidney transplantation together with liver transplantation is usually performed through a separate standard iliac fossa approach.

Surgical complications

Fluid collections – vascular

After kidney transplantation, fluid collections may form due to bleeding or leakage of lymph. Significant postoperative hemorrhage should be addressed by re-exploration. Large, stable hematomas may cause pain, become infected, or cause compression symptoms, and should be evacuated. Although mycotic aneurysm formation is rare after renal transplantation, the condition will lead to hemorrhage and carries a high mortality rate (>50%) if not repaired expeditiously. Complete excision of the arterial anastomosis and vein patch repair of the iliac artery are mandatory. When treating severe vascular infections, the limb and life of the patient are always the priority. Infrequently, severe bleeding may occur as a result of parenchymal fracture due to acute rejection. If difficult to control it may require graft removal.

The rich lymphatic network surrounding the iliac vessels is routinely divided at the time of transplantation. Suture ligation of these channels is routine, but leakage of lymph fluid occurs in 5–15% of patients. Although incidental asymptomatic collections do not require intervention, lymphoceles that partially occlude the ureter or renal vein, leading to renal dysfunction or ipsilateral leg swelling (by compressing the iliac vein), require drainage. Percutaneous drainage can be used to confirm the presence of lymphocytes, establish the association with infection, and drain the collection. In up to 30% of cases a more definitive approach is required. This is usually achieved by marsupialization of the lymphocele into the peritoneal cavity by a laparoscopic or open approach.

Fluid collections – urologic

Early urine leak occurs in 1–3% of cases. With small leaks, prolonged bladder catheterization, percutaneous drainage of the urinoma, and ureter stenting may lead to spontaneous healing. When repair is necessary, repeat implantation into the bladder is the preferred technique, but a ureter-to-ureter reconstruction utilizing the distal recipient ureter, or a bladder flap, may be required. Ureter implantation into a very small, spastic bladder may increase the risk of a high-output leak and surgical repair is required. Bladder augmentation in addition to prolonged drainage (J stent and nephrostomy tube) will provide a low-pressure system that will enhance healing.

Key points 7.5 Most common causes of perinephric fluid collections after kidney transplantation

Seromas

Hematomas

Lymphoceles

Urinomas

Case

A 49-year-old man received a deceased donor kidney transplant after being on hemodialysis for 12 years. The bladder was atrophic but a standard ureteral anastomosis was performed. A Jackson–Pratt drain was placed adjacent to the transplanted kidney. The allograft functioned immediately and serum creatinine concentration fell from 8.2 mg/dL to 2.3 mg/dL by postoperative day 3. The patient's Foley catheter was removed 4 days after transplantation. During the next 12 h, there was an abrupt increase in output of the drain and laboratory analysis of the drainage fluid indicated that the concentration of creatinine was threefold higher than a simultaneous serum creatinine concentration, confirming a urine leak. The Foley catheter was replaced with prompt reduction in output from the drain. The patient was discharged; 10 days later the Foley catheter was removed. Drainage from the Jackson–Pratt drain remained low and the drain was removed 2 days later with no further evidence of a urine leak.

Decreased diuresis – vascular

Early arterial thrombosis occurs in 1–2% of patients; it may be caused by technical errors, hypercoagulable states, or poor inflow from a stenotic/thrombosed native vessel used for reconstruction. Immediate recognition is paramount for successful salvage of the graft. Sudden development of anuria is highly suggestive of arterial thrombosis and must be investigated immediately. As delayed graft function or acute cellular rejection can have a similar presentation, an ultrasound evaluation is readily indicated. If ultrasonography is not available, return to the operating room should be considered because arterial thrombosis requires urgent thrombectomy, infusion of thrombolytic agents, and correction of any technical error. In most cases, renal function will not be restored, and transplant nephrectomy will be necessary. Isolated renal vein thrombosis may present initially with hematuria before anuria ensues. Similar to arterial thrombosis, it is rarely reversible and will often mandate allograft nephrectomy.

Decreased diuresis – urologic
Decreased urinary output may also be caused by external compression of the ureter, urinary leak, or obstruction of the urinary track at any level. If the urinary catheter is in place, it should be flushed to clear it of any obstruction. If the urinary catheter has been removed an "in-and-out" bladder catheterization may prove to be useful. High residuals may be due to bladder dysfunction or prostatic hypertrophy. Urinary stents, if used, are removed 2–4 weeks after transplantation. Late ureter stenosis may be due to ischemia, cellular or humoral rejection, or scarring from prolonged stenting, or as a consequence of a technical error. This is manifested by renal dysfunction associated with hydronephrosis. Anatomic definition of the stenotic segment is accomplished by percutaneous antegrade contrast study or by endoscopic ureterography. Focal stenoses may be amenable to transluminal dilation and stenting although long stenotic segments usually require surgical reconstruction. The latter is usually corrected by native ureter-to-graft pyelostomy.

Infectious surgical complications
Surgical site infections after kidney transplantation are not common. However, when they occur, recognition may be delayed because the inflammatory manifestations of the infection may be blunted by immunosuppressive therapy. The use of sirolimus as an immunosuppressant may compromise wound healing and promote infection due to its antiproliferative and antiangiogenic properties. Wound infections above the fascia are treated by opening of the wound, administering systemic antibiotics, and local wound care. Deep space infection must be adequately drained and aggressively controlled to avoid breakdown of any of the vascular anastomoses. Usually this requires surgical debridement and drainage.

Transplant nephrectomy

Kidney graft removal early after transplantation is rarely required. Uncontrolled accelerated/acute rejection, unremitting graft hemorrhage, arterial/venous thrombosis, and mycotic aneurysm formation are the most common indications. Late transplant nephrectomy, after the patient has returned to dialysis, is performed most often because of severe pain, persistent fever, chronic infection, hematuria, proteinuria, and/or difficult management of hypertension. Nonfunctioning renal grafts may also be removed to accommodate a new transplant or to prevent the formation of antibodies in patients who stop immunosuppression. The development of a neoplasm in the graft is a rare reason for graft removal.

Late transplant nephrectomy is best accomplished through a limited incision directly over the allograft. The renal capsule is entered and the graft is shelled out to the hilum. Significant hemorrhage is occasionally encountered, and expeditious cross-clamping at the hilum allows for rapid excision of the kidney. Vessels are individually sutured when possible. Intracapsular dissection avoids injury to the iliac vessels and other recipient structures.

Immunosuppression

Antibodies used for induction therapy

The incidence of acute rejection is greatest in the first few months after transplantation. Thus, the intensity of immunosuppression delivered is typically highest during the perioperative and early postoperative periods. An immunosuppressive strategy known as "induction therapy" is employed when the early posttransplant protocol includes antibodies against specific or multiple antigenic targets. The benefits of using such induction antibodies to reduce the risk of early acute rejection must be weighed against the cost of these agents and the potential risk of over-immunosuppression, manifested by infection or malignancy. Induction antibodies can generally be classified as either lymphocyte depleting or non-depleting agents. Within each category, there are both monoclonal agents directed against specific antigenic targets of lymphocytes and polyclonal agents containing a pool of antibodies directed against multiple antigens. Monoclonal antibodies are created with murine hybridoma techniques and are sometimes genetically engineered to create chimeric or humanized modifications. Polyclonal agents are generally produced by harvesting serum from animals previously inoculated with human thymocytes or lymphocytes. The use of induction antibody therapy varies around the world but has become increasingly popular in the USA over the past 15 years, such that more than 70% of patients currently receive one of the agents described below.

Lymphocyte-depleting antibodies

Over the years, a number of polyclonal anti-lymphocyte antibodies have been generated using a variety of animals. The only polyclonal agents currently used in the USA are rabbit antithymocyte globulin (rabbit ATG; Thymoglobulin) and ATGAM, an agent produced in horses. As Thymoglobulin proved to be superior to ATGAM for the treatment of acute rejection in a randomized trial, it has become the predominant polyclonal agent used in the USA. However, it is important to note that rabbit ATG is approved by the Food and Drug Administration (FDA) only for treatment of rejection and is technically used off-label as an induction therapy. When compared with no induction antibody therapy, this and other polyclonal agents have been shown to reduce the incidence of acute rejection and to prolong graft survival. Moreover, a randomized trial suggested that rabbit ATG is superior to basiliximab, a non-depleting antibody, in preventing acute rejection in patients deemed to be at high risk for immune graft injury. Lymphocytes are cleared from the circulation during active administration of the drug, which is usually slowly infused daily for 3–10 days post-transplantation. Thrombocytopenia and leukopenia are common side effects, often resulting in the need for dose modification. Fever, chills, and myalgias are commonly observed with the initial infusion, but can be mollified by concomitant administration of corticosteroids. Anaphylactic reactions occur rarely.

Alemtuzumab (Campath-1H) is an anti-CD52, humanized, monoclonal antibody that binds to all T and B lymphocytes, as well as most macrophages, monocytes, and natural killer cells. It was approved in the 1980s as an agent for the treatment of B-cell chronic lymphocytic leukemia and is currently used off-label in transplantation. Alemtuzumab produces significant leukopenia, probably by antibody-dependent lysis of the lymphocytes that leads to depletion of T and B cells in the peripheral circulation for >12 months. The drug is easily administered peripherally, given in a single (30 mg) or double dose in the perioperative period. Some centers have reported a relatively high incidence of humoral (antibody-mediated) acute rejection in patients treated with alemtuzumab, and repeated courses of therapy have been associated with the emergence of autoantibodies and autoimmune disorders.

Another depleting monoclonal antibody, OKT3 (Orthoclone Muromonab-CD3), targets the CD3 complex of T cells causing endocytosis of its constituent peptides and profound impairment of both T-cell activation and proliferation. Although this drug proved to be useful as an induction agent in the 1980s, it is rarely employed for induction in the USA in the modern era, mostly because of its cost and toxicities.

Non-depleting antibodies

The major agents in this category are the monoclonal antibodies directed against the α chain of the interleukin-2 (IL-2) receptor (also known as CD25). Binding to this receptor blocks the proliferative signals normally mediated by IL-2 without causing profound depletion of lymphocyte counts. Basiliximab (Simulect) is a chimeric anti-CD25 antibody (30% murine, 70% human). Daclizumab (Zenepax) is a humanized version (10% murine, 90% human). Together, the anti-CD25 antibodies are currently the second most frequently prescribed induction antibodies in the USA. However, Zenepax is no longer be produced. When compared with placebo, treatment with either of these antibodies has been associated with lower rates of early acute rejection. Basiliximab is typically administered intraoperatively and again on the fourth postoperative day.

Maintenance immunosuppression

Herein we describe the mechanisms of action and dosing strategies for maintenance immunosuppressants commonly prescribed to kidney and pancreas transplant recipients. The pharmacokinetics and side effects of these agents are discussed in greater detail in Chapter 2.

Corticosteroids

Corticosteroids exert two principal effects on the immune system. First, within 4–8 hours of administration, they alter the distribution of lymphocytes, causing their sequestration in the reticuloendothelial system. Second, corticosteroids inhibit the proliferation and function of lymphocytes by blocking the expression of various lymphokines and cytokines. Glucocorticoids easily diffuse into cells and bind to cytoplasmic receptors that exist in association with a heat shock protein. Corticosteroids also inhibit the action of transcription factors such as activating protein-1 (AP-1) and nuclear factor-κB (NF-κB). In the case of NF-κB, activated glucocorticoid receptors may bind to activated NF-κB and prevent it from binding to κB sites on proinflammatory genes. The major consequence of these intracellular effects of corticosteroids is an inhibition of the production of IL-1 and IL-6 by antigen-presenting cells such as macrophages and monocytes. As IL-1 is a primary co-stimulus for helper T-cell activation and IL-6 is a major inducer of B-cell activation, corticosteroid administration has the potential to inhibit both the cellular and humoral arms of the immune response.

Corticosteroids are most often prescribed according to fixed and empiric dose-tapering schedules. In the modern era, many centers use doses of prednisone as low as 5 mg daily beyond the several months after transplantation. These agents have been employed to prevent and treat acute allograft rejection for more than 40 years. However, the well-known side effects of steroids have led to steroid-sparing regimens and, although somewhat controversial, complete withdrawal of these agents in low-risk patients has become the standard of practice in many transplant centers.

Calcineurin inhibitors

Calcineurin inhibitors (CNIs) have formed the backbone of solid-organ transplant immunosuppressive regimens since the introduction of cyclosporine in the early 1980s. Cyclosporine is a small cyclic polypeptide of fungal origin. The other available CNI is tacrolimus, a macrolide antibiotic compound that became available in the USA in the mid-1990s. Tacrolimus has emerged as the most commonly used CNI in the USA. As described below, cyclosporine and tacrolimus have different side effects. Whether the two agents are comparably efficacious in preventing rejection or prolonging graft survival remains a subject of great debate. Calcineurin is an intracellular phosphatase that is found in T cells and functions to dephosphorylate certain nuclear regulatory proteins, allowing them to pass through the nuclear membrane. These regulatory proteins then activate the transcription of several cytokines (IL-2, IL-4, IFN-α and tumor necrosis factor α [TNF-α]) that promote T-cell activation. Cyclosporine binds to the cytoplasmic receptor, cyclophilin, whereas tacrolimus binds to the cytoplasmic receptor, FK-binding protein (FKBP) (Figure 7.9). Both the cyclosporine–cyclophilin and tacrolimus–FKBP compounds bind to calcineurin, preventing its normal function and thereby blocking T-cell activation.

The original oral formulation of cyclosporine was Sandimmune, which exhibits relatively poor bioavailability with great within- and between-patient pharmacokinetic variability. A newer microemulsion formulation, Neoral, was later developed to improve absorption and minimize variation in bioavailability. Several generic forms of cyclosporine are now available. Tacrolimus is currently available as Prograf, but generic forms of tacrolimus are now available. As a result of variations in absorption and genetic differences in the expression and function of the cytochrome P450 3A4 (CYP3A4) system responsible for metabolism of CNIs (see below), drug level monitoring is still considered necessary for optimal management of all the available CNIs. Due to subtle variations in pharmacokinetics between different formulations, it is best to avoid switching from brand name compounds to generics. However, if conversion is necessary, close monitoring of drug levels and renal function is suggested in the short term. Both CNIs are excreted in the bile with minimal renal excretion, so there is no need for dose adjustment in the presence of renal impairment. Cyclosporine can be administered intravenously, generally using 30% of the oral dose as a constant infusion over 24 h. Intravenous

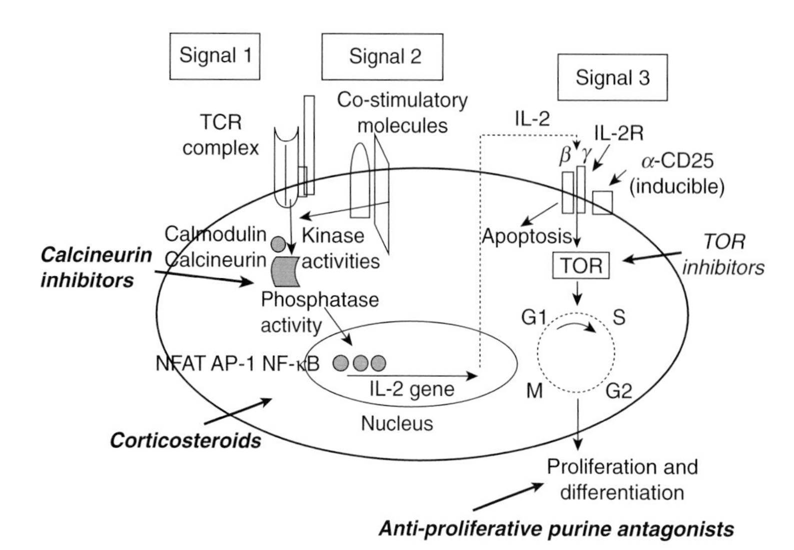

Figure 7.9 Schematic representation of intracellular signaling events associated with T-cell activation, organized according to three sets of signals: (1) antigen recognition, (2) co-stimulation, and (3) cell cycle progression. The sites of action of immunosuppressive drug classes are shown in italics. AP, activator protein; CTLA4-Ig, cytotoxic T-lymphocyte antigen 4-immunoglobulin; IL, interleukin; NFAT, nuclear factor of activated T-cells; NF-κB, nuclear factor-κB; TCR, T-cell receptor; TOR, target of rapamycin.

tacrolimus is extremely toxic and should be used with great caution.

Typical starting dose of cyclosporine is 8–12 mg/kg per day with maintenance dose of 3–5 mg/kg per day in twice daily doses. For tacrolimus, the typical starting dose is 0.15–0.3 mg/kg per day in twice daily doses. There is a reasonably good correlation between trough blood levels of tacrolimus and overall drug exposure. This correlation is less reliable with cyclosporine. Nevertheless, due to convenience and cost, trough drug levels are most commonly used in monitoring all CNIs. There are two general methods for measuring whole blood concentration of CNIs. High-performance liquid chromatography (HPLC) is the most specific method, but is also more expensive and labor intensive. Whole blood immunoassays are cheaper and more readily available for use in automated analyzers. Lower starting doses of CNIs and lower trough target levels are used when these agents are prescribed with a target for rapamycin (TOR) inhibitor, because the combination of agents increases the risk of nephrotoxicity.

CNIs are metabolized by CPY3A4 enzyme system located in the liver and gastrointestinal tract. As many drugs can up- or downregulate the cytochrome P450 enzyme system, vigilance is needed to avoid potential drug interactions between CNIs and commonly prescribed medications. Drugs that reliably decrease CNI concentration by inducing the cytochrome P450 enzyme system include rifampin and anticonvulsants such as barbiturates and phenytoin. If these drugs are required, the dose of CNI often needs to be increased to maintain therapeutic levels. Other drugs that decrease CNI levels less predictably include nafcillin, trimethoprim, imipenem, cephalosporins, and ciprofloxacin. St John's wort, a herbal mood enhancer, can also induce the cytochrome P450 enzyme system. Whenever any of these medications are used, CNI trough levels should be monitored closely. Lastly, corticosteroids are also inducers of the cytochrome P450 enzyme system. When steroids are tapered, CNI levels should be monitored closely to determine the need for dose reduction.

Drugs that increase CNI concentration by inhibiting cytochrome P450 activity include non-dihydropyridine calcium channel blockers, such as diltiazem and verapamil, the azole antifungal agents, such as ketoconazole, itraconazole, voriconazole, and fluconazole, and erythromycin and its analogs (except azithromycin). Drugs such as diltiazem and ketoconazole are occasionally prescribed together with CNIs in an effort to lower the CNI dose and reduce cost. Other medications that inhibit cytochrome P450 activity less predictably include isoniazide, oral contraceptives, amiodarone, and carvediol. With the advent of HAART, some centers are now providing organ transplants to HIV-positive patients. Therefore, it is worth noting that protease inhibitors

– particularly ritonavir – are potent inhibitors of the cytochrome P450 enzyme. Lastly, a special dietary concern for all patients on a CNI is grapefruit juice which can result in higher drug levels from increased absorption. Non-cytochrome P450 enzyme-related drug interactions can occur with cholestyramine and GoLYTELY which may interfere with absorption of CNIs. Concomitant use of CNIs and HMG-CoA (hydroxymethylglutaryl coenzyme A) reductase inhibitors alter the pharmacokinetics of the "statin," resulting in a longer half-life and a greater risk for rhabdomyolysis.

Key points 7.6 Drugs that exert predictable interactions with immunosuppressants metabolized by the cytochrome P450 3A4 enzyme system (cyclosporine, tacrolimus, sirolimus)

Drugs that increase levels:

- Erythromycin and its congeners (except azithromycin)
- Azole antifungals
- Diltiazem, verapamil
- Protease inhibitors

Drugs that decrease levels

- Phenytoin
- Barbiturates
- Rifampin

Antiproliferative agents

There are three available agents or classes of antiproliferative immunosuppressant medications: azathioprine, mycophenolic acid derivatives, and the TOR inhibitors.

Azathioprine The oldest of the antiproliferative agents is azathioprine, first introduced in the 1960s. Azathioprine is a metabolite of 6-mercaptopurine which is processed intracellularly into purine analogs that inhibit purine synthesis from both the direct and the salvage pathways. In so doing, the drug suppresses gene replication and cell proliferation via inhibition of RNA and DNA synthesis. Although it is more selective for T lymphocytes, it can also suppress promyelocytes in the bone marrow, resulting in leukopenia, thrombocytopenia, and/or anemia.

Azathioprine is available in both oral and intravenous formulations as Imuran or in generic formulation. However, only half of the orally administered azathioprine is absorbed; therefore, the equivalent intravenous dose is half that of the oral dose. The starting oral dose of azathioprine is 1–2 mg/kg administered once daily. There is no need for blood level monitoring because its effectiveness is not blood-level dependent. It is also not excreted by the kidney, so there is no need for dose reduction during episodes of acute renal insufficiency. Dose adjustments are based on toxicity. Azathioprine is metabolized by xanthine oxidase; treatment with allopurinol inhibits xanthine oxidase. Therefore, when combined with azathioprine, there can be prolonged azathioprine activity resulting in significant pancytopenia. To prevent this, the azathioprine dose should be reduced by 75–80% and blood counts should be followed closely.

Mycophenolic acid derivatives MMF (CellCept) is a prodrug of mycophenolic acid (MPA). It was approved for use in 1995 and has essentially replaced azathioprine as the antiproliferative agent of choice, given its relatively few side effects and superior effects in preventing acute rejection. An enteric-coated form of mycophenolate sodium (ECMPS or Myfortic) became available in 2004. MPA is a reversible inhibitor of inosine monophosphate dehydrogenase (IMPDH), which is a critical rate-limiting enzyme in new purine synthesis. MMF achieves its antiproliferative effect by blocking nucleic acid synthesis. However, its effect is relatively selective for lymphocytes, because not only do lymphocytes have a more susceptible isoform of IMPDH, but they also rely more heavily on new purine synthesis whereas other cell types have an alternative salvage pathway.

MMF is available as capsules in either 250 mg or 500 mg dosages. The standard dose when used together with cyclosporine is 1 g administered twice daily; African–American individuals may need a higher dose of 1.5 g twice daily to achieve adequate suppression when used with cyclosporine. ECMPS is available in 180 mg and 360 mg capsules and the standard dose is 720 mg administered twice daily, which is equivalent to 1 g twice daily of MMF. Only MMF is available as an intravenous formulation and intravenous dosing that is identical to the oral dose. MMF is hydrolyzed to MPA in the liver, producing an initial peak drug concentration in 1–2 h followed by a second peak in 5–6 h through enterohepatic cycling. It is believed that the gastrointestinal side effects of MMF stem from this cycling. Therefore, not surprisingly, ECMPS has been shown to have a similar lower gastrointestinal side-effect profile as MMF. To minimize the side effects, the daily dose can be split into three to four doses a day. Similar to azathioprine, therapeutic drug monitoring is not mandatory, although some centers measure trough levels of mycophenolic acid in an effort to individualize dosing.

There are few significant drug interactions with MMF. However, concomitant administration of other antiproliferative agents, such as azathioprine or TOR inhibitors, should be done with caution to avoid excessive myelosuppression. Drugs that can decrease intestinal absorption of MMF include antacids, cholestyramine, and oral ferrous sulfate. Cyclosporine can also decrease MMF concentrations by interfering with the enterohepatic cycling, an effect not seen with tacrolimus. This explains the higher dose of MMF sometimes needed when used together with cyclosporine compared with tacrolimus.

TOR inhibitors The newest antiproliferative agents are the TOR inhibitors. Target of rapamycin is an important regulatory kinase involved in cell cycle progression. There are two medications in this class. Sirolimus (Rapamune), also known as rapamycin, is a macrolide antibiotic compound structurally related to tacrolimus. Everolimus (Certican or Zortress) is a chemical variant of sirolimus and was approved by the FDA in 2010. Initially, there was great enthusiasm for using sirolimus as an alternative to CNIs. However, as the side-effect profile of TOR inhibitors emerged, enthusiasm for new uses of this TOR inhibitor have waned. As sirolimus is structurally similar to tacrolimus, it also binds the FKBP. However, the sirolimus–FKBP ligand does not block calcineurin, but instead blocks the effects of TOR (see Figure 7.9). As mentioned, TOR is a key regulatory kinase in cell division, hence its blockade leads to the inhibition of cellular proliferation. The TOR pathway also has an angiogenic effect, so, unlike other antiproliferative agents, sirolimus has unique antiangiogenic properties.

Sirolimus was initially formulated as an oral solution but it has now been replaced by the more convenient oral form that comes in 1 mg and 5 mg capsules. Its usual dose is 2–5 mg daily. Sometimes an initial loading dose (up to 15 mg daily for 3 days) is used to more rapidly reach a steady state. Similar to the CNIs, sirolimus is metabolized by the cytochrome P450 enzyme and has the same variations in between- and within-patient bioavailability. Therefore, blood level monitoring is required. The target level ranges from 10 ng/mL to 20 ng/mL, with a lower target of 8–12 ng/mL in stable patients. As sirolimus has a long half-life, averaging 62 h, drug levels do not need to be checked until several days after a dose adjustment.

Given that both CNIs and sirolimus are metabolized by cytochrome P450, there is a potential interaction when these two classes of medication are given together. It has been shown that, when sirolimus is given with cyclosporine, there can be a significant increase in sirolimus levels. However, this effect can be avoided if the sirolimus is given 4 h after cyclosporine. A similar interaction has not been demonstrated with tacrolimus. And like CNIs, sirolimus has similar drug interactions with increased drug levels from concomitant use of non-dihydropyridine calcium channel blockers, azole antifungal agents, erythromycin, and grapefruit juice, whereas decreased drug levels are observed with anticonvulsants such as phenytoin and carbamazepine.

Maintenance drug combinations

It should be obvious that the increased number of available maintenance immunosuppressants for transplant recipients has greatly increased the number of potential drug combinations that can be used to prevent allograft rejection. The most popular combination of drugs currently used in the USA consists of tacrolimus and a mycophenolic acid derivative with or without prednisone. Cyclosporine-based regimens have declined in popularity. As mentioned above, donor use of sirolimus is no longer common, although some centers convert patients from a CNI to sirolimus several months after transplantation. Azathioprine is most often reserved for patients who are intolerant of the side effects or costs of the other antiproliferative agents.

Case

A 26-year-old man with diabetic nephropathy received a deceased donor kidney transplant 9 months earlier and has been maintained on tacrolimus, enteric-coated mycophenolic acid, and prednisone. Between 4 and 9 months after transplantation, serum creatinine concentration rose from1.3 mg/dL to 2.1 mg/dL despite trough tacrolimus levels deemed to be in a therapeutic range. A 24-hour urine collection contained 320 mg protein. A biopsy was performed and showed patchy interstitial fibrosis and mild arteriolar hyalinosis. Based on the concern for chronic nephrotoxicity from his calcineurin inhibitor, he was converted from tacrolimus to sirolimus. Six months later, serum creatinine concentration is slightly improved (1.9 mg/dL) but repeat 24-hour urine protein has increased to 540 mg/day.

Treatment of acute rejection

Most centers prefer to obtain a percutaneous renal transplant biopsy to facilitate treatment decisions in patients with suspected rejection. Cases of acute cellular rejection that are deemed to be clinically or histologically mild are often treated initially with large "pulse" doses of corticosteroids (typically methylprednisolone in doses ranging from 250 mg to 1000 mg intravenously daily for 3–5 days, or oral prednisone 200–500 mg per day for 3–5 days). Patients who do not respond to pulse steroid therapy, and those with clinically or histologically severe rejection, are treated with anti-lymphocyte preparations including rabbit anti-thymocyte globulin or OKT3. The use of OKT3 for treatment of acute rejection has decreased greatly in the past decade, largely owing to its cost and significant first-dose side effects, including a "cytokine storm" syndrome consisting of fever, headache, flu-like symptoms, and, more rarely, acute respiratory failure. Traditional anti-lymphocyte antibodies are often employed to treat antibody-mediated rejection, based on the concern for simultaneous cellular rejection. However, treatment with plasmapheresis, anti-CD20 antibodies, and/or IVIG is now commonly used as either primary or adjunctive therapy for humoral rejection.

Diagnosis of allograft rejection

Although the cumulative incidence of early acute rejection has decreased dramatically in recent years, acute rejection continues to exert a detrimental impact on allograft survival. An episode of rejection – particularly if severe, recurrent, or late (>1 year post-transplantation) – significantly increases the risk of chronic allograft nephropathy, a major cause of long-term graft loss. Advances in molecular diagnostics, proteomics, and microarray analyses promise to generate non-invasive means for detecting early signs of immune injury. However, the diagnosis of renal allograft rejection currently continues to depend on the detection of changes in renal function (most often by changes in serum creatinine concentration) and on biopsy of the transplanted kidney. It is understood that deterioration of kidney function is a relatively late development in the course of an acute rejection episode, usually detected after significant histologic injury has already occurred.

Acute rejection

Acute cellular rejection

Acute cellular rejection occurs most commonly in the first few days to months after transplantation The immune events leading to this form of rejection center around activation and proliferation of T cells, and are described in detail in Chapter 1. Fever, allograft tenderness, oliguria, or hypertension may be present, but in the era of modern immunosuppression such symptoms are unusual. Often, the transplant recipient is asymptomatic during a rejection episode, and it is an increase in serum creatinine concentration that triggers concern.

The Banff consortium was established to standardize interpretation of renal allograft pathology in clinical trials. With further evolution, the Banff grading system has proved to be useful in guiding therapy and in establishing prognoses. According to revised Banff 2007 criteria, acute cellular rejection is characterized by the presence of tubulitis and arteritis. Leukocyte (usually lymphocyte) infiltration of the tubular epithelium is called "tubulitis," whereas disruption of the arterial intima is referred to as "arteritis." Both the intensity of interstitial infiltrate and the severity of tubulitis and intimal arteritis categorize the grade of rejection as either mild (I), moderate (II), or severe (III) (Table 7.6). Chronic allograft arteriopathy, which encompasses arterial intimal fibrosis and formation of neointima, is the hallmark of chronic cell-mediated rejection. Histopathologic findings suspicious for acute cellular rejection, but insufficient for a firm diagnosis, are deemed "borderline" or "suspicious." Decisions about treatment in these cases are based on the clinical setting.

Table 7.6 Banff 1997 classification system – revised in 2007

Category	Histology
Normal	Normal biopsy
Antibody-mediated rejection	
Acute	Type I: minimal inflammation, acute-tubular necrosis like (C4d positive) Type II: capillary–glomerulitis (C4d positive) Type III: arterial–transmural inflammation/fibrinoid change (C4d positive)
Chronic active	Glomerular double contours, lamellar peritubular capillary basement membrane, interstitial fibrosis, tubular atrophy, arterial fibrous intimal thickening (C4d positive)
Borderline	Findings suspicious for acute T-cell-mediated rejection, but non-diagnostic
T-cell-mediated rejection	
Acute	Significant interstitial inflammation (>25% of parenchyma) with: Type IA: moderate tubulitis (more than four mononuclear cells/tubular section) IIB: severe tubulitis (>10 mononuclear cells/tubular section) Type IIA: mild-to-moderate arteritis IIB: severe arteritis (>25% loss of luminal area) Type III: transmural arteritis/fibrinoid change, necrosis of medial smooth muscle in association with lymphocytic inflammation of the vessel
Chronic active	Chronic allograft arteriopathy (arterial intimal fibrosis with mononuclear cell infiltration and formation of neointima)
Interstitial fibrosis and tubular atrophy	Grade I: mild (<25% of cortical area) Grade II: moderate (25–50% of cortical area) Grade III: severe (>50% of cortical area)
Other	

Adapted from Racusen LC, Solez K, Colvin RB, et al. The Banff 97 working classification of renal allograft pathology. *Kidney Int* 1999;55:713–23 and Solez K, Colvin RB, Racusen LC, et al. Banff '05 meeting report: Differential diagnosis of chronic allograft injury and elimination of chronic allograft nephropathy ("CAN"). *Am J Transplant* 2007;7:518–26.

Antibody-mediated rejection

As many as 25–30% of acute rejection episodes have an antibody-mediated component. In general, identification of antibody-mediated rejection (AMR) portends a worse prognosis, because such cases tend to be refractory to conventional treatment. Donor HLA antigens are the predominant targets. Endothelium-associated donor antigens or ABO isoagglutinins are involved less commonly. The mechanisms leading to antibody-mediated damage to the allograft are discussed in Chapter 1. The discovery that endothelial deposition of the complement split product, C4d, is a footprint for antibody-mediated rejection, has greatly aided the diagnosis of AMR.

Catastrophic rejection within minutes to hours of transplantation, termed "hyperacute rejection," is the result of transplantation across donor-incompatible blood groups or in the presence of high titers of pre-formed donor-specific antibodies. Recipient presensitization, from prior transplantation, pregnancy, blood transfusions, or other antigenic exposures, is required to form the donor-specific antibody so quickly and typically results in a positive complement-dependent cytotoxic cross-match before transplantation. Antibody-mediated endothelial injury leads to a cascade of complement activation, vascular thrombosis, and eventual ischemic necrosis. Grossly, the transplanted kidney is mottled and cyanotic. Marked edema and rupture of the allograft may occur, so that immediate nephrectomy is usually required.

An anamnestic immune response accounts for some cases of AMR that occur days to weeks after transplantation. Such patients usually have evidence of sensitization before transplantation. However, antibody titers are presumably low at the time of transplantation, resulting in a negative complement-dependent cytotoxic cross-match. Antibody titers rise post-transplantation in the presence of an antigenic stimulus (the donor allograft). Accelerated or acute vascular rejection may ensue, presenting as an acute rise in serum creatinine with or without allograft tenderness, oliguria, and hypertension.

AMR also can occur in non-sensitized patients. In most cases, the primary cell-mediated immune response serves as the mechanism for B-cell activation. The severity of the rejection episode varies with antibody titer and relative binding affinity, as well as with the intensity of expression of HLA and other donor-specific antigens within the allograft. Such episodes can occur at any time post-transplantation, particularly during periods of inadequate immunosuppression. Either accelerated or acute vascular rejection may result. Late in the post-transplant course, antibodies may play a role in the development of chronic allograft damage. Numerous studies have documented C4d deposition preceding biopsy findings of transplant glomerulopathy (see below), suggesting an important role for anti-donor antibody and complement activation. Notably, circulating new anti-HLA antibodies can precede renal allograft loss by many months or years.

The Banff classification outlines four features fundamental to the identification of AMR:

1. Allograft dysfunction
2. Morphologic evidence of tissue injury (from minimal inflammation/acute tubular necrosis-like histology to capillary glomerulitis to transmural arterial inflammation and fibrinoid change)
3. Immunopathologic evidence for antibody-mediated action (C4d deposition in the peritubular capillaries)
4. Serologic evidence of circulating antibodies to donor HLA or to other donor endothelial antigens.

Definitive diagnosis requires the presence of three of the four criteria (see Table 7.6). Chronic active AMR is suggested by C4d deposits and glomerular double contours and/or multilayering of the peritubular capillary basement membrane, with or without interstitial fibrosis, tubular atrophy, or arteriolar fibrous intimal thickening.

Case

A 56-year-old multiparous woman had a prior kidney transplant that failed 5 years earlier as a consequence of acute and chronic rejection. Thereafter she became highly sensitized with panel-reactive antibody levels consistently >60% for both class I and class II HLA antigens. Her 28-year-old daughter wished to donate a kidney and was haploidential to her mother. A standard CDC cross-match and anti-human globulin-augmented cross-match were negative but flow cytometry cross-matching revealed a strongly positive T-cell cross-match. The daughter is otherwise healthy and deemed to be a suitable donor. The mother was treated with three courses of plasmapheresis followed by infusions of IVIG. A repeat flow cytometry cross-match was negative, and the living donor transplant was performed with initial success and excellent allograft function. Four weeks after the transplantation, serum creatinine concentration rose and a percutaneous biopsy showed leukocytes in peritubular capillaries with heavy deposits of C4d. The patient was treated with three additional courses of plasmapheresis and IVIG and also received two doses of rituximab. Serum creatinine concentration decreased but never returned to baseline. One year later, a slow rise in serum creatinine concentration and the development of proteinuria (3.5 g/day) prompted a second biopsy that showed glomerular basement membrane duplication compatible with transplant glomerulopathy.

Chronic allograft nephropathy

Renal allograft failure is a common cause of ESRD, and accounts for up to 30% of patients awaiting renal transplantation The most common cause of renal allograft failure is a poorly understood entity, variably referred to as chronic allograft nephropathy, transplant glomerulopathy, chronic renal allograft dysfunction, chronic rejection, or transplant nephropathy. The 2007 Banff consortium re-named chronic allograft nephropathy "interstitial fibrosis and tubular atrophy, without evidence of any specific etiology." Confusion surrounds this disorder because of its complex, multifactorial pathogenesis and the lack of universally accepted diagnostic criteria. In general, chronic allograft nephropathy is characterized by slowly progressive renal allograft dysfunction that usually begins 3 months or more after transplantation, in the absence of active rejection, acute drug toxicity, or another disease. Clinically, recipients develop slowly worsening azotemia, proteinuria (occasionally in the nephrotic range), and worsening hypertension.

Both immune and non-immune mechanisms of injury are implicated in the pathogenesis of chronic allograft nephropathy. The importance of cell-mediated and humoral immunity, HLA mismatch, inflammatory cytokines, anti-inflammatory cytokines, growth factors, and endothelin has been demonstrated both in vitro and in vivo. Hypertension, glomerular hyperfiltration, delayed graft function, ischemia–reperfusion injury, hyperlipidemia, proteinuria, and chronic CNI toxicity are also known contributors. Emerging data suggest that a number of donor factors (age, donor source, and comorbidities) also play a role. Histological changes are similarly diverse, involving all components of the renal parenchyma. Endothelial inflammation leading to fibrous intimal thickening is hypothesized to be one of the initial pathologic events. The glomerular capillary walls thicken with an occasional double-contour appearance, termed "transplant glomerulopathy." This is the most specific finding for chronic allograft nephropathy within the Banff classification scheme. Variable degrees of tubular atrophy and patchy interstitial fibrosis are present. Splitting and lamination of the tubular capillary basement membrane have also been described.

Although glomerular and vascular histologic findings may be more diagnostically specific, Banff criteria grades disease severity according to the amount of interstitial fibrosis and tubular atrophy (see Table 7.6), a better correlate of late graft failure. Another commonly cited index of disease severity is the chronic allograft disease index (CADI) score, which takes into account the percentage of sclerotic glomeruli and vascular change. In some studies, the CADI score from protocol renal biopsies at 2 years are predictive of graft function at 6 years.

Key points 7.7 Factors associated with the development of chronic allograft nephropathy

Immune factors
- Acute rejection episodes
- Recipient-donor HLA mismatching
- Pre-existing or new anti-HLA antibodies
- Inadequate immunosuppression

Non-immune factors
- Hypertension
- Glomerular hyperfiltration
- Ischemia–reperfusion injury
- Delayed graft function
- Hyperlipidemia
- Cytomegalovirus infection
- Calcineurin inhibitor toxicity
- BK polyoma infection

Protocol biopsies

As changes in serum creatinine tend to occur after histologic injury has been initiated, the benefit of surveillance biopsies at defined points after transplantation offers some appeal. Protocol biopsies attempt to identify pathologic changes before allograft dysfunction occurs, at a time when renal injury may be more amenable to treatment. Numerous studies suggest that detection of tubulitis (i.e., subclinical acute rejection) or chronic allograft nephropathy in early protocol biopsies predicts subsequent graft function and loss. Other studies suggest that prompt treatment of subclinical rejection may improve graft survival. However, there are few prospective data about the effect that increasing immunosuppression for subclinical rejection has on long-term clinical outcomes. Many aspects of the natural history of subclinical rejection are simply not known, e.g., the significance of persistent histologic but clinically resolved rejection, and the significance of C4d staining in patients with stable allograft function. In addition, the optimal timing of biopsies is unclear.

Moreover, early enthusiasm for protocol biopsies was based on studies from the cyclosporine era in which the incidence of subclinical rejection in the first 6 months after transplantation was as high as 30%. More recent studies in patients receiving tacrolimus-based immunosuppression suggest rates of <10%, raising serious questions as to whether the benefits of protocol biopsies outweigh their cost and risk. Nevertheless, protocol biopsies may still be valuable in high-risk populations (e.g., recipients with delayed graft function or patients in drug minimization protocols) and currently remain an important tool in research studies.

Molecular diagnosis of rejection

In the search for urinary or serum markers that allow non-invasive and rapid diagnosis of ongoing or imminent immune injury, advancements in molecular technology have allowed for the measurement of candidate molecules or their corresponding genes or messenger RNAs. The molecules studied most extensively are cytotoxic T-cell products such as perforin, granzyme B, and Fas ligand. Peripheral blood leukocyte cytokine production, recipient T-cell responses to donor-specific HLA antigens, and urinary proteomic profiling have all shown correlations with immune injury but require further validation in large scale studies. Quantitative reverse transcriptase polymerase chain reaction (RT-PCR) and DNA microarray assays derived from peripheral blood, urine, or the allograft itself show great promise as non-invasive approaches to detect early immune injury. At this time, all of these assays are used primarily as research tools.

Pancreatic rejection

Pancreas allografts can fail for a variety of reasons. Early graft loss, occurring within hours to days of surgery, is usually secondary to technical failure (thrombosis, leak, bleeding, or pancreatitis). Acute rejection of the pancreas can occur at any time, but typically occurs in the same time frame as described for renal allografts. The diagnosis of acute pancreatic rejection can be difficult using non-invasive tests. Elevations in serum lipase and amylase are non-specific, whereas a rise in fasting serum glucose can occur under conditions of physiologic stress (e.g., infection) or as a late indicator of allograft dysfunction. In simultaneous kidney–pancreas transplantation, rejection of the pancreas allograft alone is uncommon (<15% of cases) and an increase in serum creatinine concentration is often relied on as the earliest indication of concomitant pancreas rejection. In recipients with bladder-drained pancreatic allografts, a serially decreasing urinary amylase has been used as a crude sign of rejection. Some but not all centers perform percutaneous pancreatic biopsies routinely as the definitive means for diagnosing pancreatic rejection. However, biopsy may be technically difficult in some patients, depending on the exact placement of the organ. After the first 6 months post-transplantation, the most common cause of pancreatic graft loss is chronic rejection, with progressive allograft sclerosis (increasing fibrosis and atrophy of the glandular components) secondarily leading to endocrine failure.

Long-term complications

Cardiovascular disease, diabetes mellitus, and hyperlipidemia

Cardiovascular disease remains highly prevalent in kidney transplant recipients and is the most frequent cause of late allograft loss. Traditional risk factors such as smoking and diabetes mellitus influence the risk of cardiovascular disease after transplantation. Additional risk is derived from the presence of CKD before transplantation, particularly in patients with prolonged exposure to dialysis. Some reduction of GFR is common after transplantation and further contributes to cardiac risk. Persistent proteinuria after transplantation is an independent risk factor for cardiovascular disease, and elevations in C-reactive protein and homocysteine are also associated with increased risk.

Specific immunosuppressive agents independently increase cardiovascular risk through an array of side effects that contribute to the metabolic syndrome (Table 7.7). Corticosteroids increase serum lipids, blood pressure, obesity, glucose intolerance, and vascular atherogenesis. Cyclosporine also increases lipids, blood pressure, and glucose intolerance, and can lead to progression of CKD. Tacrolimus appears to have a favorable side-effect profile relative to cyclosporine in terms of lipid elevation and endothelial dysfunction, but is associated with a greater risk

Table 7.7 Semiquantitative associations between various immunosuppressants and cardiovascular risk factors

	Hypertension	Diabetes mellitus	Hyperlipidemia	Nephrotoxicity
Corticosteroids	++	+++	++	–
Cyclosporine	++	+	++	++
Tacrolimus	±	+++	±	++
Sirolimus	–	+	+++	+

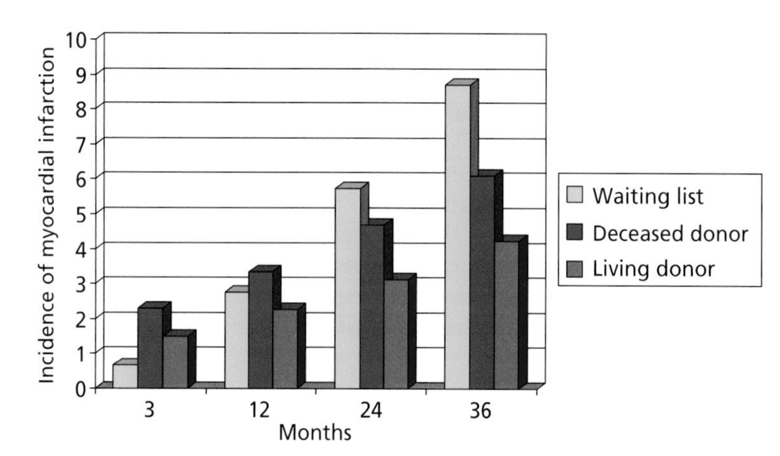

Figure 7.10 Incidence of myocardial infarction over time in wait-listed transplant candidates, deceased donor kidney transplant recipients, and living donor transplant recipients. (Adapted from Kasiske BL, Maclean JR, Snyder JJ. Acute myocardial infarction and kidney transplantation. *J Am Soc Nephrol* 2006;**17**:900–7.)

of glucose intolerance and diabetes mellitus. A randomized trial of 682 patients comparing tacrolimus and cyclosporine therapy found the incidence of new-onset diabetes after transplantation (NODAT) to be 34% versus 26% in *tacrolimus- and cyclosporine-treated* recipients, respectively ($p = 0.05$). However, low-density lipoprotein (LDL)-cholesterol and triglyceride levels were higher in the cyclosporine group.

Sirolimus increases total cholesterol, LDL-cholesterol, and triglycerides relative to other agents, related to a decrease in the metabolism of apoB100-containing lipoproteins. Emerging data have also linked sirolimus to increased insulin resistance and decreased insulin production. Therapy with this TOR inhibitor has also been associated with an increase in proteinuria, further contributing to cardiovascular risk. Despite these risks, sirolimus and other TOR inhibitors have putative antiatherogenic effects mediated, in part, by inhibition of vascular smooth muscle proliferation, as evidenced by the observation that sirolimus-coated stents decrease neointimal proliferation after coronary intervention. It remains to be proven whether systemic therapy with TOR inhibitors conveys protection against cardiovascular disease despite their negative influence on multiple risk factors.

Screening for cardiovascular disease is integral to the evaluation for kidney transplantation, although the benefit gained by preoperative revascularization is unclear (see "Recipient evaluation" above). Adverse cardiovascular events remain highly prevalent after transplantation relative to the general population, but the risk of disease declines over time relative to that of patients remaining on the transplant waiting list. When Kasiske et al. compared analyzed cardiovascular mortality rates after kidney transplantation to rates in wait-listed patients, the adjusted relative cumulative risk of myocardial infarction at 3 years post-transplantation was 0.83 ($p < 0.001$) (see Further reading). Living donor recipients had a greater benefit, with a relative risk of 0.69 ($p < 0.001$). However, the risk of myocardial infarction during the perioperative period exceeded the rate of wait-listed patients (Figure 7.10).

Transplant-associated hyperglycemia and NODAT are common and contribute to cardiovascular and overall mortality after transplantation. The risk of NODAT is roughly 15% in the first post-transplant year, and is followed by a roughly 5% incidence per year for subsequent years. In a Mayo Clinic experience, prediabetic hyperglycemia, defined as fasting glucose between 100 and 125 mg/dL, was present at 1 year in a third of patients who were euglycemic pretransplantation. Considering the significant percentage of transplant recipients with diabetes mellitus at baseline, glucose impairment after kidney transplantation is the norm rather than the exception, particularly in the USA. Pretransplant diabetes mellitus, NODAT, and even pretransplant hyperglycemia are all associated with an increased risk for cardiovascular disease after transplantation. NODAT is also a risk factor for mortality and death-censored graft failure post-transplantation.

Risk factors for NODAT have been elucidated and include non-modifiable and modifiable risks (Table 7.8). One key modifiable risk factor is weight gain, which is typical after transplantation and is associated with black race, poor socioeconomic status, female gender, and younger age. Weight gain is accelerated in the first year post-transplantation and may relate in part to higher steroid doses during this interval. One study of over 600 kidney recipients found that progression to obesity after transplantation increased the risk of diabetes mellitus, hypertension, cardiovascular disease, and deterioration of allograft function.

Table 7.8 Risk factors for development of new-onset diabetes after transplantation

Non-modifiable	Modifiable
Older age	Greater body weight/obesity
Race/ethnicity	Immunosuppressive therapy
Black	Corticosteroids
Hispanic	Tacrolimus
Native American	Cyclosporine
Asian Indian	Sirolimus
Genetic risk/family history	Hepatitis C infection
Impaired glucose tolerance pre-transplantation	
Time post-transplantation	

Adapted from Rodrigo E, Fernandez-Fresnedo G, Valero R, et al. New-onset diabetes after kidney transplantation: risk factors. *J Am Soc Nephrol* 2006;**17**, S291–5.

Hyperlipidemia is common after transplantation and is associated with specific immunosuppressive agents as described above. Over 2000 cyclosporine-treated kidney transplant recipients from Europe and Canada were analyzed in the Assessment of Lescol in Renal Transplantation (ALERT) trial. This double-blinded study randomized patients to fluvastatin (40–80 mg/day) or placebo and monitored outcomes for 5 years. Fluvastatin effectively lowered LDL-cholesterol by a third. The primary endpoint of cardiac death, myocardial infarction, or coronary intervention was not significantly different between groups, but the risk ratio for cardiac death or myocardial infarction was 0.65 ($p = 0.005$) in the fluvastatin group. Treatment was well tolerated with no difference in side effects compared with placebo. In the placebo group, cholesterol level was an independent risk factor for myocardial infarction, further strengthening the argument for statin usage in the kidney transplant population.

Malignancy

Recent data indicate that most types of cancer occur at increased frequency after kidney transplantation compared with the general population. In particular, risk of malignancies related to certain viral infections is increased severalfold. These include EBV-related post-transplant lymphoproliferative disease (PTLD), as well as cervical, skin and lip cancers related to human papillomavirus (HPV). Kaposi's sarcoma is linked to human herpes virus 8 (HHV-8) and has a 10- to 20-fold incidence in transplant recipients relative to the general population (Table 7.9).

Certain cancers such as myeloma, and kidney or urinary tract malignancies are associated with kidney disease and thus are more prevalent in kidney transplant failure patients compared with the general population. Acquired cystic disease is common in ESRD and is a risk factor for renal cell carcinoma. One analysis of kidney recipients found a 1.2%

incidence of renal cell carcinoma at 2–7 years post-transplantation, a rate approximately 10-fold that of the general population.

PTLD represents a spectrum of disease ranging from benign polyclonal proliferation of EBV-positive lymphocytes to a monoclonal non-Hodgkin's B-cell lymphoma that requires aggressive chemotherapeutic treatment (see Chapter 5). PTLD occurs in 1–5% of kidney transplant recipients with the highest incidence observed within the first year after transplantation. It is more commonly seen in children due to the risk related to EBV antibody mismatch with a seronegative recipient. PTLD may present with fever, pharyngitis, and lymphadenopathy. Solid lymphomatous tumors may be found in the chest, gastrointestinal tract, or the kidney allograft. PTLD in the gastrointestinal tract may present with abdominal pain, bleeding, or obstruction.

One study of 25 000 Medicare kidney recipients transplanted between 1996 and 2000 found that PTLD developed in 344 (1.4%). Risk factors for PTLD included antibody induction therapy or rejection treatment with OKT3 or anti-thymocyte globulin, but not with IL-2 receptor antibody-induction therapy. Other risks included absence of serologic evidence for prior exposure to EBV, younger age, pre-transplantation malignancy, and maintenance therapy with tacrolimus.

Recent reports utilizing Medicare data forms have identified an increased risk for most cancers post-transplantation even in the absence of a known viral association (Table 7.9). Kasiske et al. examined US Renal Data System (USRDS) and Medicare data and found that common solid tumors including colon, lung, prostate, and breast cancers were increased roughly twofold within 3 years of transplantation (see Further reading). An analysis of the Canadian Organ Replacement Register database measured the standardized incidence ratio of malignancy, excluding non-melanoma skin cancers. The overall ratio was 2.5 relative to the general population, and no type of cancer was less common after transplantation. Risk of malignancy progressed over time, with a cumulative incidence of >10% after 15 years. A German analysis tracked patients up to 25 years post-transplantation and found a 49.3% incidence of malignancy, compared with a 21% rate for the general population matched for sex and age. Patients who survived longer on immunosuppressive therapy had a greater risk of new malignancy. In an Australian registry analysis, the average time to cancer after transplantation was 9.4 years.

Table 7.9 Relative risk of specific cancer types after kidney transplantation relative to the general population

>10–100	Non-melanoma skin cancer Lip cancer Non-Hodgkin's lymphoma Renal carcinoma Cervical and uterine cancer Penile cancer Anal cancer Kaposi's sarcoma
>1–10	Hodgkin's lymphoma Leukemia Melanoma Esophageal cancer Gastric cancer Hepatic cancer Biliary carcinoma Colon cancer Lung cancer Thyroid carcinoma Head and neck cancer Bladder cancer Pancreatic cancer Breast cancer Testicular cancer

Screening for malignancy in patients with reasonable life expectancy is clearly warranted after kidney transplantation. Skin surveillance with an annual examination by the transplant surgeon or a dermatologist is recommended. Women should have annual pelvic examinations and cytological studies, and women aged >40 or with a first-degree family history of breast cancer at age <50 should undergo yearly mammography and self-breast examinations. Colonoscopy is warranted in patients aged >50 or with a primary family history of malignancy. Digital rectal examination along with serum prostate specific antigen should be considered in all men aged >50 years. Annual chest radiographs may be considered in smokers. Lung cancer is increased approximately twofold in transplant recipients, and smoking cessation must be stressed. Patients with chronic liver disease or viral hepatitis should be screened with liver ultrasonography every 6–12 months.

Increased risk of cancer is thought to be related to potent immunosuppressive therapy. However, sirolimus appears to have unique anti-neoplastic properties. The drug inhibits the TOR which prevents downstream activation of cellular translation through inhibition of Akt and p79S6 kinase, and secondarily inhibits angiogenic growth factors such as vascular endothelial growth factor (VEGF). Animal models have demonstrated a reduction in tumor progression of kidney cancer cells. A study of 33 249 deceased donor kidney recipients reported to the OPTN database showed that the incidence rates of malignancy were 0.6% with sirolimus-based therapy compared with 1.8% in patients on cyclosporine or tacrolimus-based treatment. Sirolimus may have a particular benefit in the treatment of Kaposi's sarcoma. Fifteen transplant recipients converted from cyclosporine to sirolimus showed complete resolution of Kaposi's sarcoma lesions. Other case reports have demonstrated similar success, although a recent series did not show uniform resolution, particularly in more severe cases.

Bone disease

Bone disease is common after kidney transplantation, and risk for fracture increases over time with a rate greater than that seen in dialysis patients. Risk is related in part to osteoporosis, with a higher incidence of fractures in postmenopausal women. Although guidelines exist for monitoring bone mineral density (BMD) after transplantation, low BMD does not consistently correlate with the risk of fracture. Risk factors for fracture after transplantation include older age, diabetic status, and previous fractures before transplantation. Steroid usage likely contributes to bone demineralization and low bone turnover after transplantation, although BMD has been shown to decline in a similar fashion early post-transplantation even in the absence of corticosteroids. Steroid usage has been clearly linked to the development of osteonecrosis, a severe adverse event that typically involves the femoral head and typically requires surgical repair.

Studies incorporating bone biopsy in kidney recipients show a mixture of low bone turnover disease and increased bone resorption, making treatment decisions difficult in the absence of histologic analysis. Although studies have used BMD as a surrogate outcome, few have analyzed fracture rates between groups. Vitamin D supplementation increases BMD, and can help control hyperparathyroidism early after transplantation. Bisphosphonates have also been shown to increase BMD, but their use may contribute to low bone turnover disease. Furthermore, is not clear whether bisphosphonates prevent fracture after kidney transplantation.

Post-transplant hyperparathyroidism is common, and parathyroid hormone (PTH) levels tend to fall gradually but remain elevated in most transplant recipients. The implications of persistent hyperparathyroidism after kidney transplantation are unclear. One report identified tubulointerstitial calcification of the renal allograft in 18% of protocol biopsies at 6 months, and patients with calcification had higher PTH and serum calcium levels. High PTH in the face of calcification also predicted inferior graft function at 1 year. However, over 60% of patients in this cohort received phosphorus supplementation, which may have contributed to the risk of calcium phosphate calcification in the allograft. A second study analyzed bone biopsy and urinary calcium in kidney recipients with high PTH and hypercalcemia. These patients had a surprising mix of high and low bone turnover disease, with most demonstrating low-to-normal levels of urinary calcium excretion, suggesting an increase in renal tubular calcium uptake. This study brings into question the benefit of parathyroidectomy, which may be inappropriate in patients with low bone turnover disease. Current guidelines recommend waiting 1 year for PTH levels to fall, and considering parathyroidectomy only when serum calcium levels remain >11.5 mg/dL. Calcimimetic therapy with cinacalcet has been used with some success after kidney transplantation. Both parathyroidectomy and cinacalcet have been associated with a reduction in renal allograft function, perhaps related to an increase in hypercalcuria.

Current status of islet cell transplantation

The field of islet cell transplantation was revolutionized in 2000 when investigators from the University of Alberta in Edmonton described a small group of patients with type 1 diabetes who remained insulin independent for more than 1 year after receiving intrahepatic injections of islet cells.

Notably, the major indication for islet cell transplantation was hypoglycemic unawareness, and none of the patients in this landmark trial had advanced complications of diabetic microvascular disease at the time of transplantation. The success of this protocol was attributed to the use of advanced techniques for isolating and preparing islets from human pancreata, the fact that most patients in the series required islets from two or more separate donor organs, and the then novel immunosppressive protocol that completely avoided corticosteroids, but included an anti-IL-R antibody for induction and maintenance therapy with "low-dose" tacrolimus and sirolimus. The unexpected short-term success of this protocol spawned the initiation of a National Institute for Health (NIH)-sponsored multicenter study in the USA, originally intended to use the "Edmonton protocol" to facilitate successful islet cell transplantation. Outside the NIH study, a number of other centers were motivated to begin islet cell transplant programs based on the Edmonton experience.

However, long-term outcomes of islet cell transplant recipients treated with the Edmonton protocol or closely related protocols have been disappointing. Almost 80% of patients have returned to insulin dependence after 5 years. Some of these patients continue to show evidence of islet cell activity, as evidenced by the presence of detectable C-peptide levels, and may still be protected from hypoglycemic unawareness. Even more concerning, however, is the observation that the vast majority of islet cell transplants develop evidence of HLA sensitization, especially when the islets fail and immunosuppression is withdrawn. These high rates of sensitization could reflect both the use of multiple donors in most cases and the robust presence of antigen-presenting cells in islet cell preparations. As mentioned earlier in this and other chapters, both tacrolimus and sirolimus are diabetogenic, so it remains possible that some long-term islet cell failures may reflect drug toxicity and not immune injury. Whatever the mechanisms, investigators in the field are currently studying new immunosuppressants, including a number of new biologic agents, in an effort to improve long-term outcomes and to minimize the numbers of donor pancreata needed to acquire insulin independence. In the meantime, islet cell transplantation is regarded by many to remain an experimental treatment for type 1 diabetes mellitus.

References

Adams PL, Cohen DJ, Danovitch GM, et al. The nondirected live-kidney donor: ethical considerations and practice guidelines: A National Conference Report. *Transplantation* 2002;**74**:582–9.

Ahsan N, Holman MJ, Jarowenko MV, et al. Limited dose monoclonal IL-2R antibody induction protocol after primary kidney transplantation. *Am J Transplant* 2002; **2**:568–73.

Alejandro R, Barton FB, Hering BJ, et al. 2008 update from the Collaborative Islet Transplant Registry. *Transplantation* 2008;**86**:1783–8.

Andres A, Morales JM, Herrero JC, et al. Double versus single renal allografts from aged donors. *Transplantation* 2000;**69**:2060–9.

Ardoli A, Lampertico P, Montagnino G, et al. Natural history of hepatitis B and C in renal allograft recipients. *Clin Transplant* 2005;**19**:364–6.

Augustine JJ, Bodziak KA, Hricik DE. Use of sirolimus in solid organ transplantation. *Drugs* 2007;**67**:369–91.

Augustine JJ, Hricik DE. Steroid sparing in kidney transplantation: changing paradigms, improving outcomes, and remaining questions. *Clin J Am Soc Nephrol* 2006;**1**: 1080–9.

Baid-Agrawal S, Delmonico FL, Tolkoff-Rubin NE, et al. Cardiovascular risk profile after conversion from cyclosporine A to tacrolimus in stable renal transplant recipients. *Transplantation* 2004;**77**:1199–202.

Bakir N, Sluiter WJ, Ploeg RJ, et al. Primary renal graft thrombosis. *Nephrol Dial Transplant* 1996;**11**: 140–7.

Ball AM, Gillen DL, Sherrard D, et al. Risk of hip fracture among dialysis and renal transplant recipients. *JAMA* 2002;**288**:3014–18.

Balupuri S, Buckley P, Snowden C, et al. The trouble with kidneys derived from the non heart-beating donor: a single center 10-year experience. *Transplantation* 2000; **69**:842–6.

Bloom DD, Hu H, Fechner JH, et al. T-lymphocyte alloresponses of Campath 1-H treated kidney transplant patients. *Transplantation* 2006;**81**:81–7.

Borchhardt K, Sulzbacher I, Benesch T, et al. Low-turnover bone disease in hypercalcemic hyperparathyroidism after kidney transplantation. *Am J Transplant* 2007;**7**:2515–21.

Boulware LE, Troll MU, Wang NY, et al. Public attitudes toward incentives for organ donation: a national study of different racial/ethnic and income groups. *Am J Transplant* 2006;**6**:2774–85.

Brekke IB, Lien B, Sodal G. Aortoiliac reconstruction in preparation for renal transplantation. *Transplant Int* 1993;**6**:161–3.

Brennan DC, Daller JA, Lake KD, et al. Rabbit antithymocyte globulin versus basiliximab in renal transplantation. *N Engl J Med* 2006;**355**:1967–77.

Briganti EM, Russ GR, McNeil JJ, Atkins RC, Chadban SJ. Risk of renal allograft loss from recurrent glomerulonephritis. *N Engl J Med* 2002;**347**:103–9.

Bustami RT, Ojo AO, Wolfe RA, et al. Immunosuppression and the risk of post-transplant malignancy among cadaveric first kidney transplant recipients. *Am J Transplant* 2004;**4**:87–93.

Caillard S, Dharnidharka V, Agodoa L, et al. Posttransplant lymphoproliferative disorders after renal transplantation in the United States in era of modern immunosuppression. *Transplantation* 2005;**80**:1233–43.

Cameron JI, Whiteside C, Katz J, Devins GM. Differences in quality of life across renal replacement therapies: a meta-analytic comparison. *Am J Kidney Dis* 2000;**35**:629.

Chan GLC, Canafax DM, Johnson CA. The therapeutic use of azathioprine in renal transplantation. *Pharmacotherapy* 1987;**7**:165–77.

Chapman JR, O'Connell PJ, Nankivell BJ. Chronic renal allograft dysfunction. *J Am Soc Nephrol* 2005;**16**: 3015–26.

Cherikh WS, Kauffman HM, McBride MA, et al. Association of the type of induction immunosuppression with post-transplant lymphoproliferative disorder, graft survival, and patient survival after primary kidney transplantation. *Transplantation* 2003;**76**:1289–93.

Clemens KK, Thiessen-Philbrook H, Parikh CR, et al. Psychosocial health of living kidney donors: a systematic review. *Am J Transplant* 2006;**6**:1965–77.

Clunk JM, Lin CY, Curtis JJ. Variables affecting weight gain in renal transplant recipients. *Am J Kidney Dis* 2001; **38**:349–53.

Coco M, Glicklich D, Faugere MC, et al. Prevention of bone loss in renal transplant recipients: a prospective, randomized trial of intravenous pamidronate. *J Am Soc Nephrol* 2003;**14**:2669–76.

Cohen D, Galbraith C. General health management and long-term care of the renal transplant recipient. *Am J Kidney Dis* 2001;**38**(suppl 6):10–24.

Cosio FG, Kudva Y, van der Velde M, et al. New onset hyperglycemia and diabetes are associated with increased cardiovascular risk after kidney transplantation. *Kidney Int* 2005;**67**:2415–21.

Cueto-Manzano AM, Konel S, Hutchison AJ, et al. Bone loss in long-term renal transplantation: histopathology and densitometry analysis. *Kidney Int* 1999;**55**:2021–9.

Curtis JJ. Cyclosporine and posttransplant hypertension. *J Am Soc Nephrol* 1992;**2**(12 suppl):243–5.

D'Alessandro AM, Odorico JS, Knechtle SJ, et al. Simultaneous pancreas-kidney (SPK) transplantation from controlled non-heart beating donors (NHBDs). *Cell Transplant* 2000;**9**:889–93.

Danovitch GM, Leichtman AB. Kidney vending: The "Trojan Horse" of organ transplantation. *Clin J Am Soc Nephrol* 2006;**1**:1133–5.

De La Vega LS, Torres A, Bohorquez HE, et al. Patient and graft outcomes from older living kidney donors are similar to those from younger donors despite lower GFR. *Kidney Int* 2004;**66**:1654–61.

De Lima JJ, Sabbaga E, Vieira ML, et al. Coronary angiography is the best predictor of events in renal transplant candidates compared with noninvasive testing. *Hypertension* 2003;**42**:263–8.

Delmonico FL. Exchanging kidneys–advances in living-donor transplantation. *N Engl J Med* 2004;**350**:1812–14.

Dimeny EM. Cardiovascular disease after renal transplantation. *Kidney Int Suppl* 2002;**80**:78–84.

Drachenberg CB, Papadimitriou JC. Spectrum of histopathological changes in pancreas allograft biopsies and relationship to graft loss. *Transplant Proc* 2007;**39**:2326–8.

Drafts HH, Anjum MR, Wynn JJ, Mulloy LL, Bowley JN, Humphries AL. The impact of pre-transplant obesity on renal transplant outcomes. *Clin Transplant* 1997;**11**: 493–6.

Dreno B. Skin cancers after transplantation. *Nephrol Dial Transplant* 2003;**18**:1052–8.

Ducloux D, Kazory A, Chalopin JM. Predicting coronary heart disease in renal transplant recipients: a prospective study. *Kidney Int* 2004;**66**:441–7.

Dunn CJ, Wagstaff AJ, Perry CM, et al. Cyclosporin: an updated review of the pharmacokinetic properties, clinical Efficacy and tolerability of a microemulsion-based formulation (neoral) in organ transplantation. *Drugs* 2001;**61**: 1957–2016.

EBPG (European Expert Group on Renal Transplantation); European Renal Association (ERA-EDTA); European Society for Organ Transplantation. European Best Practice Guidelines for Renal Transplantation (part 1). *Nephrol Dial Transplant* 2000;**15**(suppl 7):1–85.

el-Agroudy AE, Wafa EW, Gheith OE, et al. Weight gain after renal transplantation is a risk factor for patient and graft outcome. *Transplantation* 2004;**77**:1381–5.

Fehrman-Ekholm I, Elinder CG, Stenbeck M, et al. Kidney donors live longer. *Transplantation* 1997;**64**:976–8.

Fernández-Fresnedo G, Escallada R, Rodrigo E, et al. The risk of cardiovascular disease associated with proteinuria in renal transplant patients. *Transplantation* 2002;**73**: 1345–8.

First MR. Improving long-term renal transplant outcomes with tacrolimus: speculation vs evidence. *Nephrol Dial Transplant* 2004;**19**(suppl 6):17–22.

Friedman JS, Meier-Kriesche HU, Kaplan B, et al. Hypercoagulable states in renal transplant candidates: impact on anticoagulation upon incidence of renal allograft thrombosis. *Transplantation* 2001;**72**:1073–8.

Fung JJ. Tacrolimus and transplantation: a decade in review. *Transplantation* 2004;**77**(9 suppl):41–3.

Gaston RS, Danovitch GM, Epstein RA, et al. Limiting financial disincentives in live organ donation: a rational solution to the kidney shortage. *Am J Transplant* 2006;**6**: 2529–30.

Gill JS, Abichandani R, Kausz AT, Pereira BJ. Mortality after kidney transplant failure: the impact of non-immunologic factors. *Kidney Int* 2002;**62**:1875–83.

Gjertson DW, Cecka JM. Living unrelated donor kidney transplantation. *Kidney Int* 2000;**58**:491–9.

Gloor JM, Sethi S, Stegall MD, et al. Transplant glomerulopathy: subclinical incidence and association with alloantibody. *Am J Transplant* 2007;**7**:2124–32.

Glotz D, Antoine C, Julia P, et al. Desensitization and subsequent kidney transplantation of patients using intravenous immunoglobulins (IVIg). *Am J Transplant* 2002;**2**: 758–60.

Go AS, Chertow GM, Fan D, et al. Chronic kidney disease and the risks of death, cardiovascular events, and hospitalization. *N Engl J Med* 2004;**351**:1296–305.

Grotz WH, Mundinger FA, Gugel B, et al. Bone fracture and osteodensitometry with dual energy X-ray absorptiometry in kidney transplant recipients. *Transplantation* 1994;**58**: 912–15.

Gruessner RWG, Nakhleh R, Tzardis P et al. Rejection patterns after simultaneous pancreaticoduodenal-kidney transplants in pigs. *Transplantation* 1994;**57**:756.

Guba M, von Breitenbuch P, Steinbauer M, et al. Rapamycin inhibits primary and metastatic tumor growth by antiangiogenesis: involvement of vascular endothelial growth factor. *Nature Med* 2002;**8**:128–35.

Gutierrez-Dalmau A, Campistol JM. Immunosuppressive therapy and malignancy in organ transplant recipients: a systematic review. *Drugs* 2007;**67**:1167–98.

Gwinner W, Suppa S, Mengel M, et al. Early calcification of renal allografts detected by protocol biopsies: causes and clinical implications. *Am J Transplant* 2005;**5**: 1934–41.

Haajanen J, Saarinen O, Laasonen L, et al. Steroid treatment and aseptic necrosis of the femoral head in renal transplant recipients. *Transplant Proc* 1984;**16**:1316–19.

Hariharan S. Recurrent and de novo disease after renal transplantation. *Semin Dial* 2000;**13**:195–9.

Hariharan S, Johnson CP, Bresnahan BA, Taranto SE, McIntosh MJ, Stablein D. Improved graft survival after renal transplantation in the United States, 1988 to 1996. *N Engl J Med* 2000;**342**:605–12.

Heimbach JK, Taler SJ, Prieto M, et al. Obesity in living kidney donors: clinical characteristics and outcomes in the era of laparoscopic donor nephrectomy. *Am J Transplant* 2005;**5**:1057–64.

Henderson AJ, Landolt MA, McDonald MF, et al. The living anonymous kidney donor: lunatic or saint? *Am J Transplant* 2003;**3**:203–13.

Hochleitner BW, Kafka R, Spechtenhauser B, et al. Renal allograft rupture is associated with rejection or acute tubular necrosis, but not with renal vein thrombosis. *Nephrol Dial Transplant* 2001;**16**:124–7.

Hoogeveen RC, Ballantyne CM, Pownall HJ, et al. Effect of sirolimus on the metabolism of apoB100- containing lipoproteins in renal transplant patients. *Transplantation* 2001;**72**:1244–50.

Huston J, Torres VE, Sullivan PP, Offord KP, Wiebers DO. Value of magnetic resonance angiography for the detection of intracranial aneurysms in autosomal dominant polycystic kidney disease. *J Am Soc Nephrol* 1993;**3**: 1871–7.

Ibrahim HN, Foley RF, Tan L, et al. Long-term consequences of kidney donation. *N Engl J Med* 2009;**360**: 459–69.

Infectious Disease Committee of the American Society of Transplantation. Solid organ transplantation in the HIV-infected patient. *Am J Transplant* 2004;**4**(suppl 10):83–8.

Ishani A, Ibrahim HN, Gilberstson D, Collins AJ. The impact of residual renal function on graft and patient survival rates in recipients of preemptive renal transplants. *Am J Kidney Dis* 2003;**42**:1275–82.

Isoniemi H, Taskinen E, Hayry P. Histological chronic allograft damage index accurately predicts chronic renal allograft rejection. *Transplantation* 1994;**58**:1195–8.

Jardine AG, Fellström B, Logan JO, et al. Cardiovascular risk and renal transplantation: post hoc analyses of the Assessment of Lescol in Renal Transplantation (ALERT) Study. *Am J Kidney Dis* 2005;**46**:529–36.

Jassal SV, Schaubel DE, Fenton SSA. Baseline comorbidity in kidney transplant recipients: A comparison of comorbidity indices. *Am J Kidney Dis* 2005;**46**:136–42.

Johnson EM, Anderson JK, Jacobs C, et al. Long-term follow-up of living kidney donors: quality of life after donation. *Transplantation* 1999;**67**:717–21.

Jordan SC, Tyan D, Stablein D, et al. Evaluation of intravenous immunoglobulin as an agent to lower allosensitization and improve transplantation in highly sensitized adult patients with end-stage renal disease: report of the NIH IG02 trial. *J Am Soc Nephrol* 2004;**15**:3256–62.

Josephson MA, Schumm LP, Chiu MY, et al. Calcium and calcitriol prophylaxis attenuates posttransplant bone loss. *Transplantation* 2004;**78**:1233–6.

Kahan BD. The era of cyclosporine: twenty years forward, twenty years back. *Transplant Proc* 2004;**36**(2 suppl): 378S–91S.

Kasiske BL, Cangro CB, Hariharan S, et al., American Society of Transplantation. The evaluation of renal transplantation candidates: Clinical practice guidelines. *Am J Transplant* 2001;**1**:3–95.

Kasiske BL, Guijarro C, Massy ZA, et al. Cardiovascular disease after renal transplantation. *J Am Soc Nephrol* 1996;**7**:158–65.

Kasiske BL, Klinger D. Cigarette smoking in renal transplant recipients. *J Am Soc Nephrol* 2000;**11**:753–9.

Kasiske BL, Maclean JR, Snyder JJ. Acute myocardial infarction and kidney transplantation. *J Am Soc Nephrol* 2006;**17**:900–7.

Kasiske BL, Snyder JJ, Gilbertson D, Matas AJ. Diabetes mellitus after kidney transplantation in the United States. *Am J Transplant* 2003;**3**:178–85.

Kasiske BL, Snyder JJ, Gilbertson DT, Wang C. Cancer after kidney transplantation in the United States. *Am J Transplant* 2004;**4**:905–13.

Kasiske BL, Snyder JJ, Matas AJ, Ellison MD, Gill JS, Kausz A. Preemptive kidney transplantation: The advantage and the advantaged. *J Am Soc Nephrol* 2002;**13**:1358–64.

Kasiske BL. Epidemiology of cardiovascular disease after renal transplantation. *Transplantation* 2001;**72**(6 suppl): 5–8.

Kauffman HM, Cherikh WS, Cheng Y, et al. Maintenance immunosuppression with target-of-rapamycin inhibitors is associated with a reduced incidence of de novo malignancies. *Transplantation* 2005;**80**:883–9.

Kok NFM, Lind MY, Hansson BME, et al. Comparison of laparosocopic and mini incision open donor nephrectomy: single blind, randomised controlled clinical trial. *BMJ* 2006;**333**:221–4.

Koo HP, Bunchman TE, Flynn JT, et al. Renal transplantation in children with severe lower urinary tract dysfunction. *J Urol* 1999;**161**:240–5.

Kumar MS, Sierka DR, Damask, et al. Safety and success of kidney transplantation and concomitant immunosuppression in HIV-positive patients. *Kidney Int* 2005;**67**: 1622–9.

Kuypers DR. Benefit-risk assessment of sirolimus in renal transplantation. *Drug Saf* 2005;**28**:153–81.

Le A, Wilson R, Douek K, et al. Prospective risk stratification in renal transplant candidates for cardiac death. *Am J Kidney Dis* 1994;**24**:65–71.

Lebbé C, Euvrard S, Barrou B, et al. Sirolimus conversion for patients with posttransplant Kaposi's sarcoma. *Am J Transplant* 2006;**6**:2164–8.

Lee PC, Terasaki PI, Takemoto SK, et al. All chronic rejection failures of kidney transplants were preceded by the development of HLA antibodies. *Transplantation* 2002; **74**:1192–4.

Lee YH, Huang WC, Chang LS, et al. The long-term stone recurrence rate and renal function change in unilateral nephrectomy urolithiasis patients. *J Urol* 1994;**152**: 1386–8.

Lentine KL, Brennan DC, Schnitzler MA. Incidence and predictors of myocardial infarction after kidney transplantation. *J Am Soc Nephrol* 2005;**16**:496–506.

Lindenauer PK, Pekow P, Wang K, et al. Perioperative betablocker therapy and mortality after major noncardiac surgery. *N Engl J Med* 2005;**353**:349–61.

Linne Y, Barkeling B, Rossner S. Natural course of gestational diabetes mellitus: long term follow up of women in the SPAWN study. *Br J Obstet Gynaecol* 2002;**109**: 1227–31.

Luan FL, Ding R, Sharma VK, et al Rapamycin is an effective inhibitor of human renal cancer metastasis. *Kidney Int* 2003;**63**:917–26.

McFalls EO, Ward HB, Moritz TE, et al. Coronary-artery revascularization before elective major vascular surgery. *N Engl J Med* 2004;**351**:2795–804.

Maes BD, Vanrenterghem YF. Cyclosporine: advantages versus disadvantages vis-à-vis tacrolimus. *Transplant Proc* 2004;**36**(2 suppl):40S–9S.

Matas AJ, Bartlett ST, Leichtman AB, et al. Morbidity and mortality after living kidney donation, 1999–2001: survey of United States transplant centers. *Am J Transplant* 2003;**3**:830–4.

Matas AJ. Why we should develop a regulated system of kidney sales: a call for action! *Clin J Am Soc Nephrol* 2006;**1**:1129–32.

Mauiyyedi S, Pelle P, Saidman S. Chronic humoral rejection: Identification of antibody mediated chronic renal allograft rejection by C4d deposits in peritubular capillaries. *J Am Soc Nephrol* 2001;**12**:574–82.

Meier-Kriesche HU, Blaiga R, Kaplan B. Decreased renal function is a strong risk factor for cardiovascular death after renal transplantation. *Transplantation* 2003;**75**: 1291–5.

Meier-Kriesche HU, Kaplan B. Waiting time on dialysis as the strongest modifiable risk factor for renal transplant outcomes: a paired donor kidney analysis. *Transplantation* 2002;**27**:1377–81.

Meier-Kriesche HU, Schold JD, Kaplan B. Long-term renal allograft survival: have we made significant progress or is it time to rethink our analytic and therapeutic strategies? *Am J Transplant* 2004;**4**:1289–95.

Meier-Kriesche HU, Steffen BJ, Hochberg AM et al. Mycophenolate mofetil versus azathioprine therapy is associated with a significant protection against long-term renal allograft function deterioration. *Transplantation* 2003;**75**:1341–6.

Melvin WS, Bumgardner GL, Davies EA, et al. The laparoscopic management of post-transplant lymphocele. A critical review. *Surg Endosc* 1997;**11**:245–8.

Merion RM, Ashby UB, Wolfe RA, et al. Deceased-donor characteristics and the survival benefit of kidney transplantation. *JAMA* 2005;**294**:2726–33.

Miller LW. Cardiovascular toxicities of immunosuppressive agents. *Am J Transplant* 2002;**2**:807–18.

Monier-Faugere MC, Mawad H, Qi Q, et al. High prevalence of low bone turnover and occurrence of osteomalacia after kidney transplantation. *J Am Soc Nephrol* 2000;**11**:1093–9.

Montgomery RA, Hardy MA, Jordan SC, et al. Consensus opinion from the antibody working group on the diagnosis, reporting and risk assessment for antibody-mediated rejection and desensitization protocols. *Transplantation* 2004;**78**:181.

Montgomery RA, Simpkins CE, Segey DL. New options for patients with donor incompatibilities. *Transplantation* 2006;**82**:164–5.

Montgomery RA, Zachary AA, Racusen LC, et al. Plasmapheresis and intravenous immune globulin provides effective rescue therapy for refractory humoral rejection and allows kidneys to be successfully transplanted into cross-match-positive recipients. *Transplantation* 2000;**70**:887–95.

Montgomery RA, Zachary AA, Ratner LE, et al. Clinical results from transplanting incompatible live kidney donor/recipient pairs using kidney paired donation. *JAMA* 2005;**294**:1655–63.

Morales JM, Campistol JM. Transplantation in the patient with hepatitis C. *J Am Soc Nephrol* 2000;**11**:1343–53.

Nashan B, Moore R, Amlot P, et al. Randomized trial of basiliximab versus placebo for control of acute cellular rejection in renal allograft recipients. *Lancet* 1997;**i**:1193.

Neuzillet Y, Lay F, Luccioni A, et al. De novo renal cell carcinoma of native kidney in renal transplant recipients. *Cancer* 2005;**103**:251–7.

Nicolau C, Torra R, Badenas C, et al. Autosomal dominant polycystic kidney disease types 1 and 2: assessment of US sensitivity for diagnosis. *Radiology* 1999;**213**:273–6.

Nogueira JM, Cangro CB, Fink JC, et al. A comparison of recipient renal outcomes with laparoscopic versus open live donor nephrectomy. *Transplantation* 1999;**67**:722–8.

O'Connor KJ, Delmonico FL. Increasing the supply of kidneys for transplantation. *Semin Dialysis* 2005;**18**: 460–462.

Ojo AO, Hanson JA, Meier-Kriesche H, et al. Survival in recipients of marginal cadaveric donor kidneys compared with other recipients and wait-listed transplant candidates. *J Am Soc Nephrol* 2001;**12**:589–97.

Opelz G, Döhler B. Lymphomas after solid organ transplantation: a collaborative transplant study report. *Am J Transplant* 2004;**4**:222–30.

O'Shaughnessy EA, Dahl DC, Smith CL, Kasiske BL. Risk factors for fractures in kidney transplantation. *Transplantation* 2002;**74**:362–6.

Palmer SC, McGregor DO, Strippoli GF. Interventions for preventing bone disease in kidney transplant recipients. *Cochrane Database Syst Rev* 2007;(3):CD005015.

Peng LW, Logan JL, James SH, et al. Cinacalcet-associated graft dysfunction and nephrocalcinosis in a kidney transplant recipient. *Am J Med* 2007;**120**:e7–9.

Penn I. The effect of immunosuppression on pre-existing cancers. *Transplantation* 1993;**55**:742–7.

Pilmore H. Cardiac assessment for renal transplantation. *Am J Transplant* 2006;**6**:659–65.

Pirsch JD. Medical evaluation for pancreas transplantation: Evolving concepts. *Transplant Proc* 2001;**33**:3489–91.

Pirsch JD, D'Alessandro AM, Sollinger HW, et al. Hyperlipidemia and transplantation: etiologic factors and therapy. *J Am Soc Nephrol* 1992;**2**(12 suppl):238–42.

Polyak MM, Arrington BO, Stubenbord WT, et al. The influence of pulsatile preservation on renal transplantation in the 1990s. *Transplantation* 2000;**69**:249–58.

Rabbat CG, Treleaven DJ, Russell JD, et al. Prognostic value of myocardial perfusion studies in patients with end-stage renal disease assessed for kidney or kidney-pancreas transplantation: a meta-analysis. *J Am Soc Nephrol* 2003; **14**:431–9.

Racusen LC. Protocol transplant biopsies in kidney allografts: why and when are they indicated? *Clin J Am Soc Nephrol* 2006;**1**:144–7.

Racusen LC, Solez K, Colvin RB, et al. The Banff 97 working classification of renal allograft pathology. *Kidney Int* 1999;**55**:713–23.

Rana A, Robles S, Russo MJ, et al. The combined organ effect; protection against rejection? *Ann Surg* 2008; **248**:871–9.

Ratner LE, Ciseck LJ, Moore NG, et al. Laparoscopic live donor nephrectomy. *Transplantation* 1995;**60**:1047–9.

Ratner LE, Kavoussi LR, Sroka M, et al. Laparoscopic assisted live donor nephrectomy – a comparison with the open approach. *Transplantation* 1997;**63**:229–33.

Redman JF. An anterior extraperitoneal incision for donor nephrectomy that spares the rectus abdominis muscle and anterior abdominal wall nerves. *J Urol* 2000;**164**:1898–900.

Reese PP, Beckman J. Cardiac assessment for renal transplantation should be evidence based. *Am J Transplant* 2006;**6**:659–65.

Rizvi SA, Nagvi SA, Jawad F, et al. Living kidney donor follow-up in a dedicated clinic. *Transplantation* 2005; **79**:1247–51.

Rodrigo E, Fernandez-Fresnedo G, Valero R, et al. New-onset diabetes after kidney transplantation: risk factors. *J Am Soc Nephrol* 2006;**17**, S291–5.

Rubin NE, Williams WW, Cosimi AA, et al. Chronic humoral rejection: Identification of antibody mediated chronic renal allograft rejection by C4d deposits in peritubular capillaries. *J Am Soc Nephrol* 2001;**12**:574–82.

Rush D. Protocol Transplant biopsies: an underutilized tool in kidney transplantation. *Clin J Am Soc Nephrol* 2006;**1**:138–43.

Schaub S, Rush D, Wilkins J, et al. Proteomic-based detection of urine proteins associated with acute renal allograft rejection. *J Am Soc Nephrol* 2004;**15**:219–27.

Schold JD and Meier-Kriesche HU. Which renal transplant candidates should accept marginal kidneys in exchange for a shorter waiting time on dialysis? *Clin J Am Soc Nephrol* 2006;**1**:532–8.

Schwaiger JP, Lamina C, Neyer U, et al. Carotid plaques and their predictive value for cardiovascular and all-cause mortality in hemodialysis patients considering renal transplantation: A decade follow-up. *Am J Kidney Dis* 2006; **47**:888–97.

Schwartz J, Stegall MD, Kremers WK, et al. Complications, resource utilization, and cost of ABO-incompatible living donor kidney transplantation. *Transplantation* 2006;**82**: 155–63.

Schwarz A, Rustien G, Merkel S, et al. Decreased renal transplant function after parathyroidectomy. *Nephrol Dial Transplant* 2007;**22**:584–91.

Scott LJ, McKeage K, Keam SJ, et al. Tacrolimus: a further update of its use in the management of organ transplantation. *Drugs* 2003;**63**:1247–97.

Shapiro AM, Lakey JR, Ryan EA, et al. Islet cell transplantation in seven patients with type 1 diabetes mellitus using a glucocorticoid-free immunosuppressive regimen. *N Engl J Med* 2000;**343**:230–8.

Shapiro R, Basu A, Tan H, et al. Kidney transplantation under minimal immunosuppression after pretransplant lymphoid depletion either thymoglobulin or campath. *J Am Coll Surg* 2005;**200**:505–15.

Solez K, Colvin RB, Racusen LC, et al. Banff '05 meeting report: Differential diagnosis of chronic allograft injury and elimination of chronic allograft nephropathy ("CAN"). *Am J Transplant* 2007;**7**:518.

Sollinger H. Enteric-coated mycophenolate sodium: therapeutic equivalence to mycophenolate mofetil in de novo renal transplant patients. *Transplant Proc* 2004;**36**(suppl):S517–20.

Sousa JE, Costa MA, Abizaid A, et al. Lack of neointimal proliferation after implantation of sirolimus-coated stents in human coronary arteries: a quantitative coronary angiography and three-dimensional intravascular ultrasound study. *Circulation* 2001;**103**:192–5.

Srinivas TR, Schold JD, Womer KL, et al. Improvement in hypercalcemia with cinacalcet after kidney transplantation. *Clin J Am Soc Nephrol* 2006;**1**:323–6.

Stallone G, Schena A, Infante B, et al. Sirolimus for Kaposi's sarcoma in renal-transplant recipients. *N Engl J Med* 2005;**352**:1317–23.

Stegall MD, Gloor J, Winters JL, et al. A comparison of plasmapheresis versus high-dose IVIG desensitization in renal allograft recipients with high levels of donor specific alloantibody. *Am J Transplant* 2006;**6**:346–51.

Steinbrook R. Public solicitation of organ donors. *N Engl J Med.* 2005;**353**:441–4.

Strey C, Grotz W, Mutz C, et al. Graft survival and graft function of pediatric en bloc kidneys in paraaortal position. *Transplantation* 2002;**73**:1095–9.

Swanson SJ, Kirk AD, Ko CW, Jones CA, Agodoa LY, Abbott KC. Impact of HIV seropositivity on graft and patient survival after cadaveric renal transplantation in the United States in the pre highly active antiretroviral therapy (HAART) era: an historical cohort analysis of the United States Renal Data System. *Transplant Infect Dis* 2002;**4**:144–7.

Szczech LA, Berlin JA, Aradhye S, et al. Effect of antilymphocyte induction on renal allograft survival: a meta-analysis. *J Am Soc Nephrol* 1997;**8**:1771–7.

Tanabe K. Calcineurin inhibitors in renal transplantation. *Drugs* 2003;**63**:1535–48.

Teutonico A, Schena PF, Di Paolo S. Glucose metabolism in renal transplant recipients: effect of calcineurin inhibitor withdrawal and conversion to sirolimus. *J Am Soc Nephrol* 2005;**16**:3128–35.

Textor SC, Taler SJ, Driscoll N, et al. Blood pressure and renal function after kidney donation from hypertensive living donors. *Transplantation* 2004;**78**:276–82.

Textor SC, Taler SJ, Larson TS, et al. Blood pressure evaluation among older living kidney donors. *J Am Soc Nephrol* 2003;**14**:2159–67.

Torres A, Rodríguez AP, Concepción MT, et al. Parathyroid function in long-term renal transplant patients: importance of pre-transplant PTH concentrations. *Nephrol Dial Transplant* 1998;**13**(suppl 3):94–7.

Truog RD. The ethics of organ donation by living donors. *N Engl J Med.* 2005;**353**:444–6.

Vajdic CM, McDonald SP, McCredie MR, et al. Cancer incidence before and after kidney transplantation. *JAMA* 2006;**296**:2823–31.

Valapour M, Kahn JP, Rogers TB, et al. How voluntary is consent for living donation? *Am J Transplant* 2006;**6**(suppl 2):465–6[A].

Valente JF, Hricik DE, Weigel K, et al. Comparison of sirolimus versus mycophenolate mofetil on surgical complications and wound healing in adult kidney transplantation. *Am J Transplant* 2003;**3**:1128–34.

van den Akker JM, Wetzels JF, Hoitsma AJ. Proteinuria following conversion from azathioprine to sirolimus in renal transplant recipients. *Kidney Int* 2006;**70**:1355–7.

van den Ham EC, Kooman JP, Christiaans ML, van Hooff JP. The influence of early steroid withdrawal on body composition and bone mineral density in renal transplantation patients. *Transplant Int* 2003;**16**:82–7.

Van Paassen P, Van Breda Vriesman PJ, Van Rie H, et al. Signs and symptoms of thin basement membrane nephropathy: a prospective regional study on primary glomerular disease – The Limburg Renal Registry. *Kidney Int* 2004;**66**:909–13.

van Roijen JH, Kirkels WJ, Zietse R, et al. Long-term graft survival after urological complications of 695 kidney transplantations. *J Urol* 2001;**165**:1884–7.

Vasconcellos LM, Asher F, Schachter D, et al. Cytotoxic lymphocyte gene expression in peripheral blood leukocytes correlates with rejecting renal allografts. *Transplantation* 1998;**66**:562.

Vautour LM, Melton LJ 3rd, Clarke BL, et al. Long-term fracture risk following renal transplantation: a population-based study. *Osteoporos Int* 2004;**15**:160–7.

Vella JP, Spadafora-Ferreira M, Murphy B et al. Indirect allorecognition of major histocompatibility complex allopeptides in human renal transplant recipients with chronic graft dysfunction. *Transplantation* 1997;**64**: 795.

Villeneuve PJ, Schaubel DE, Fenton SS, et al. Cancer incidence among Canadian kidney transplant recipients. *Am J Transplant* 2007;**7**:941–8.

Vincenti F, Friman S, Scheuermann E, et al. Results of an international, randomized trial comparing glucose metabolism disorders and outcome with cyclosporine versus tacrolimus. *Am J Transplant* 2007;**7**:1506–14.

Vincenti F, Kirkman R, Light S, et al. Interleukin-2 receptor blockade with daclizumab to prevent acute rejection in renal transplantation. *N Engl J Med* 1998;**338**: 161–5.

Vongwiwatana A, Gourishankar S, Campell PM, et al. Peritubular capillary changes and C4d deposits are associated with transplant glomerulopathy but not IgA nephropathy. *Am J Transplant* 2004;**4**:124–9.

Walker BR. Glucocorticoids and cardiovascular disease. *Eur J Endocrinol* 2007;**157**:545–59.

Watson CJ, Bradley JA, Friend PJ, et al. Alemtuzumab (Campath-1H) induction therapy in cadaveric kidney transplantation – efficacy and safety at five years. *Am J Transplant* 2005;**5**:1347–53.

Webb AT, Franks PJ, Reaveley DA, Greenhalgh RM, Brown EA. Prevalence of intermittent claudication and risk factors for its development in patients on renal replacement therapy. *Eur J Vasc Surg* 1993;**7**:523–7.

Webster AC, Lee VW, Chapman JR, et al. Target of rapamycin inhibitors (sirolimus and everolimus) for primary immunosuppression of kidney transplant recipients: a systematic review and meta-analysis of randomized trials. *Transplantation* 2006;**81**:1234–48.

Weisinger JR, Carlini RG, Rojas E, Bellorin-Font E. Bone disease after renal transplantation. *Clin J Am Soc Nephrol* 2006;**1**:1300–13.

Wilkinson A. Protocol Transplant biopsies: are they really needed? *Clin J Am Soc Nephrol* 2006;**1**:130–7.

Wimmer CD, Rentsch M, Crispin A, et al. The janus face of immunosuppression – de novo malignancy after renal transplantation: the experience of the Transplantation Center Munich. *Kidney Int* 2007;**71**:1271–8.

Wissing KM, Broeders N, Moreno-Reyes R, et al. A controlled study of vitamin D3 to prevent bone loss in renal-transplant patients receiving low doses of steroids. *Transplantation* 2005;**79**:108–15.

Wolf JS, Merion RM, Leichtman AB, et al. Randomized controlled trial of hand-assisted laparoscopic versus open surgical live donor nephrectomy. *Transplantation* 2001; **72**:284–90.

Wolfe RA, Ashby VB, Milford EL, et al. Comparison of mortality in all patients on dialysis, patients on dialysis awaiting transplantation, and recipients of a first cadaveric transplant. *N Engl J Med* 1999;**341**:1725–30.

Wood K. Outlook for longer lasting islets. *Nature Med* 2008;**14**:1156–7.

Woodward RS, Schnitzler MA, Baty J, et al. Incidence and cost of new onset diabetes mellitus among U.S. wait-listed and transplanted renal allograft recipients. *Am J Transplant* 2003;**3**:590–8.

Wrenshall LE, McHugh L, Felton P, et al. Pregnancy after donor nephrectomy. *Transplantation* 1996;**62**:1934–6.

Wynn JJ, Distant DA, Pirsch JD, et al. Kidney and pancreas transplantation. *Am J Transplant* 2004;**4**(suppl 9):72–80.

Zahr E, Molano RD, Pileggi A, et al. Rapamycin impairs in vivo proliferation of islet beta-cells. *Transplantation* 2007;**84**:1576–83.

Zenios SA, Woodle ES, Ross LF. Primum non nocere: avoiding harm to vulnerable wait list candidates in an indirect kidney exchange. *Transplantation* 2001;**72**:648–54.

8 Heart transplantation

Maryl R Johnson, Walter G Kao, Elaine M Winkel, Joseph L Bobadilla, Takushi Kohmoto, and Niloo M Edwards
University of Wisconsin School of Medicine and Public Health, Madison, Wisconsin, USA

The past four decades have seen remarkable improvements in the medical and surgical treatment of end-stage heart disease, including cardiac transplantation. Advances in surgical techniques, immunosuppression and medical management have improved transplant survival with each passing year. Improved outcomes and experience have resulted in expanded eligibility for transplantation. Advancements in assist devices and the medical management of heart failure have resulted in an increased need for organs as more patients survive to need transplantation. Consequently, over the last 20 years of the previous century (Figure 8.1), there was a rapid increase in the number of transplantations performed worldwide. However, the advent of other technologies and societal changes has resulted in fewer suitable cardiac donors and correspondingly declining numbers of transplantations performed in the past 10 years. This has occurred despite a better understanding of donor suitability that has allowed the use of donors that would have never been considered appropriate a few years ago.

According to the International Society for Heart and Lung Transplantation (ISHLT) Registry, from January 1, 2004 to June 20, 2006, both adult heart transplant recipients and donors have gradually increased in age, with the average recipient age being 50.7 ± 12.5 years and donor age 38.5 ± 13.0 years. The majority of heart transplant recipients are male (77.1% in the most recent ISHLT Registry report).

Survival after cardiac transplantation has progressively improved (Figure 8.2). Risk factors for mortality within the first year include temporary circulatory support pretransplant, a pretransplant diagnosis of congenital heart disease, the use of a ventricular assist device pretransplant, recipient history of diabetes mellitus, ventilator support pretransplant, dialysis pretransplant, cerebrovascular event pretransplant, recipient previous pregnancy, recipient with infection requiring IV antibiotics within 2 weeks pretransplant, long-term pulsatile device support pretransplant, recipient prior sternotomy, and donor cytomegalovirus (CMV) +/recipient CMV-status. Continuous variables that increase mortality in the first year include recipient age, recipient weight, donor age, ischemic time, center volume (inverse relationship to survival), recipient pretransplant pulmonary artery systolic pressure and pulmonary vascular resistance, recipient pretransplant bilirubin, and recipient pretransplant creatinine. Risk factors for mortality within 5 years following transplantation, conditional on survival to 1 year, include re-transplantation, cardiac allograft vasculopathy within the first year, ventilator at time of transplant, diabetes mellitus, treatment for rejection prior to discharge, treatment for infection prior to transplant discharge, rejection between discharge and first year, total HLA mismatches (0-4 vs 5-6), panel reactive antibody (PRA) >10%, other surgical procedures (excluding cardiac reoperation) prior to transplant discharge, and diagnosis of ischemic heart disease vs. cardiomyopathy. Continuous risk factors for mortality at 5 years include recipient age, donor age, and donor/recipient body mass index ratio (inverse relationship).

Early mortality after transplantation often relates to the severity of illness in the recipient. Therefore, transplantation is a balance between the increased mortality risk of transplanting sicker patients and the improved survival seen in this cohort. Conversely,

Primer on Transplantation, 3rd edition.
Edited by Donald Hricik.

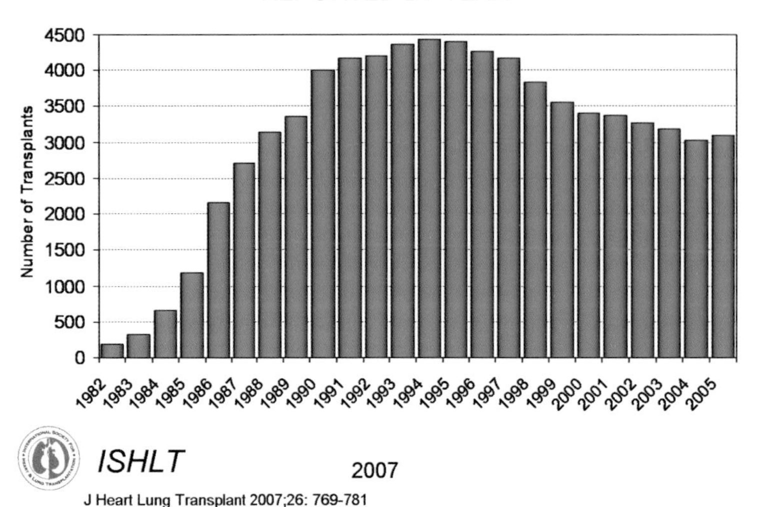

Figure 8.1 Number of heart transplantations performed annually worldwide as reported to the Registry of the International Society for Heart and Lung Transplantation. (Reprinted with permission from Taylor DO, Edwards LB, Boucek MM, et al. Registry of the International Society for Heart and Lung Transplantation: twenty-fourth official adult heart transplant report – 2007. *J Heart Lung Transplant* 2007;**26**:769–81.)

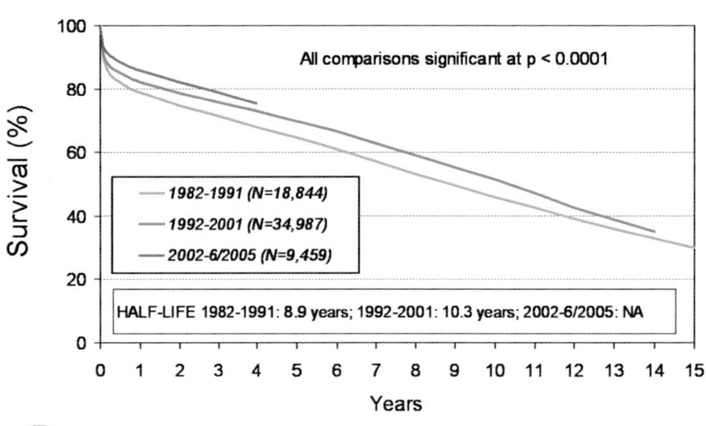

Figure 8.2 Heart transplant survival by era. (Reprinted with permission from Taylor DO, Edwards LB, Boucek MM, et al. Registry of the International Society for Heart and Lung Transplantation: twenty-second official adult heart transplant report – 2007. *J Heart Lung Transplant* 2007;**26**:769–81.)

with the improvement in medical management of heart failure, the survival advantage of transplanting status 2 (see status descriptions later in this chapter) patients has been questioned. This is important because, in the USA in 2004, 36% of patients were status 1A at transplantation, 36% were status 1B, and 28% were status 2. Status 2 patients still accrue a survival advantage from transplantation, although it may take at least 2 years before this survival benefit becomes evident.

Recipient selection

The pretransplant evaluation of a potential recipient (Table 8.1) must not only determine whether the cardiac disease is significant enough to warrant trans-

Table 8.1 Evaluation for heart transplantation

Complete history and physical examination
Chest radiogram
EKG
Echocardiogram
Coronary angiogram
Cardiopulmonary exercise test
Right heart catheterization (with vasodilator challenge when indicated)
Screening laboratory studies (chemistry, hematology, coagulation, endocrine, blood type, lipid panel, HbA1c in patients with diabetes, PSA in males)
Serologic studies (hepatitis A, B, and C; HIV, CMV, EBV, *Toxoplasma* spp., VDRL, varicella)
PPD and anergy testing
Urinalysis
24-hour urine collection (creatinine clearance, protein)
Pulmonary function testing
Carotid artery Doppler study
Lower extremity ankle–brachial indices
Dental radiogram and examination
Ophthalmologic consultation (if has diabetes or aged >50 years)
Abdominal ultrasound examination
Colonoscopy (age ≥50)
Panel-reactive antibody screen
HLA typing
Social work consult
Nutrition consult
Gynecologic exam in females
Mammogram in females aged >40 years
Chest CT if patient aged >40 years, has smoking history, or has had previous chest surgical procedure

CMV, cytomegalovirus; CT, computed tomography; EBV, Epstein–Barr virus; HbA1c, glycated hemoglobin; PPD, purified protein derivative; PSA, prostate-specific antigen; VDRL, Venereal Disease Reference Laboratory.

plantation, but also define the presence of other medical conditions that might compromise outcome after transplantation. Abnormalities discovered on screening should be evaluated definitively before listing, although the presence of severe heart failure can often render it difficult to distinguish between primary end-organ disease and reversible organ dysfunction due to low cardiac output and/or increased venous pressure. This dilemma is particularly manifest in organs such as the kidney and lung, the functions of which reflect perturbations in hemodynamics. In some cases, biopsy may be required to discriminate between reversible dysfunction related to heart failure and permanent parenchymal damage.

Evaluation for heart transplantation revolves around establishment of a survival benefit of transplantation over optimized medical and non-transplant surgical therapies. The current 1-year survival rate after heart transplantation is over 80%, so transplant candidates should be expected to have a worse survival with other surgical or medical options. An in-depth heart failure cardiology evaluation is indicated before consideration for transplantation. Until the patient has failed optimal conventional medical and surgical management, consideration for heart transplantation should remain secondary. The most common reason for referral for heart transplant evaluation is left ventricular systolic dysfunction (regardless of etiology), although patients with angina refractory to maximal medical therapy, life-threatening arrhythmias, right ventricular failure, hypertrophic cardiomyopathy, etc. may also benefit from transplantation. The evaluation must be individualized, because prognostic characteristics vary with the underlying pathology.

Conventional therapy encompasses treatment of underlying myocardial ischemia, valvular dysfunction, arrhythmias, and conduction disorders. Medical therapy should be optimized (addressing neurohumoral and hemodynamic variables), circulatory consequences of other medical conditions (i.e. thyroid disease, anemia) treated, and patient behaviors that adversely affect the heart failure syndrome corrected. In some cases, the full benefit of interventions (i.e., revascularization of ischemic myocardium, β-blocker therapy, and resynchronization therapy) may be delayed and ample time must be allowed to demonstrate their benefits before deciding whether an individual is a candidate for transplantation.

Key points 8.1 If the patient's condition permits it, heart failure should be optimally treated before evaluation and listing for heart transplantation. Optimal therapy includes:

Treatment of myocardial ischemia by percutaneous or surgical revascularization, if indicated and possible

Treatment of valvular heart disease surgically if appropriate

Optimized medical therapy including:
- Angiotensin-converting enzyme (ACE) inhibitor (or angiotensin receptor blocker [ARB])
- β Blocker
- Aldosterone antagonist
- Hydralazine and nitrates (if intolerant of ACE inhibitors and [ARBs])
- Diuretics (as indicated by volume status)

Prevention of sudden death by implantation of implantable cardioverter–defibrillator

Restoration of sinus rhythm in patients with atrial fibrillation or atrial flutter, if possible

Resynchronization therapy in patients with left ventricular dyssynchrony

Optimal treatment of non-cardiac diseases that adversely affect cardiac performance (i.e., thyroid disease, anemia)

Confirmed abstinence from alcohol, smoking, and recreational drug use

Intensive education and counseling in patients with a history of non-compliance

An important component of the transplant evaluation is the assessment of the patient's risk of mortality associated with medical or non-transplant surgical treatment options. This includes an assessment of functional capacity based on cardiopulmonary exercise testing (typically expressed as peak exercise oxygen consumption or $VO_{2\ max}$), the presence of ventricular arrhythmias, measurement of neurohormonal factors (e.g., plasma levels of brain natriuretic peptide and norepinephrine), estimation of ejection fraction, and assessment of the New York Heart Association (NYHA) functional class. Frequently, a consensus prognosis can be estimated. However, many patients exhibit conflicting profiles, with certain parameters suggesting an ominous prognosis whereas others are more reassuring. Reconciling disparate findings is challenging and may mandate additional assessment and/or observation. Some transplant programs calculate a heart failure survival score (as described by Aaronson and Mancini) that incorporates $VO_{2\ max}$, left ventricular ejection fraction, serum sodium, QRS duration, presence or absence of coronary artery disease, and heart rate to stratify patient mortality risk. Patients defined as high risk by the heart failure survival score are considered for listing if they do not have other contraindications to transplantation.

Key points 8.2 The typical profile of a patient listed for heart transplant (as assessed after optimization of heart failure therapy)

Functional classes IIIB–IV

Left ventricular ejection fraction <30%

Cardiac index <2.5 L/min per m^2 (in a euvolemic state)

Peak exercise oxygen consumption <14 mL/kg per min (or even lower in patients clinically stable on β-blocker therapy)

Plasma brain natriuretic peptide level >500 pg/mL

The timing of listing for heart transplantation has been altered by two recent advances:

1. The routine implementation of implantable cardioverter–defibrillators (ICDs) for primary prevention of sudden death
2. The use of mechanical circulatory support devices to support patients as a "bridge" to heart transplantation.

Both technologies allow clinicians a greater margin of safety when dealing with patients whose mortality risk was underestimated, because they allow for the possibility of "rescue to transplant" interventions.

Sudden cardiac death contributes substantially to mortality of patients with heart failure. Although there is a paucity of data in patients with advanced disease, ICDs have been shown to reduce mortality in patients with mild-to-moderate heart failure. In addition, cardiac resynchronization therapy (biventricular pacing) has been shown to improve the functional status and survival of patients with left ventricular systolic dysfunction and dyssynchronous contraction. With further refinement of these therapies, conventional assessments of pretransplant and heart failure mortality will need to be revisited to better determine optimal listing time for heart transplant.

Patients are also screened for conditions that affect perioperative mortality after transplantation. Recent pulmonary embolism, active peptic ulcer disease, smoking or alcohol abuse within 6 months, and active infection are examples of conditions that might preclude transplantation at the time of assessment, but may not be absolute contraindications to transplantation. Other conditions such as multiple prior mediastinal operations, chest wall radiation, or limited venous access must be considered on an individual basis.

In addition, the non-cardiac evaluation for heart transplantation identifies conditions that impact prognosis independent of cardiac status and complicate post-transplant management or compromise outcome. Although the contraindications to heart transplantation (Table 8.2) have evolved to allow consideration of transplantation of increasingly compromised patients, the limited donor supply suggests that centers remain mindful of individual long-term survival and other patients on the transplant wait list. The decision not to list a patient is typically due to multiple coexistent contraindications. Even so, occasionally, combined solid organ transplants (i.e., heart–kidney, heart–liver, heart–lung) can address complicating conditions previously considered preclusive of heart transplant.

Case: recipient selection

A 56-year-old man developed severe left ventricular dysfunction after a myocardial infarction 7 years ago, but with appropriate management with an angiotensin-converting enzyme (ACE inhibitor and a β blocker he had remained functional class II. Six months ago, despite no new clinical events, his symptoms progressed to functional class III. Coronary angiography revealed an occluded left anterior descending artery (LAD) but MRI revealed an infarcted anterior wall. His EKG revealed a QRS duration of 150 ms, so he underwent biventricular pacer/AICD (automatic implantable cardioverter defibrillator) implantation. He was also started on spironolactone. His condition improved for 1–2 months, but over the last few months he has been hospitalized three times for heart failure, despite compliance with his dietary regimen and increasing diuretic therapy. His BNP at his last hospital discharge was 1200 and on

Table 8.2 Possible contraindications to heart transplantation

Condition	Outcomes of concern
Age >65 years	Decreased survival benefit
Primary renal insufficiency	Decreased survival, accelerated progression
Hepatic insufficiency	Decreased survival, abnormal pharmacokinetics
Active peptic ulcer disease	Exacerbation with corticosteroids
Chronic inflammatory bowel disease	Increased infectious risk
Pulmonary vascular disease	Right ventricular failure, decreased survival
Chronic lung disease	Decreased survival, functional limitation, infectious risk
Peripheral vascular disease	Functional limitation, accelerated progression, infectious risk
Stroke (recent)	Hemorrhagic transformation
Pulmonary embolism (recent)	Hemorrhagic transformation, infection
Malignancy	Premature mortality, accelerated progression with immunosuppression
Infection	Spread with immunosuppression
Diabetes mellitus	Premature mortality, end-organ compromise
Amyloid	End-organ compromise, allograft recurrence
Sarcoid	End-organ compromise, allograft recurrence
Obesity	Decreased survival benefit
Medical non-compliance	Inadequate follow-up care, decreased survival
Smoking	Infectious risk, accelerated pulmonary and vascular disease

cardiopulmonary exercise testing his $VO_{2\,max}$ was 9.8 mL/kg per min with a respiratory exchange ratio of 1.15. Transplant evaluation revealed no contraindications to transplantation and the patient was placed on the waiting list.

The waiting list

Once a patient is designated a heart transplant candidate by a program approved by the United Network for Organ Sharing (UNOS), the patient's name is entered on the UNOS heart waiting list with the prospective recipient's ABO blood type and center-established acceptable donor weight range. The patient's transplant priority must also be indicated, using the UNOS priority system (Table 8.3). Donor hearts are allocated based on ABO type, weight range compatibility, acuity, and accumulated waiting time at the designated status for recipients within the local organ procurement organization (OPO). If no local recipients are identified, the organ is offered regionally and then nationally, again discriminating between potential recipients based on ABO type, weight range, status, and time at status. Waiting time depends on a number of factors, including priority status, body size, ABO type, region, and recipient sensitization. As a result of the shortage of donor organs, the interval between listing and transplantation may be long.

When a patient's acuity of illness does not conform to the designated criteria, the transplant center may petition to list the individual at a higher priority that more accurately reflects disease acuity. Examples would include patients with recurrent life-threatening arrhythmias or refractory myocardial ischemia. Such a request is forwarded to a regional review board representing other transplant centers in the region. If the review board agrees, the patient's status is upgraded. At the time of writing, centers may list the patient at the higher status pending the review, but are then subject to review and/or disciplinary action if the review board finds insufficient evidence to justify the higher listing status.

Heart failure management seeks to maximize survival and quality of life, although survival takes precedence for a listed patient. Interventions that may improve quality of life at the expense of mortality risk should be avoided if possible, e.g., the use of outpatient inotropic therapy should be minimized, particularly in the absence of an ICD, because this approach may increase mortality. Patients refractory to oral agents and whose characteristics predict a prolonged wait until transplantation should be considered for mechanical circulatory support with a left ventricular-assist device (VAD), right VAD, or total artificial heart (Figure 8.3). Mechanical circulatory support as a "bridge to transplant" results in improved systemic perfusion and end-organ function, and allows patient rehabilitation, thus optimizing post-transplant outcome. Hospital discharge, which decreases costs

Table 8.3 Heart transplant candidate listing status

UNOS waiting list status (in order of priority)	Patient/Management description
1A	(a) Mechanical circulatory support[a] (excepting LVAD or RVAD)[b] (b) Mechanical circulatory support (including LVAD or RVAD) with complications (c) Continuous mechanical ventilation (d) Continuous infusion of high dose intravenous inotropic agent[c] with continuous invasive hemodynamic monitoring
1B	(a) RVAD and/or LVAD, uncomplicated (b) Continuous infusion of intravenous inotropic agent
2	Patients actively awaiting heart transplant not meeting criteria as 1A or 1B
7	Patients temporarily unsuitable to undergo transplantation

[a]Total artificial heart, intra-aortic balloon pump, or extracorporeal membrane oxygenator.
[b]Patients with an LVAD and/or RVAD (uncomplicated) are allowed 30 days time at 1A status designated at the discretion of the transplant center.
[c]Dobutamine ≥7.5 μg/kg per min, milrinone ≥0.5 μg/kg per min.
LVAD, left ventricular assist device; RVAD, right ventricular assist device.

(a)

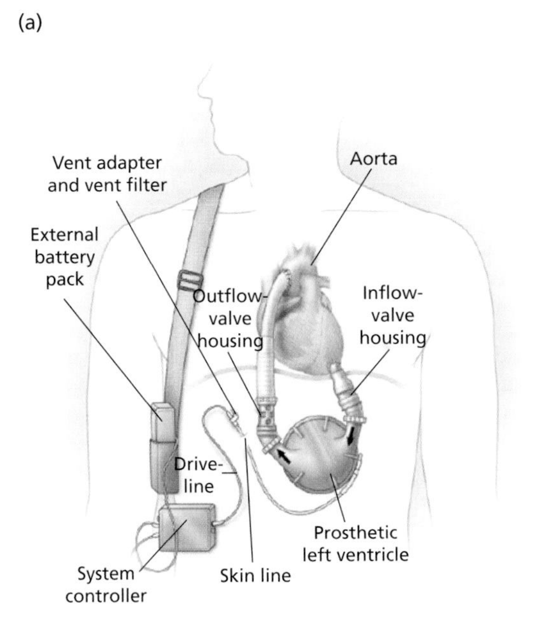

(b)

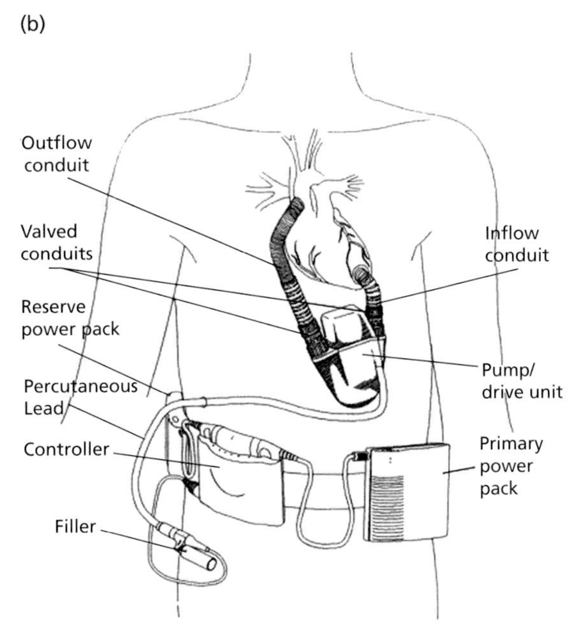

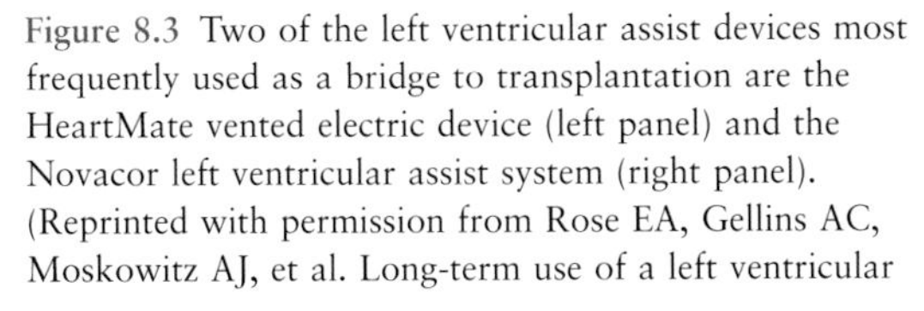

Figure 8.3 Two of the left ventricular assist devices most frequently used as a bridge to transplantation are the HeartMate vented electric device (left panel) and the Novacor left ventricular assist system (right panel). (Reprinted with permission from Rose EA, Gellins AC, Moskowitz AJ, et al. Long-term use of a left ventricular assist device for end-stage heart failure. *N Engl J Med* 2001;**345**:1435–43 (left panel) and Deng MC, Loebe M, El-Banayosy A, et al. Mechanical circulatory support for advanced heart failure: effect of patient selection on outcome. *Circulation* 2001;**103**:231–7 (right panel).)

and encourages rehabilitation, is possible using many of these devices. This alternative must be weighed against the additional surgery and risk of sensitization. If recipient and region characteristics are predictive of a short pretransplant wait, inotropic support in hospital may be considered. However, prolonged hospitalizations result in exposure to nosocomial organisms, end-organ dysfunction, and increased costs.

Case: the waiting list

A 35-year-old woman was referred to the clinic with a 1-month history of progressive fatigue and abdominal complaints, including nausea, vomiting, and right upper quadrant pain. Her lab work was unremarkable. Her symptoms did not improve with a proton pump inhibitor. An abdominal ultrasound scan revealed a large, congested liver, so an echocardiogram was performed which revealed severe diffuse left ventricular dysfunction. On arrival in clinic, she is pale and diaphoretic with cool extremities, a pulse of 120 and regular and blood pressure of 80/64 mmHg. She is euvolemic on examination. It is immediately apparent that she requires hospital admission for aggressive evaluation and therapy. Emergent catheterization and heart biopsy reveal a cardiac index of 1.5 L/min per m^2, pulmonary capillary wedge pressure (PCWP) 20 mmHg, systemic vascular resistance (SVR) 2500 dyn·s/cm^5, normal coronary arteries, and no evidence of myocarditis. Milrinone therapy is begun with no improvement and a slight decrease in blood pressure. The patient is unable to tolerate even 6.25 mg captopril and develops progressive renal insufficiency and increased liver function tests along with increasing ventricular ectopy. Although heart transplant evaluation has not been completed, no obvious contraindications are apparent. The patient undergoes emergency implantation of a HeartMate left VAD as a bridge to allowing complete evaluation for heart transplantation. Her condition stabilizes with left VAD support and, after clinical rehabilitation, she is evaluated for transplantation and placed on the waiting list.

Infections should be treated aggressively because systemic infection constitutes a contraindication to transplantation. This can be problematic in patients with indwelling devices such as assist devices or catheters utilized for chronic intravenous infusions. In the absence of bacteremia or distant seeding, local device or catheter infections are not necessarily a contraindication to transplantation.

Pretransplant blood product transfusions should be avoided if possible to avoid the possibility of sensitization. Leukocyte depletion may decrease the risk of sensitization, and should be used if blood products must be given to transplant candidates. However, because sensitization can render transplantation difficult or impossible, exposure to blood products should still be minimized. This can be problematic because anemia is common in heart failure patients. Patients should be instructed to report all transfusions to the transplant center to allow follow-up testing for sensitization.

Patients with a panel-reactive antibody (PRA) >10% or those demonstrating reactivity to common antigens should undergo prospective cross-matching before transplantation, although "virtual" cross-matching (avoiding unacceptable donor antigens) may be possible. The time constraints imposed by traditional cross-matching can be problematic, especially with distant or unstable donors or recipients in whom an extended explantation is anticipated. When the degree of sensitization renders transplantation unlikely, desensitization should be considered. This entails antibody removal or binding coupled with suppression of antibody production. Serial PRA screening is performed every 4–8 weeks in patients sensitized at the time of evaluation or on VADs (as sensitization can occur, even without additional antigen exposure), and 2 and 4 weeks after transfusion of any blood products.

Routine pretransplant follow-up with the listing transplant center, usually at 4- to 8-week intervals, is recommended. However, in practice, status 2 patients are often followed up less frequently based on the reduced likelihood of imminent transplantation compared with patients who are status 1A or 1B. Close follow-up permits early intervention for conditions that would complicate or preclude transplantation (e.g. infection, pulmonary hypertension), and also allows modification of care and change in status if heart failure worsens. To accurately monitor pulmonary vascular disease, serial right heart catheterizations with vasodilator challenge (if appropriate) are performed at least every 3–6 months. A pulmonary vascular resistance of ≤2.5 Wood units and/or a transpulmonary gradient of ≤15 mmHg on optimized medical therapy (including vasodilator infusions) portends a low risk of post-transplant right ventricular failure and mortality. Resistant pulmonary vascular disease, especially with elevated left-sided filling pressures, may respond to left VAD support, but is generally not regarded as an indication for mechanical support in the absence of advanced clinical disease.

The benefit of optimized medical and surgical pretransplant management is incremental over time, so serial prognostic assessments of listed patients should be performed, particularly measurement of functional capacity by cardiopulmonary exercise testing and contractility by echocardiography. Patients who experience clinical improvement can be removed from the waiting list, either temporarily or permanently, if updated prognostic evaluation suggests a declining benefit of transplantation. More importantly, delisting should be considered for patients who no longer meet the criteria for transplantation. This is often a difficult conversation but can be made easier by taking the time to discuss this possibility with patients and their families at the time of listing/evaluation.

Key points 8.3 The close follow-up by the transplant center needed by patients listed for transplantation

Clinical assessment at least every 4–8 weeks

Right heart catheterizations every 3–6 months

Plasma reactive antibody levels every 4–8 weeks if positive at the time of evaluation or for patients on ventricular assist devices and 2 and 4 weeks after transfusion of any blood products

Cardiopulmonary exercise testing and echocardiography every 6–12 months for clinically stable patients

Donor selection and management

General donor criteria

The first step in defining a potential donor is confirmation of brain death. The organ/tissue donation consent form must then be completed and signed. When the organ procurement team arrives at the donor hospital, the responsible surgeon reviews the chart and confirms the declaration of brain death and consent. It is also crucial to confirm the donor blood type and the UNOS ID. Currently, US centers have instituted at least two separate checks of donor/recipient ABO compatibility, as mandated by UNOS. It is important to confirm ABO type in donors who have had multiple blood transfusions, because massive type O transfusions at resuscitation have resulted in false ABO typing.

Certain factors are a contraindication to donation of any organ, including HIV positivity and major extracranial malignancy. Factors that specifically preclude heart donation include penetrating cardiac trauma, known cardiac disease, or prolonged cardiac arrest with intracardiac injections, although cardiopulmonary resuscitation (CPR) is not an absolute contraindication to organ use.

In 1971, criteria describing the ideal cardiac donor included age <30, no significant medical problems, no history of substance abuse, ischemic time <2 h, and no evidence of infection. Over time, significant changes have been made to these criteria based on experience and the realities of the donor shortage. Heart donor selection criteria vary among centers, but expanded donor criteria at some centers include age >60 years, echocardiographic abnormalities, ischemic time up to 7 h, donor/recipient size mismatch up to 70%, positive donor urine/sputum cultures, significant pressor/inotrope requirements, donor substance abuse, and longstanding diabetes mellitus. Judgments need to be carefully made when evaluating marginal donors, and additional evaluation may be required to assure donor suitability. It is important to realize that donor selection is as much a function of the recipient's medical condition as it is that of the donor.

Tests routinely performed to evaluate the suitability of a donor heart include the following:

- Blood tests, including CBC, chemistry, coagulation, blood type, serology.
- 12-lead EKG (non-specific ST changes associated with brain death do not preclude donation)
- Cardiac enzymes, including creatine phosphokinase MB and troponin (positive cardiac enzymes do not preclude use of the heart, but warrant more careful evaluation)
- Chest radiograph
- Echocardiogram (transthoracic or transesophageal, if needed); echocardiography is used to eliminate donors with abnormalities such as valvular pathology or septal defects; if the donor has a regional wall motion abnormality or ventricular hypertrophy, donor suitability needs to be carefully evaluated; if there is mild, diffuse hypocontractility in a young donor with no history of or reason for cardiac dysfunction, heart donation can still be considered
- Coronary angiography: we recommend coronary angiography for male donors >40 years and female donors >45 years, particularly if the donor has a history of hypertension, smoking, diabetes, cocaine use, or focal EKG or echocardiographic abnormalities. If coronary angiography is not available, direct palpation for plaques by an experienced donor surgeon may represent the only, albeit unreliable, method to evaluate the coronary arteries.

Donor suitability

Whether or not to accept older donors needs to be determined case by case, depending on the recipient's age and urgency for transplantation. The predicted ischemic time also plays a role in determining the suitability of a potential donor. Currently, most centers accept an ischemic time up to 4 h. Although reports indicate that longer ischemic times can be tolerated, especially by younger heart donors, this needs to be assessed individually, particularly in donors considered "marginal" for other reasons. It is not completely elucidated to what extent longer ischemic times affect outcomes because a longer ischemic time may result not only in primary graft failure but also in the need for prolonged inotropic support, a prolonged intensive care unit (ICU) stay, and an increase in cardiac allograft vasculopathy.

Frequently, donors are on inotropic and/or vasopressor support. The need for such support should be carefully assessed. It is helpful to have experienced on-site clinicians to evaluate and manage potential donors. Optimizing volume status, acid–base status, serum electrolytes (especially calcium), body temperature, oxygenation, and hematocrit often reduces the need for inotropic or vasoconstrictor medications.

Donor hearts with cardiac damage such as cardiac contusion or that have received open cardiac massage are not suitable for transplantation. However, it is difficult to diagnose cardiac contusion before opening the chest. Therefore, careful evaluation in the donor operating room is essential. A history of brief closed chest CPR does not preclude the heart from transplantation.

The most common substance abuse is cigarette smoking. If there is a significant history of tobacco use, particularly in an older donor, coronary angiography may be warranted. The second most common substance abuse is alcohol abuse. Caution is suggested as preclinical alcoholic cardiomyopathy could lead to postoperative graft dysfunction.

Illicit drug use includes primarily marijuana and cocaine. Marijuana use by the donor does not preclude heart donation. However, cocaine can cause vasospastic coronary disease and needs particular attention. Various poisons, such as carbon monoxide and cyanide, can cause brain death. The transplant team needs to carefully evaluate such donors, although successful heart transplantations from donors with these exposures have been reported.

It is relatively common to find a positive culture, especially urine or sputum, in donors. However, transmission of bacterial infection from the donor to a heart recipient is rare. When the results of the donor culture and sensitivity tests become available, perioperative antibiotic coverage of the recipient should be modified appropriately. Currently, the use of hepatitis B- and C-positive donors is not recommended, except perhaps for critically ill transplant candidates felt not to have other options.

Donor/Recipient matching

The donor and recipient must be of compatible blood type. If a patient waiting for heart transplantation has a PRA >10%, a prospective cross-match or "virtual" cross-match is mandatory before transplantation. Donor size is matched to recipient size on a weight and height basis. Many centers avoid discrepancies >20%, although successful transplants have resulted with mismatches as great as 50%. Size match crudely estimates that the donor heart is large enough to generate adequate cardiac output to support the recipient, but not so large as to preclude sternal closure or promote tamponade. Many transplant recipients have dilated hearts and, therefore, the pericardial cavity is large enough to accept a larger heart. Although weight and height are the current standards used to assess donor/recipient size compatibility, donor weight is a poor surrogate of heart size or function, and the transplant team needs to recognize this limitation and evaluate each donor/recipient combination case by case.

To prevent post-transplant right heart failure, some centers purposefully use larger donors for recipients with pulmonary hypertension. Although this strategy is theoretical, there are no data to support the practice. On the other hand, use of a smaller donor for recipients with known high pulmonary vascular resistance can be problematic because the donor right heart is not conditioned to pump against high afterload and may develop severe right heart failure early after transplantation.

Donor management

The management of potential deceased donors is discussed in detail in Chapter 3. Continuous monitoring of the donor, including use of an arterial line, central venous pressure monitoring (CVP), and pulse oximetry is recommended. A pulmonary artery (Swan–Ganz) catheter may be helpful in the management of an unstable donor. Attempts should be made to maintain a systolic arterial pressure of 100 mmHg and a mean arterial pressure of 60–65 mmHg. Brain death involves an initial catecholamine surge, followed by depletion, resulting in hypotension related to vasodilation. Hypotension should be treated by replacing fluids (colloid, crystalloid, or packed red blood cells if the hematocrit falls to <25%); if hypotension persists despite apparent euvolemia (CVP = 10–15 mmHg), low-dose inotropic or vasopressor support may be needed. Due to the relative deficiency of vasopressin in brain death, intravenous arginine vasopressin (1–4 units/h) can be effective in maintaining hemodynamic stability in donors. In addition, because of a relative thyroid hormone deficiency in brain death, intravenous levothyroxine (T_4, 20 μg bolus and 40–80 μg/h) may also help reduce inotrope and vasopressor requirements.

Urine output should be maintained at >2 ml/kg per h. Frequently, due to brain death and diabetes insipidus, urine output exceeds 500 mL/h. In such cases, CVP monitoring is essential and desmopressin acetate (a single bolus of 0.5 μg i.v. or infusion at 0.05–0.1 units/min) is given. Fluid replacement should match hourly urine output plus 100 mL, and electrolytes should be monitored and replaced aggressively.

Serial arterial blood gases define the adequacy of ventilation and acid–base status. When managing a donor for multiorgan recovery, a careful balance considering each solid organ is mandatory. Although hydration maintains cardiac and renal function, it is harmful for the lungs; on the other hand, vasoconstriction compromises abdominal organs. Ultimately, striking a balance between hemodynamic stability and end-organ perfusion, while maintaining adequate fluid balance, is the best approach to allow successful recovery of all possible organs.

Case: donor selection and management

A 20-year-old man is declared brain dead 1 day after admission to the neuro-ICU following a rollover car accident. Upon initial declaration of brain death, he is tachycardic with a blood pressure 82/30 mmHg on dobutamine 5 μg/kg per min, dopamine 20 μg/kg per min, norepinephrine 6 μg/kg per min, and vasopressin 6 units/h with a CVP of 1 cmH_2O. There is no evidence of chest wall trauma, no history of cardiac disease, and the troponin is normal. Echocardiogram reveals mild diffuse left ventricular (LV) dysfunction with an LV ejection fraction (LVEF) of 40%. The heart has been turned down for transplantation by three centers but it is requested that the OPO optimize donor volume status, wean the inotropic and vasopressor support as much as possible, and repeat an echocardiogram in 6 h. Six hours later, with a CVP of 7 cmH_2O, the potential donor's blood pressure is 100/60 mmHg on only dobutamine 5 μg/kg per min and vasopressin 4 units/h and the echocardiogram reveals an LVEF of 55%. The heart is transplanted into a 40-year-old man who has been waiting for a heart for more than a year with recent clinical deterioration. The transplant recipient does well and is discharged from the hospital 8 days post-transplantation.

Surgical techniques/perioperative management/early complications

Preparation of the recipient

Recipient preparation begins long before an organ becomes available. A complete history and physical examination with frequent monitoring and updating are important because many transplantations occur off-hours when personnel are at a minimum. Nevertheless, an updated history and physical examination should be completed on admission for transplantation, along with routine laboratory evaluation including: complete blood count (CBC) with differential, coagulation profile with platelet count, electrolytes, creatinine, liver function tests, and a type and cross-match. A chest radiograph should be obtained and the patient made nil by mouth. When time is a concern, the patient may be admitted directly to the operating room with labs drawn at the time of line placement and the chest radiograph obtained there.

Upon donor team confirmation of organ suitability, the recipient can be intubated and anesthesia induced, based on estimated donor organ arrival time and estimated recipient surgical time. Central venous access is obtained and a Swan–Ganz catheter floated into the pulmonary artery. Although it is helpful to know the immediate preoperative pulmonary artery pressures, sometimes the large right atrium and right ventricle make it difficult to float the Swan–Ganz catheter. In these patients, the Swan–Ganz catheter may be floated into the right atrium, where the surgeon can find it and place it under direct vision into the pulmonary artery at the time of implantation. Arterial pressure monitoring should begin, and a Foley catheter should be inserted. Some surgeons opt to dissect out the femoral vessels in patients who have undergone previous thoracic operations to allow cannulation should there be a need to go on emergency bypass. Routine femoral dissection should not, however, be performed, because it can be a source of complications including seroma, wound infection, pain, and restriction of mobility.

Timing of recipient explantation is variable. Some centers wait until the donor heart has arrived in the operating room and others time the explantation so that implantation may occur immediately as the donor heart arrives (Figure 8.4). Dissection in the naive chest can take as little as 45 min. However, complex reoperative dissection, including that performed in patients with a VAD *in situ*, may require more than 2 h. After sternotomy, a pericardial well is created by retracting the pericardium laterally and attaching it to the sternal retractor with 2/0 silk stay sutures. Bone wax should be avoided on the sternotomy edges because it could produce an infectious nidus in the postoperative period.

Aortic cannulation is best done high on the lesser curvature of the arch, allowing excision of the proximal aorta if prior bypass graft sites exist. The cavae

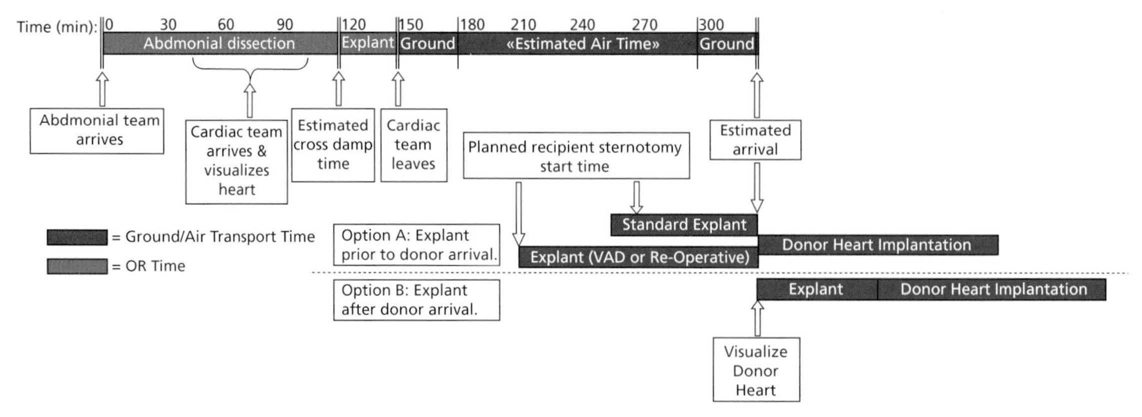

Figure 8.4 Timelines for donor and recipient surgeries for cardiac transplantation. Close coordination and communication between recipient and donor teams is essential.

should be cannulated as far distally as possible and secured with umbilical tape snares around the vessel and cannula. Right-angled metal-tipped cannulae are preferred because they allow smaller purse-string suturing.

The great vessels are dissected free and the aorta is transected just above the sinotubular junction, care being taken while dividing the back wall of the aorta to avoid injuring the right pulmonary trunk. This allows the surgeon to trim the aorta based on donor aortic length and possible excision of prior graft sites. The pulmonary artery is divided just distal to the pulmonary valve. Care must be taken to keep the plane of dissection parallel with the orifice of the pulmonary valve to prevent foreshortening of the pulmonary artery cuff, which leads to a technically difficult anastomosis.

If a biatrial implantation is planned, the left atrial dome is incised just below the aorta and the incision is carried around in a counterclockwise fashion into the atrial septum. Next, the right atrium is incised at the base of the appendage and this incision extended through the septum to the base of the coronary sinus. The remainder of the left atrial cuff is then excised from the atrial dome to the coronary sinus in a clockwise direction (Figure 8.5a). If bicaval implantation is planned, the left atrial resection proceeds as described above. However, the right atrium is divided at the cavoatrial junctions, leaving a short cuff of atrium for later anastomosis (Figure 8.5b). A longer cuff is preferable on the inferior vena cava (IVC), because it tends to retract toward the diaphragm after transection. Finally, the left atrium should be inspected for thrombus and hemostasis of the posterior pericardial space should be achieved before implantation because this region is difficult to visualize after implantation.

Explantation techniques

Donor

Donor heart explantation is performed via a median sternotomy. Communication between the abdominal and thoracic teams is essential for successful procurement on both sides. Upon sternotomy, the donor heart is examined for contusion, infarction, congenital anomalies, aneurysmal disease, or vascular anomalies. The coronary arteries are palpated for plaques and global function is assessed. Once suitability is confirmed, communication to the recipient team as to the expected cross-clamp time must occur (see Figure 8.4).

We recommend that the donor team call the recipient team on arrival at the donor hospital to confirm that there are no delays in the organ procurement. The second call is usually after visualization to confirm the condition of the organ; a third call should be made upon leaving the donor operating room to confirm arrival time at the recipient center.

After the abdominal team has completed dissection, 300 U/kg of heparin is administered and the aorta is cannulated for delivery of cold preservation solution. It is our preference to use 1000–2000 mL of the UW

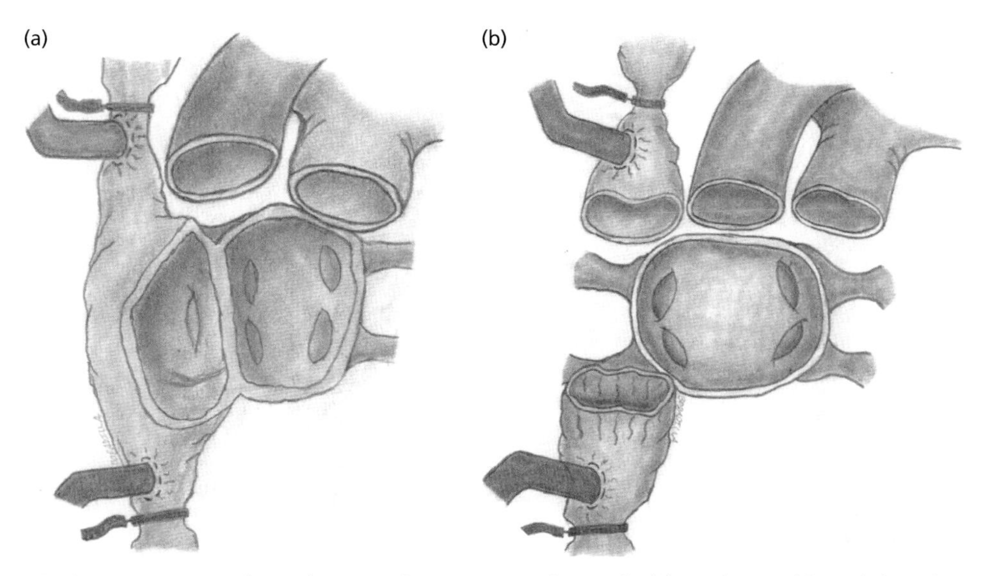

Figure 8.5 Recipient preparation for cardiac transplantation using the standard biatrial (a) and bicaval (b) techniques.

solution. When the anesthesia, abdominal, and thoracic teams are prepared, the heart is decompressed by incising the IVC and left inferior pulmonary vein, the aorta is cross-clamped and the cold preservation solution is infused via the aortic root cannula. Vigorous suction is applied to keep the pericardial well clear and rapid transection of the IVC, pulmonary veins, aorta, superior vena cava (SVC), and pulmonary artery at its bifurcation occurs.

Back-table procedures

Upon return to the recipient institution, back-table dissection prepares the donor heart for implantation. The heart is again inspected for defects – specifically, the foramen ovale is probed for patency. If a patent foramen ovale is found, it is closed in two layers using 4/0 monofilament non-absorbable suture. Next, the pulmonary vein fossae are connected to form a single left atrial cuff for anastomosis. If a biatrial procedure is planned, the SVC is ligated using silk ties and oversewn with a 3/0 or 4/0 monofilament, and the right atrium is incised from the lateral-most portion of the IVC to the base of the right atrial appendage, avoiding the sinus node. If the left atrial appendage was incised to vent the heart during pulmoplegia for simultaneous lung procurement, this should be repaired at this time.

Implantation techniques

Heterotopic transplantation

Heterotopic transplantation is mostly of historical interest. This technique leaves the native heart in place and implants the donor heart in the right chest. This technique was utilized in cases of significant donor-recipient size mismatch or irreversibly elevated pulmonary vascular resistance.

Total excision of recipient atria

Total excision of recipient atria (TERA) and pulmonary vein implantation were first described in 1991. This technique required total excision of the donor atria along with extra lengths of the cavae. With TERA, the donor superior and inferior pulmonary veins are resected on the back table to form a single orifice for the right and left veins. Implantation then proceeds with the left then right pulmonary vein islands, the IVC and SVC, and finally the aorta and pulmonary artery. The added anastomotic time and technical difficulty have prevented widespread acceptance of this technique.

Standard (classic–biatrial) technique

Implantation starts at the base of the left atrial appendage and extends clockwise toward the atrial septum, using a double-armed 3/0 monofilament. Once the septum is reached inferiorly, the second arm is used to complete the superior portion of the left atrial anastomosis. The right atrial anastomosis is completed starting at the mid-portion of the donor right atrium, again with a double-armed 3/0 monofilament. This anastomosis proceeds inferiorly, then superiorly, incorporating the previous septal suture line. Finally, the pulmonary artery and aorta are anastomosed end to end using a running 4/0 monofilament suture.

This biatrial procedure results in a "snowman" or hourglass-shaped atrium. This disruption of atrial geometry may lead to tricuspid and mitral valvular dysfunction and sinus node dysfunction.

Bicaval technique

Concerns over valvular dysfunction and atrial dysfunction resulted in the development of an implantation technique to better preserve atrial anatomy. Sievers and colleagues were among the first to describe the bicaval implantation technique in 1991. Recipient cardiectomy proceeds as previously described, and implantation begins with the left atrial cuff as in the standard technique. Care should be taken to evert the cut edges of the atrial wall to avoid exposed free wall inside the atrial chamber – a potential source of postoperative thrombus. After the left atrial anastomosis is completed, some centers vent the left atria via the appendage and run ice-cold saline to de-air the heart and prevent premature rewarming. It is our practice to wrap the heart in a cold, saline-soaked laparotomy pad and use continuous carbon dioxide flow over the pericardial well to aid in de-airing. At this point, a Swan–Ganz catheter may be manually placed under direct visualization through the SVC and into the pulmonary artery. Attention is then turned to the caval anastomoses, performed end to end using 4/0 monofilament suture; care must be taken not to purse-string the anastomoses. The pulmonary artery is then trimmed and an end-to-end anastomosis performed with 4/0 monofilament; care must be taken here to avoid rotation of the anastomosis. Finally, the aortic anastomosis is performed using 4/0 monofilament as well; however, as the medial wall of the aorta is often stripped of adventitia from the separation from the pulmonary artery, we routinely use reinforcing bovine or autologous pericardial strips.

Since its introduction, the bicaval technique has become the procedure of choice, because of its ability to preserve right atrial conformation, and thus minimize tricuspid regurgitation and nodal arrhythmias. A survey by Aziz et al. in 1999 showed that, among 210 transplant centers worldwide, the bicaval technique was preferred. Multiple groups have documented various benefits to the bicaval technique including:

- improved cardiac output/index, ejection fraction, and exercise tolerance
- lower pulmonary artery pressures and atrial volumes and improved right ventricular function
- lower incidence of atrial arrhythmias/blocks
- reduced mitral and tricuspid regurgitation.

Perioperative management

Once all anastomoses are completed, the patient is placed in the Trendelenburg position, the aortic cross-clamp removed, and the heart de-aired via an aortic root vent. Transesophageal echo (TEE) is instrumental in confirming the removal of all air from the cardiac chambers, as well as for assessing graft function. After de-airing and return of sinus rhythm, the patient is weaned from cardiopulmonary bypass. We utilize inotropic support in all patients, either dobutamine or milrinone, because cardiac function tends to transiently decline 6–8 h post-transplant. After successful weaning of cardiopulmonary bypass, temporary pacing wires are placed in the right atrium and right ventricle, and mediastinal/pericardial drains are placed.

The immediate postoperative period provides many challenges. Vasodilatory hypotension, bleeding, early allograft dysfunction, sinus node dysfunction, right heart failure, and acute renal failure are only a few of the obstacles in the early postoperative period. Continuous invasive hemodynamic monitoring of arterial and pulmonary arterial pressure and back-up pacing are essential. Slow weaning of vasopressor and inotropic support should be attempted over the first 24–48 h. Typically, our institution weans vasoconstrictors first and maintains inotropic support for at least 24 h. It also monitors mixed venous oxygen content. Mixed venous O_2 monitoring allows a physiologic measure of adequacy of systemic perfusion. Attempts should be made to extubate early after return from the operating room.

Early complications

Hypotension

Hypotension can be multifactorial, but tamponade must always be considered. The use of aprotinin and meticulous attention to hemostasis during implantation are of utmost importance. Special attention should be paid to the medial wall of the aorta and the cut edges of the recipient atrial cuffs, as these tend to be foci of bleeding. Given that the mediastinal drains are not obstructed and output is minimal, other causes of hypotension should be considered. Often, systemic inflammatory response syndrome-like conditions evolve as a result of cytokine activation from cardiopulmonary bypass use. Treatment with vasoactive catecholamines, such as norepinephrine, should be initiated if this is suspected. We advocate the use of arginine vasopressin, because it may serve to replace depleted stores, especially in the decompensated heart failure patient.

Early allograft dysfunction

Early allograft dysfunction may also cause postoperative hypotension, characterized by poor cardiac output/index and reduced mixed venous oxygenation. This phenomenon may account for a third of transplant-related deaths, and may be due to ischemia–reperfusion injury, prolonged ischemic times (>4 h), unanticipated donor heart dysfunction, and/or hyperacute rejection. Recent evidence has implicated an inhibitory G-protein-associated pathway, which impairs cardiac contractility and is unregulated in ischemia–reperfusion conditions. Inotropic support is, however, usually enough to maintain patients through the period of ischemia–reperfusion injury-related graft dysfunction, which peaks at 6–8 h post-transplantation. If inotropic support is inadequate to maintain end-organ perfusion, mechanical circulatory assistance (left VAD, right VAD, bi-VAD) should be initiated early.

Hyperacute rejection, which may present as a "stone heart," is a more daunting complication, seen more commonly in people with elevated PRAs. Donor-recipient cross-matching has helped reduce hyperacute rejection in the current era.

Arrhythmias

Bradycardia is the most common postoperative rhythm disturbance. As the resting rate of the denervated heart varies from 90–115 beats/min, rates less than this are often due to sinus node injury or ischemia. Other implications of the denervated heart are discussed later in this chapter. We recommend back-up use of a pacemaker targeted to 90–110 beats/min, especially in the immediate postoperative period. Atrial fibrillation or flutter is uncommon, and may be a sign of graft rejection.

Right heart failure

Right heart failure (RHF) may develop due to right-sided susceptibility to poor myocardial preservation, recipient pulmonary hypertension, and/or ischemia–reperfusion injury. RHF is suspected in the setting of an elevated CVP and/or poor cardiac index. If the patient is intubated, TEE allows optimal visualization of the right heart, compared with standard transthoracic echo. Inotropic support with milrinone is preferred because it also dilates the pulmonary vascular bed. If pulmonary hypertension is present, inhaled nitric oxide may be added to decrease right ventricular afterload. Tight control of volume status guided by pulmonary artery catheter data is essential, and excess fluid should be eliminated with diuretics or continuous venovenous hemofiltration (CVVH).

Renal failure

Acute renal dysfunction may be related to ischemia from cardiopulmonary bypass, thromboemboli, perioperative hypotension, nephrotoxic medications, or intrinsic renal disease. Unfortunately, many cardiac transplant recipients also have dysregulation of normal natriuretic responses, and do not respond appropriately to volume overload. Aggressive volume control with diuresis is needed to prevent right heart strain, especially in the early postischemic phase. In patients whose urine output cannot be matched to the fluid infusion associated with administration of vasopressors, inotropes, and blood products, renal replacement therapy must be entertained. CVVH allows for removal of large volumes of fluid and may serve as a bridge until renal function returns.

Physiology of the denervated heart

During donor heart implantation, the nerve supply is not anastomosed, and therefore the transplanted heart is denervated, at least early after transplantation. This denervation results in an increased resting heart rate (due to lack of vagal tone) and an altered physiologic response to exercise. The increase in cardiac output produced by the transplanted heart early in exercise depends on an increase in venous return due to peripheral muscle pumping of blood back to the heart and the Frank–Starling mechanism. The increase in heart rate with exercise is delayed and prolonged, as it is related to an increase in circulating catecholamines rather than a withdrawal and later increase in vagal tone. With time after transplantation there is partial sympathetic reinnervation, as shown by an increase in coronary sinus norepinephrine in response to intravenous tyramine (which causes degranulation of neural vesicles containing norepinephrine) or sustained handgrip, MIBG (^{131}I-labeled *meta*-iodobenzylguanidine) cardiac uptake on nuclear scanning, PET (positron emission tomography), and an improved heart rate response to exercise. Although partial vagal reinnervation has been suggested, this has not been confirmed to be of clinical relevance.

Early after cardiac transplantation, due to the denervated state, symptoms of myocardial ischemia may be absent or atypical. However, later after transplantation angina may occur. Another clinically relevant implication of the denervated state is that digoxin is relatively ineffective for treating supraventricular tachycardia because the drug usually works in this regard by inhibiting vagal tone. Similarly, atropine is ineffective for treating bradycardia. Supraventricular tachycardia should be treated with direct-acting drugs, including procainamide (which is relatively safe if LV function is normal, and, as vagal tone is not withdrawn, an increase in ventricular response does not occur) or amiodarone. As the denervated heart is exquisitely sensitive to adenosine, adenosine should be used cautiously and in low doses, if at all. Isoproterenol or other direct β stimulants should be used for acute treatment of bradycardia.

Immunosuppression after heart transplantation

Immunosuppressive management after heart transplantation epitomizes the art of medicine. The transplant physician starts with an immunosuppressive protocol that is largely driven by the endomyocardial biopsy grade, and then individualizes therapy based on time since transplantation, risk of rejection, prior rejection history, the presence of hemodynamic compromise, and the presence of cardiac allograft vasculopathy. Standard immunosuppression consists of a combination of drugs in doses that lessen individual toxic effects but together inhibit the immune response. Most centers use triple-drug therapy with corticosteroids, a calcineurin inhibitor CNI (tacrolimus or cyclosporine), and an antiproliferative drug (mycophenolate mofetil or azathioprine), but there are almost as many immunosuppressive protocols as there are heart transplant centers.

Early rejection prophylaxis

Early rejection prophylaxis refers to immunosuppressive therapy given perioperatively and in the first 2 weeks after transplantation. The primary goal is to prevent or delay allograft rejection until ischemia-induced graft dysfunction resolves. Patients are given high doses of intravenous methylprednisolone perioperatively, combined with a CNI and mycophenolate mofetil (MMF) or azathioprine. CNI dosing is determined by whole blood levels and adjusted for creatinine because of the nephrotoxicity associated with these drugs. Initial cyclosporine doses are in the 5–10 mg/kg per day range. Target CSA levels are in the 175–350 ng/mL range, with the highest target levels immediately after transplantation. Less is known about optimal tacrolimus dosing for heart transplant recipients. Initial doses range from 0.075 mg/kg per day to 0.15 mg/kg per day with therapeutic levels of 10–20 ng/mL. MMF is dosed 1000–1500 mg twice daily and azathioprine 2 mg/kg daily. Dosing of all immunosuppressive drugs must be modified if side effects occur.

Heart transplant recipients develop some degree of allograft tolerance, regardless of the early immunosuppression protocol; however, whether tolerance is enhanced by specific protocols remains uncertain. Studies comparing triple-drug immunosuppressive prophylaxis with and without anti-lymphocyte therapy have shown that OKT3 delayed the time to first rejection, but did not confer additional immunologic benefit over triple-drug immunosuppression. A recent report from the Cardiac Transplant Research

Database (CTRD) revealed that anti-lymphocyte therapy was most beneficial in patients at high risk for rejection-mediated death (long-term VAD support, black ethnicity, and extensive HLA mismatching). However, perioperative OKT3 may increase the risk of infection, especially cytomegalovirus (CMV), and lymphoproliferative disease, especially when a cumulative dose of OKT3 exceeds 75 mg.

Antibodies to the interleukin-2 receptor (IL-R2 – daclizumab and basiliximab) have also been used as perioperative immunosuppressive prophylaxis in heart transplantation. In a randomized study, perioperative daclizumab with triple maintenance immunosuppression decreased early rejection. However, there was an increased risk of infectious death in patients who received daclizumab and also received anti-lymphocyte therapy (for renal sparing or to treat rejection). Therefore, combined use of IL-2R antibodies and anti-lymphocyte therapy is not recommended.

Triple-drug immunosuppression without perioperative antibody induction therapy yields excellent patient survival. Although data demonstrate the effectiveness of anti-lymphocyte antibodies in treating recalcitrant rejection, the value of these agents for routine perioperative use remains unclear. Anti-lymphocyte therapy provides no clear benefit compared with standard triple-drug immunosuppression and has been associated with an increased risk of infection and lymphoproliferative disorders. As these agents can produce a severe systemic inflammatory response, and as foreign proteins can induce an immune response limiting subsequent effectiveness, many centers reserve use of anti-lymphocyte agents for refractory rejection. However, perioperative anti-lymphocyte antibody therapy may be valuable to allow delayed initiation of CNIs in patients with renal insufficiency and for maximization of immunosuppression for patients at greater risk for rejection.

Maintenance immunosuppressive strategies

Steroid withdrawal Concerns about the harmful effects of chronic steroid use have stimulated interest in immunosuppressive regimens that eliminate steroids without endangering graft survival. In a review of 670 heart transplant patients from 26 centers in the USA, survival of patients on steroid-free regimens was comparable to that on maintenance steroids. Indeed, data suggest that the ability to wean patients from steroids identifies a group with a lower propensity to reject and a better long-term prognosis.

Yacoub et al. (see Further reading) introduced the concept of steroid-free immunosuppression in 1985, reporting a 1-year actuarial survival rate of 82% in 67 patients in whom steroids were stopped at 3 days while receiving perioperative anti-thymocyte globulin, and maintenance therapy with cyclosporine and azathioprine. There is currently no consensus on the optimal time to withdraw steroids, but two approaches have evolved: early withdrawal (within 1 month), usually with perioperative anti-lymphocyte therapy, or late withdrawal (>3 months post-transplantation) with or without perioperative anti-lymphocyte therapy. A prospective, randomized trial compared double (steroid free) with triple therapy in 112 patients, and reported similar 5-year survival and systolic function if recurrent rejectors in the double-therapy group were converted to maintenance steroids. The Utah program has the largest experience with early steroid withdrawal, both with and without perioperative OKT3, reporting 50–60% 1-year and 40–50% 2-year freedom from maintenance steroids. As most acute rejection occurs in the first 6 months after transplantation, many centers delay steroid withdrawal. Steroid weaning after 6 months yields success rates of 69–80%.

There is no optimum steroid withdrawal protocol or criteria for protocol entry or protocol failure. Some centers consider steroid withdrawal in patients at high risk for complications from steroids whereas others select patients at low rejection risk. Some centers consider protocol failure as one rejection episode with hemodynamic compromise, whereas others do not reinstitute maintenance steroids until up to four rejection episodes have occurred. Predictors of successful steroid withdrawal include withdrawal timing, HLA-DR match, male gender, fewer rejection episodes before steroid withdrawal, the degree of allosensitization, and older age. Late steroid withdrawal in patients with a low propensity for rejection predicts the highest success rate.

Benefits of steroid withdrawal include an improved lipid profile, easier to control hypertension, fewer gastrointestinal complications, and an increased growth velocity in children. About half of patients can be withdrawn from corticosteroids without jeopardizing patient or graft survival, given a few caveats. Perioperative anti-lymphocyte therapy should be considered if steroids are withdrawn early. One rejection episode after steroid withdrawal does not warrant return to steroid use; however, recurrent rejectors should resume steroids. Available data suggest that the greatest success in steroid withdrawal occurs with late withdrawal in patients at low risk of rejection. The low success rate of steroid withdrawal in women especially favors the late approach. Patients intolerant of MMF or azathioprine, or with progressive renal insufficiency indicating the need for lower CNI levels, are not good steroid-withdrawal candidates. Late rejection can occur and warrants surveillance endomyocardial biopsies during weaning and after steroid withdrawal. Close monitoring and optimization of CNI levels is also important.

Calcineurin inhibitors The Collaborative Transplant Study of over 12 000 patients showed superior survival with cyclosporine-based regimens compared with therapy with prednisone and azathioprine alone. In 1994, a microemulsion formulation of cyclosporine was introduced which stabilized the absorption and blood concentration of cyclosporine without increasing toxicity.

The ability of tacrolimus to reverse acute rejection led to investigation of its use as a maintenance immunosuppressive. A small early study comparing tacrolimus with cyclosporine (in combination with both azathioprine and steroids) showed no differences in early rejection or survival, suggesting that tacrolimus was at least as effective as cyclosporine. A more recent and larger study compared a tacrolimus–MMF–steroid regimen with a regimen of cyclosporine–MMF–steroids. The 12-month report from this study revealed no difference in survival between the two groups and a decrease in treated rejection (although only a trend to a decrease in hemodynamically compromising rejection) in the tacrolimus group. Longer-term follow-up data from this study are eagerly awaited. When compared with cyclosporine, tacrolimus has similar nephrotoxic and neurotoxic effects but produces less hypertension, hyperlipidemia, and gingival hyperplasia. There is a propensity for greater glucose intolerance with tacrolimus. CNIs are monitored by whole blood trough levels to guide dose adjustments, although recent data suggest that cyclosporine concentrations at 2 h after administration may better reflect drug exposure.

Antiproliferative drugs Azathioprine dosages must be decreased if leukopenia (white blood cell count or WBC $<3500/mm^3$), anemia, or thrombocytopenia occurs. Concomitant use of trimethoprim–sulfamethoxazole or allopurinol increases the risk of leukopenia. MMF has largely replaced azathioprine because of its superior efficacy in reducing rejection, mortality, and possibly cardiac allograft vasculopathy.

TOR inhibitors

Sirolimus and everolimus are members of a new class of immunosuppressants acting through inhibition of a molecular complex, the target of rapamycin (TOR), which inhibits cell proliferation. Everolimus significantly reduces the incidence of rejection and severity of cardiac allograft vasculopathy in patients at 1 and 2 years compared with azathioprine. A similar 2-year benefit was seen with sirolimus.

Treatment of rejection

Acute cellular rejection

Cellular rejection is treated with a short course of intensified immunosuppression, usually steroids. Rejection occurring up to 6 months post-transplantation is treated more aggressively, as is rejection accompanied by hemodynamic compromise or graft dysfunction. Aggressive immunosuppression may involve high doses of intravenous steroids, an anti-lymphocytic agent for 10–14 days, or an increase in CNI target level.

Refractory allograft rejection

Anti-rejection therapy may successfully reverse acute rejection, but the effects may not be sustained. Anti-lymphocyte antibodies, as discussed above, have shown been to reverse refractory rejection. Low-dose methotrexate is also effective in reversing and chronically suppressing recalcitrant rejection in heart transplant recipients. More recently, conversion to tacrolimus has been shown to reverse rejection refractory to continued therapy with cyclosporine. The addition of sirolimus to the baseline immunosuppressive regimen may also be effective. Total lymphoid radiation, plasmapheresis, and photopheresis have also been used to treat refractory rejection.

Diagnosis of rejection

Rejection surveillance

Rejection remains a lifelong threat to survival, so early recognition and treatment of rejection are a major focus of post-transplant follow-up. There is currently no reliable non-invasive method to diagnose rejection. EKG, echocardiography, radionuclide imaging, and MRI all lack sufficient sensitivity and specificity to replace endomyocardial biopsy, as do cytologic, serologic, and chemical tests. Therefore, patients undergo serial biopsies to detect rejection before loss of graft function. Endomyocardial biopsy is an invasive, yet simple, outpatient procedure with few complications when performed by experienced physicians.

The incidence of rejection is highest in the first 6 months after transplantation, and then falls dramatically (see "Acute rejection"). Therefore, biopsies are performed frequently in the first year. The incidence of rejection is low after 1 year; however, rejection does occur, so most centers continue routine surveillance with endomyocardial biopsy. A typical biopsy schedule would include biopsies weekly for 1 month, every other week for 2 months, monthly for 3 months, and then every 6–8 weeks for the remainder of the first year. During the second year biopsies are performed every 3 months, with biopsies performed every 6–12 months in subsequent years.

Histologic grading system for acute rejection

Acute cellular rejection

Acute cellular rejection manifests histologically as lymphocytic infiltration, with or without myocyte necrosis. It may be accompanied by hemodynamic compromise and can lead to temporary or permanent graft dysfunction. Macrophages and eosinophils may be present, but neutrophilic infiltration suggests a diagnosis other than rejection. Cellular rejection is classified histologically using a standardized grading system as shown in Table 8.4.

Before 1990, there were numerous grading systems for the pathologic diagnosis of rejection in cardiac biopsies. In 1990 the ISHLT developed a standardized grading system for cardiac rejection. This system was widely adopted, but was revised in 2004 to address issues that arose in the previous 15 years. A major issue in the former system concerned grade 2 rejection. As the interobserver variability in diagnosing grade 2 rejection was high and the risk of progression from grade 2 to more severe rejection low, the 1990 ISHLT grades 1A, 1B, and 2 are now combined into the 2004 ISHLT grade 1R.

Antibody-mediated rejection

Antibody-mediated rejection (AMR) is a recognized but controversial entity, associated with poor graft survival. AMR is suspected in the setting of acute graft dysfunction (ventricular systolic dysfunction with or without hemodynamic compromise) in the absence of cellular infiltrate or ischemia. Predisposing factors include prior allosensitization and VAD use. Pathologic findings include immunoglobulin and complement deposition in the coronary vasculature combined with endothelial cell swelling, with or without vasculitis. There is no consensus regarding the histologic or immunologic diagnosis of AMR; however, the revised ISHLT grading scale recommends optional immunofluorescent and immunohistochemical biopsy staining techniques (Table 8.4). If AMR is suspected on light microscopy, further immunohistochemical testing should be performed, along with a serum sample for donor-specific antibody.

Biopsy findings other than rejection

Ischemic injury, the Quilty effect, infection, and lymphoproliferative disorder all cause histologic changes that must be distinguished from rejection. Ischemic injury is classified as either perioperative or related to cardiac allograft vasculopathy. Perioperative or early ischemia refers to injury sustained during organ procurement and implantation, and is intensified by bleeding, hypotension, and inotropic agents. Commonly seen up to 6 weeks post-transplantation, early ischemia is characterized by contraction band, myocyte or fat necrosis, and myocyte vacuolization. Late ischemia refers to injury from cardiac allograft vasculopathy. As large vessels are not routinely seen on biopsy, the pathologist looks for vacuolization and microinfarcts, secondary changes from ischemic injury.

Table 8.4 ISHLT standardized cardiac biopsy grading: acute cellular rejection and antibody-mediated rejection

Grade 0 R[a] 2005	No rejection	Grade 0 1990	No rejection
Grade 1 R, mild	Interstitial and/or perivascular infiltrate with up to one focus of myocyte damage	Grade 1, mild A – focal B – diffuse Grade 2, moderate (focal)	Focal perivascular and/or interstitial infiltrate without myocyte damage Diffuse infiltrate without myocyte damage One focus of infiltrate with myocyte damage
Grade 2 R, moderate	Two or more foci of infiltrate with associated myocyte damage	Grade 3, moderate A – focal B – diffuse	Multifocal infiltrate with myocyte damage Diffuse infiltrate with myocyte damage
Grade 3 R, severe	Diffuse infiltrate with multifocal myocyte damage ± edema, ± hemorrhage, ± vasculitis	Grade 4, severe	Diffuse polymorphous infiltrate with extensive myocyte damage ± edema, ± hemorrhage, ± vasculitis
AMR 0	Negative for acute AMR No histologic or immunologic features of AMR		
AMR 1	Positive for AMR Histologic features of AMR Positive immunofluorescence or immunoperoxidase staining for AMR (positive CD68, C4d)		Humoral rejection (positive immunofluorescence, vasculitis or severe edema in absence of cellular infiltrate) recorded as additional required information

[a]R denotes revised grade to avoid confusion with 1990 scheme.
AMR, antibody-mediated rejection.

The Quilty effect refers to nodular endocardial infiltrates seen in up to 20% of biopsies. Quilty lesions are usually confined to the endocardium, but, when lesions invade the myocardium, accompanying myocyte damage makes differentiation from rejection problematic. There is no known relationship between the Quilty effect and rejection, so Quilty lesions require no treatment.

With the exception of CMV and toxoplasmosis, which may be associated with lymphocytic infiltration, infection and PTLD are not commonly seen in biopsy specimens, making confusion with acute rejection less likely.

Case: acute rejection

A 52-year-old woman, gravida 4, para 4, underwent heart transplantation in 2005 due to ischemic cardiomyopathy. Her PRA pretransplant was 0% and her initial post-transplant course was uncomplicated. She was compliant with her medical regimen and follow-up. However, at 8 months post-transplantation, she presented with a several day history of increasing fatigue, dyspnea on exertion, and an increase in her resting heart rate. Echocardiogram showed a decrease in her LVEF to 35%. Coronary angiography revealed no coronary artery disease and biopsy was grade 1R, AMR O. Due to the acute nature of the patient's decline and a strong suspicion for immune-mediated allograft dysfunction, the patient received methylprednisolone 250 mg i.v. daily for 3 days and completed a 2-week course (total of six treatments) of plasmapheresis with intravenous gammaglobulin after the third and sixth plasmaphereses. Fortunately 1 month after presentation, her ejection fraction had improved to 55% and she felt well. Of interest, a PRA drawn at the time she presented with LV dysfunction was 80% and donor-specific antibody was present. Although the patient's improvement is encouraging, she is at high risk for poor long-term outcome because of her presentation with hemodynamic compromise in the absence of cellular rejection.

Functional assessment of the cardiac allograft
Echocardiography is indispensable in the evaluation of the cardiac allograft. The rejecting cardiac allograft typically exhibits diastolic stiffness with preserved systolic function. Echocardiographic features of restrictive physiology include decreases in isovolumic relaxation time, mitral valve pressure half-time, deceleration time, and fractional shortening. Systolic dysfunction is a late finding with rejection.

The hemodynamic findings of acute rejection are also those of a restrictive cardiomyopathy, including pulmonary hypertension and increased end-diastolic pressure. Early diastolic filling tends to be slow rather than fast, so the dip-and-plateau ventricular waveform is not usually seen. Although echocardiographic and hemodynamic evaluation of the cardiac allograft should be routinely performed, neither by itself can accurately diagnose acute rejection.

Outcomes/post-transplant follow-up

Acute rejection

The frequency of rejection is highest early after transplantation; however, the risk for rejection continues throughout the life of the transplant recipient. As shown in Figure 8.6, from the Cardiac Transplant Research Database (CTRD), 62% of adult recipients have a rejection episode (defined as a clinical event requiring augmentation of immunosuppression, and usually accompanied by an abnormal biopsy) during the first year. Risk factors for recurrent rejection in the first year include a female recipient, a younger recipient, positive recipient CMV serology pretransplant, a female donor organ, OKT3 induction therapy, fewer months since transplantation, fewer months since the last rejection episode, and a greater number of previous infections. Risk factors for rejection >1 year after transplantation are similar, and include female transplant recipient, black recipient race, OKT3 induction therapy, a greater number of rejections during the first year, and prior CMV infection. Fortunately, despite the frequency of acute rejection, there is 97% freedom from death or re-transplantation due to acute rejection at 1 year.

Additional comments should be made concerning a rejection episode with hemodynamic compromise (defined as a decrease in cardiac index, a decreased ejection fraction, clinical signs of low cardiac output, or the need to use inotropic agents). In the CTRD, only 8% of recipients had a rejection episode with hemodynamic compromise in the first 3 years. Risk factors for rejection with hemodynamic compromise early after transplantation included a female or a diabetic recipient. Later after transplantation, black recipient race, older donor age, black donor race, and a diabetic donor were risk factors for the first rejection episode with hemodynamic compromise. Of importance, if rejection with hemodynamic compromise occurred in the presence of cellular rejection of

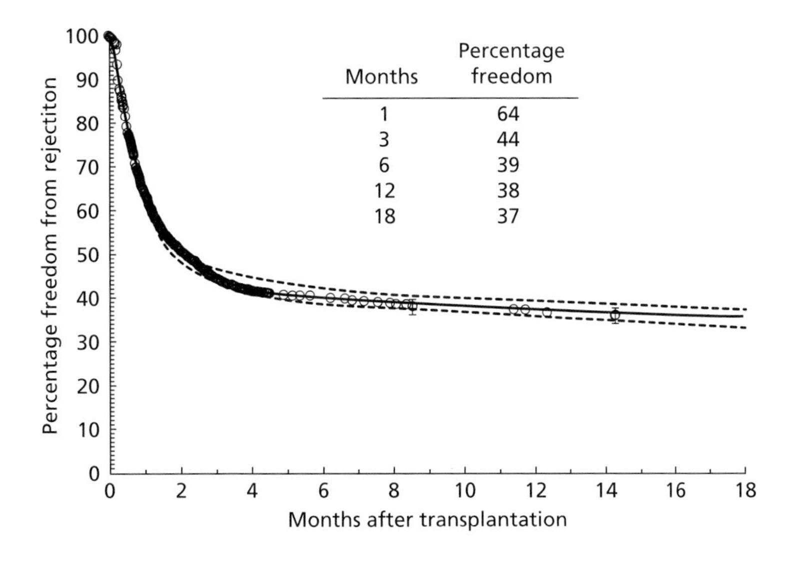

Figure 8.6 Freedom from rejection over time in cardiac transplant recipients: Jan 1990 to June 1991 – $n = 911$; patients with rejection episodes = 495. (Reprinted with permission from Kobashigawa JA, Kirklin JK, Naftel DC, et al. Pretransplantation risk factors for acute rejection after heart transplantation: a multiinstitutional study. The Transplant Cardiologists Research Database Group. *J Heart Lung Transplant* 1993;**12**:355–66.)

grade 3A or higher, outcome was better than if hemodynamic compromise occurred without cellular rejection on biopsy. It is assumed that many rejection episodes with hemodynamic compromise represent non-cellular-mediated rejection or AMR; however, this is still poorly understood. The exact definition of AMR and appropriate therapy for it still require significant clinical investigation.

Cardiac allograft vasculopathy

Cardiac allograft vasculopathy is a major cause of morbidity and mortality in heart transplant recipients more than 1 year after transplantation. Cardiac allograft vasculopathy is defined as allograft vascular injury induced by a variety of stimuli which leads to a progressive, diffuse vascular obliteration of intramural and epicardial arteries and veins, and the donor segment of the aorta. The diagnosis of cardiac allograft vasculopathy is difficult because the patient frequently has absent or atypical symptoms (due to cardiac denervation) and non-invasive testing is unsatisfactory. The most common test for cardiac allograft vasculopathy is coronary angiography, which is performed annually by most centers, especially early after transplantation. Figure 8.7 shows the angiographic development of allograft vasculopathy and some of its differences from native coronary artery disease. The left panel shows a coronary angiogram 2 years after transplantation with only minor luminal irregularities. The angiogram in the right panel was performed 3 years after transplantation, when the patient remained asymptomatic. There is significant pruning/disappearance of distal vessels, irregularities in the proximal vessels, and total disappearance of a marginal circumflex branch. As shown, cardiac allograft vasculopathy is more likely to be distal and diffuse compared with the proximal and more focal nature of native coronary artery disease.

Although the most frequent method of diagnosis of cardiac allograft vasculopathy is angiography, the angiogram is insensitive to early disease, and intracoronary ultrasound studies have shown significant intimal thickening before any angiographic abnormalities. Therefore, in studies defining methods to decrease the onset and progression of cardiac allograft vasculopathy, intracoronary ultrasonography is frequently used to quantify maximal intimal thickness and the intimal index (ratio of plaque area to vessel area) (Figure 8.8).

Cardiac allograft vasculopathy begins as smooth muscle cell proliferation followed by concentric

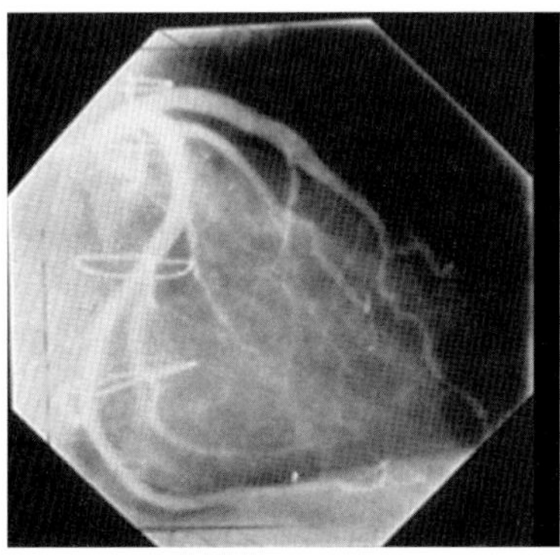

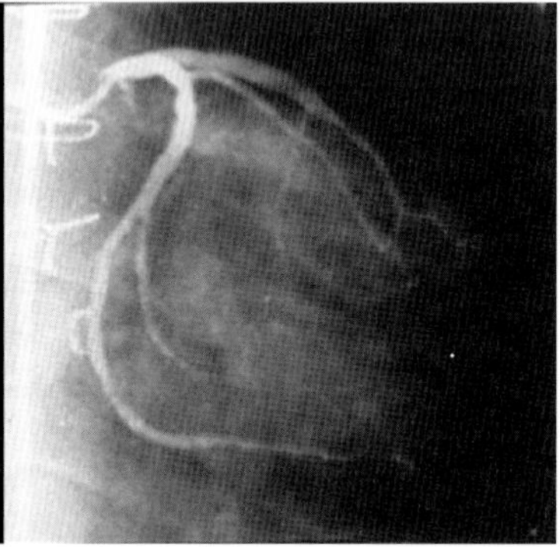

Figure 8.7 Serial coronary angiograms of a cardiac transplant recipient showing the development of cardiac allograft vasculopathy. Panel A shows a left coronary angiogram (right anterior oblique projection) 2 years after transplantation which reveals only minor luminal irregularities. Panel B is an angiogram of the same vessel 3 years after transplantation and reveals severe diffuse disease with pruning of the distal vessels. The patient was asymptomatic at the time of the 3-year angiogram but died suddenly 2 months later before a suitable donor heart for re-transplantation became available. (Reprinted with permission from Johnson MR. Principles and practice of coronary angiography. In: Skorton DJ, Schelbert HR, Wolf GL, Brundage BH, Braunwald E (eds), *Marcus' Cardiac Imaging*. Philadelphia, PA: WB Saunders Co., 1996: 220–51.)

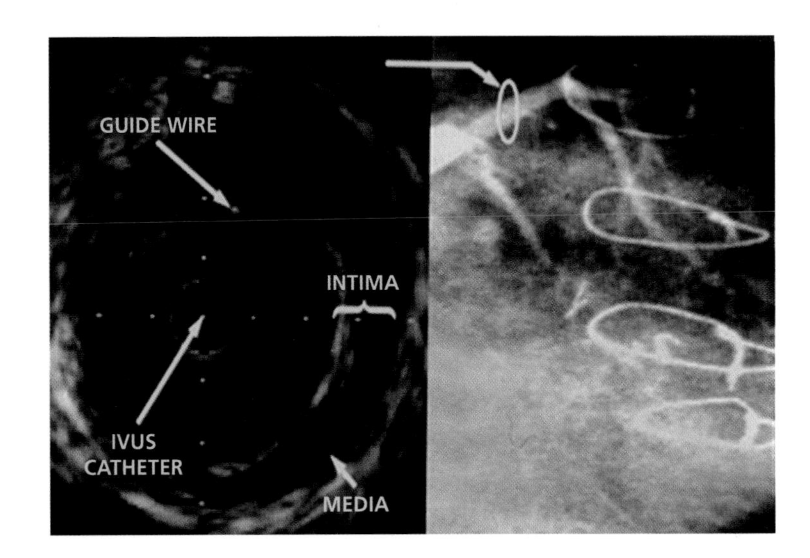

Figure 8.8 An intravascular ultrasound image (left panel) and coronary angiogram (right panel) of the left anterior descending artery in a cardiac transplant recipient. Although the angiogram appears normal, ultrasonography at the site noted shows significant intimal thickening.

intimal proliferation, with an intact internal elastic lamina. Endothelial expression of MHC (major histocompatibility complex) class II antigens is frequently present. Unlike native coronary disease where cholesterol deposition is extracellular, in allograft vasculopathy cholesterol is deposited intracellularly. Cardiac allograft vasculopathy is less likely to calcify or develop collaterals than native coronary disease. The time for development of cardiac allograft vasculopathy also tends to be months to years rather than many years, which is the situation with native coronary artery disease.

Unfortunately cardiac allograft vasculopathy is quite common. Angiographically it occurs in nearly 50% of patients at 5 years, although the incidence of moderate and severe vasculopathy is much less, and only 7% of patients die or require re-transplantation at 5 years due to cardiac allograft vasculopathy (Figure 8.9). The prognosis of a patient with cardiac allograft vasculopathy is related to disease severity, and those with severe angiographic disease or severe intimal thickening on ultrasonography are more likely to suffer a cardiac event.

The precise etiology of cardiac allograft vasculopathy remains unclear, although immune mechanisms are involved because the disease affects the transplanted vessels (coronary arteries, coronary veins, donor segment of the aorta) whereas recipient vessels, even in patients who have undergone heterotopic transplantation, are not affected. Alloimmune mechanisms and possibly immune changes after CMV infection play a role. Non-immune endothelial injury related to donor brain death, ischemia–reperfusion injury, direct injury from CMV infection in the donor or the recipient, and effects of immunosuppressive medications, particularly cyclosporine, may be contributing factors. Conventional risk factors in the donor and recipient may be risk factors for cardiac allograft vasculopathy. Donor characteristics shown to increase the risk of allograft vasculopathy include age, male gender, increased body mass index, hypertension, and pre-existing atherosclerosis (although donor lesions progress less rapidly than new lesions in the transplanted heart). Recipient characteristics shown to increase the risk of allograft vasculopathy include older age, male sex, black race, obesity, hyperlipidemia, hypertension, smoking, diabetes mellitus, and pretransplant diagnosis (although whether non-ischemic or ischemic disease increases risk varies in different studies).

Small studies have suggested factors which may prevent the onset or delay progression of allograft vasculopathy including treatment with aspirin, diltiazem, or angiotensin converting enzyme inhibitors; prophylaxis for CMV infection, and treatment of conventional risk factors. However, the clinical impact of such measures remains questionable. In a study of 40 cardiac transplant recipients randomized

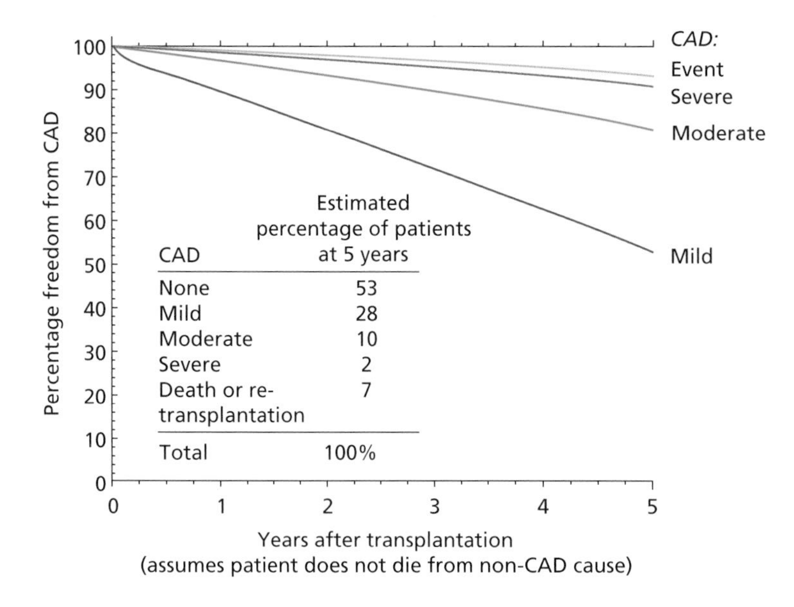

Figure 8.9 Freedom from mild, moderate, and severe cardiac allograft vasculopathy and events due to cardiac allograft vasculopathy as reported to the Cardiac Transplant Research Database: Jan 1990 to Dec 1994 – $n = 609$. CAD, coronary artery disease. (Reprinted with permission from Costanzo MR, Naftel DC, Pritzker MR, et al. Heart transplant coronary artery disease detected by coronary angiography: a multiinstitutional study of preoperative donor and recipient risk factors. Cardiac Transplant Research Database. *J Heart Lung Transplant* 1998;**17**:744–53.)

to vitamin C 500 mg plus vitamin E 400 IU twice daily versus placebo for 1 year, vitamin treatment prevented the increase in intimal index seen in the placebo group. No longer-term follow-up has been published. Further analysis of an MMF study also suggested a decrease in intimal proliferation with MMF versus azathioprine.

The first drug shown to decrease coronary intimal proliferation after cardiac transplantation was pravastatin. When patients were randomized to pravastatin versus placebo at transplantation, pravastatin not only decreased cholesterol, but also decreased the number of rejections with hemodynamic compromise, increased 1-year survival, and decreased the progression of cardiac allograft vasculopathy. A recent report confirmed increased survival and freedom from allograft vasculopathy and death in the pravastatin group after 10 years of follow-up. A similar benefit was shown with simvastatin. Of interest, an 8-year follow-up from the simvastatin study showed that patients who received placebo initially but began simvastatin at 4 years post-transplantation had an increased incidence of allograft vasculopathy compared with the group started on simvastatin at transplantation. Statins should therefore be routinely incorporated into the regimen of cardiac transplant recipients, starting at the time of transplantation. However, patients do require close follow-up of creatine kinase levels and liver function tests as the adverse effects of statins are increased by drug interactions with the CNIs.

Studies using the TOR inhibitors, everolimus and sirolimus, instead of azathioprine from the time of cardiac transplantation have shown a decrease in cellular rejection and less progression of intimal thickness. These studies should, however, be interpreted cautiously because the data available reflect only the early post-transplant period, and everolimus and sirolimus increase serum lipids, particularly triglycerides, which could have long-term negative ramifications. Another limiting factor is that the comparator drug in the studies was azathioprine and not MMF, which may itself decrease progression of allograft vasculopathy. In addition, combined use of TOR inhibitors with cyclosporine was associated with increased serum creatinine concentrations, resulting in recommendations to decrease the target cyclosporine levels later in the studies. The increase in renal insufficiency produced by combined use of TOR inhibitors and cyclosporine is not yet understood.

Treatment for cardiac allograft vasculopathy is limited. As the disease is commonly diffuse and distal, percutaneous coronary interventions and bypass graft surgery are often not possible, and, when angioplasty is performed, re-stenosis is higher than in the general population (55% at 19 months in the study by Halle et al. – see Further reading). In the small subset of patients who are candidates for bypass grafting, mortality is high. With the ability to stent coronary lesions, particularly using drug-eluting stents, outcomes of percutaneous coronary interventions in cardiac transplant recipients have improved; however, no large series have been published and long-term outcomes remain questionable. Attempts at percutaneous interventions or bypass surgery for allograft vasculopathy must be considered palliative and, in patients who are candidates for percutaneous coronary intervention or bypass surgery, distal angiographic disease predicts poor outcome.

An encouraging study randomized patients to sirolimus versus continuation of azathioprine or MMF when significant cardiac allograft vasculopathy was diagnosed. Patients randomized to sirolimus had fewer primary endpoints (death, angioplasty, bypass surgery, myocardial infarction, or an increase in angiographic coronary artery disease score) and secondary endpoints (cardiac hospitalizations, onset of heart failure, chest pain, and re-listing for transplantation) than the control group (Figure 8.10). Thus, many centers are initiating sirolimus in patients with cardiac allograft vasculopathy. However, whether the sirolimus should be substituted for the azathioprine or MMF as in the study or added to the immunosuppressive regimen is a question that remains unanswered.

The only true treatment for cardiac allograft vasculopathy is re-transplantation. However, survival after re-transplantation is decreased compared with that after initial transplantation and, with the donor shortage, re-transplantation is done selectively (see "Re-transplantation"). Survival after re-transplantation for cardiac allograft vasculopathy is better than after re-transplantation for other indications, so in selected cases re-transplantation for allograft vasculopathy should be considered. Indeed, a recent series looking at re-transplantation for cardiac allograft vasculopathy found a 1-year survival rate of 85% for those re-transplanted between 1996 and 1999, approaching the outcome after initial transplantation. However, longer-term survival after re-transplantation is still compromised compared with that after initial transplantation.

Overview of medical complications following cardiac transplantation

Although medical complications after transplantation are detailed in Chapter 5, it is appropriate to discuss the importance of some complications in cardiac transplant recipients here. Table 8.5 shows causes of death at varying periods after cardiac transplantation in a recent era, excluding deaths due to technical factors, acute rejection, and primary and non-specific graft failure. In the first year, the primary cause of death is infection, whereas, later after transplantation, an increasing number of deaths are caused by malignancy and cardiac allograft vasculopathy.

Deaths due to renal failure also increase with time after cardiac transplantation. Risk factors for death due to infection early after cardiac transplantation include younger recipient age, male recipient, being

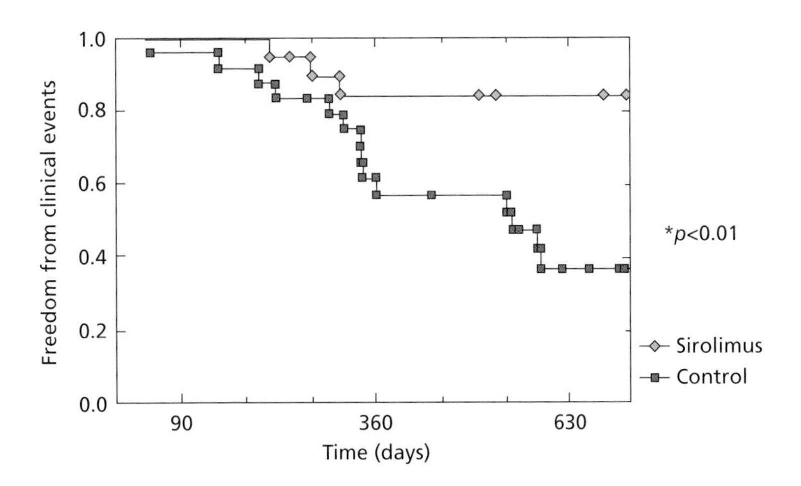

Figure 8.10 Freedom from clinical events (death, angioplasty, myocardial infarction or >25% increase in catheterization score) for patients with significant cardiac allograft vasculopathy treated with rapamycin versus control. (Reprinted with permission from Mancini D, Pinney S, Burkhoff D, et al. Use of sirolimus slows progression of cardiac transplantation vasculopathy. *Circulation* 2003;**108**:48–53.)

Table 8.5 Causes of death for adult heart transplant recipients (deaths January, 1992–June, 2003)[a]

Cause of death	0–30 days (n = 2759)	31 days–1 year (n = 2310)	>1–3 years (n = 1737)	>3–5 years (n = 1492)	>5 years (n = 4009)
Infection	374 (13.5%)	813 (35.2%)	249 (14.4%)	148 (9.9%)	397 (9.9%)
Malignancy	4 (0.2%)	97 (4.1%)	258 (14.8%)	361 (24.2%)	964 (24.0%)
CAV	43 (1.6%)	111 (4.8%)	257 (14.8%)	268 (18.0%)	651 (16.2%)
Renal failure	17 (0.6%)	19 (0.8%)	31 (1.8%)	51 (3.4%)	238 (5.9%)
Other[b]	778 (28.2%)	525 (22.7%)	345 (19.9%)	298 (20%)	906 (22.7%)

[a]Excluding deaths due to technical factors, acute rejection, primary failure, and graft failure.
[b]Including multiorgan failure, pulmonary, cerebrovascular.
CAV, cardiac allograft vasculopathy.Reprinted with permission from Taylor DO, Edwards LB, Boucek MM, et al. Registry of the International Society for Heart and Lung Transplantation: twenty-second official adult heart transplant report – 2005. *J Heart Lung Transplant* 2005;**24**:945–55 (and accompanying slide set).

on a ventilator at the time of transplantation, older donor age, and longer donor ischemic time. In long-term follow-up, older recipient age is the only significant risk factor for death from infection. Malignancy increases with time after cardiac transplantation, with non-skin malignancies affecting 5.6% of 5-year survivors and 6.5% of 7-year survivors. Chronic renal failure develops in nearly 11% of patients at 5 years after cardiac transplantation, with risk factors including age, preoperative renal function, postoperative acute renal failure, female recipient, hepatitis C infection, pretransplant hypertension, diabetes mellitus, and being transplanted more recently. Chronic renal insufficiency increases costs of care and the risk of death. As patients have a better outcome with renal transplantation than hemodialysis, and with the continued shortage of donor organs for the current renal waiting list, this becomes of societal importance. An area of active clinical investigation is defining means, particularly modifications in immunosuppression, to decrease the risk of renal failure after transplantation. Other significant morbidities that occur after cardiac transplantation and require ongoing medical attention are hypertension, hyperlipidemia, diabetes mellitus, obesity, and osteoporosis.

Prevention of complications after heart transplantation

Complications after heart transplantation challenge even the most experienced transplant physician. Complications arise primarily from chronic immunosuppression, either directly or by worsening preexisting conditions. Therefore it is incumbent to choose immunosuppressive regimens that prevent rejection but minimize side effects.

Key points 8.4 Avoiding medical complications after heart transplantation

Preventing medical problems is vital, because problems are magnified in immunosuppressed patients

Patients should participate in health maintenance by monitoring vital signs, recognizing and reporting symptoms, and adhering to a complex medical regimen

Smoking is strongly discouraged; patients who resume smoking need referral to a smoking cessation program

Regular aerobic exercise promotes physical rehabilitation and maintains functional capacity

Maintaining ideal body weight is important, because obesity is associated with glucose intolerance and dyslipidemia

Prevention of infection

Transplant recipients are at life-long risk for infection. There is a peak of bacterial and viral infections in the first post-transplant month, followed by a second peak of opportunistic infections (CMV, fungi, and protozoa) in the second to fifth months. Community-acquired infections are more common later. As the lung is the most commonly affected organ, chest radiographs are done routinely. Patients should report any fever or infectious symptoms immediately because infection can progress rapidly to death.

Prophylaxis decreases certain infections in heart transplant recipients. CMV is a common cause of infection, with donor-seropositive, recipient-seronegative (D+/R–) patients at highest risk. Two approaches to CMV prophylaxis are universal prophylaxis and pre-emptive therapy. Universal CMV prophylaxis for D+/R–, D–/R+, and D+/R+ heart transplant recipients involves valganciclovir for 3–6 months, sometimes with perioperative intravenous ganciclovir. Some centers add CMV Ig for D+/R– recipients. Pre-emptive therapy involves weekly monitoring to detect CMV viremia for the first 3 months. CMV viremia prompts treatment with intravenous ganciclovir or oral valganciclovir. Our institution uses universal prophylaxis.

Oral high-dose aciclovir and valaciclovir prevent reactivation of herpes simplex and herpes zoster. Trimethoprim–sulfamethoxazole, one single or double strength tablet daily for 1 year, prevents infection with *Pneumocystis jiroveci* (formerly *carinii*), *Toxoplasma gondii*, *Isospora belli*, and *Nocardia asteroides*. For pneumocystis prevention in patients allergic to sulfa, monthly inhaled pentamidine is an alternative.

Oral clotrimazole or nystatin (swish and swallow) prevents mucocutaneous candidiasis, although fluconazole or ketoconazole can be used. Patients need endocarditis prophylaxis before any dental, upper respiratory, gastrointestinal, or urologic procedures.

Patients should be immunized against hepatitis A, hepatitis B, pneumococcal pneumonia, influenza, diphtheria, and tetanus before transplantation. After transplantation, neither the patient nor any household contact should receive live viral vaccines, especially Sabin oral polio vaccine, because the virus is transmissible. Immunization with influenza vaccine after transplantation is controversial because of concerns about increased rejection. The transplant physician should be consulted before administration of any vaccine after transplantation.

Key points 8.5 Principles of prevention of infection after heart transplantation

- As most infections are acquired by direct contact or inhalation, frequent hand washing with an antimicrobial soap and avoidance of crowded areas, tobacco smoke, construction sites, and exposure to people with respiratory illnesses are recommended
- Food safety involves avoidance of unpasteurized, raw, or undercooked food, soft cheeses, and unpeeled vegetables and fruits
- Patients should wash their hands thoroughly after contact with pets and should avoid animals with diarrhea, stray animals, reptiles, chicks, ducklings, cats aged <1 year, and monkeys
- Sexually active patients should use latex condoms during sexual activity
- Travel to developing countries involves substantial infectious risk and should be discussed with the transplant physician at least 2 months before departure

Prevention and detection of malignancy

There is a progressive linear increase in malignancies after transplantation, especially virally driven cancers. Cancer screening recommendations by the American Cancer Society include flexible sigmoidoscopy every 3–5 years starting at age 50, annual stool tests for occult blood, routine gynecologic examinations and mammography for women, and regular prostate examinations and prostate-specific antigen levels for men.

Surveillance for skin cancer and post transplant lymphoproliferative disorder (PTLD) are mandatory in transplant recipients. Sun protection and regular skin examinations are recommended. In a report from the Israel Penn International Transplant Tumor Registry, heart transplant patients had a higher incidence of PTLD and worse prognosis than other solid organ transplant recipients. An interesting finding in this series was that non-ischemic cardiomyopathy was the primary cardiac disease in 75% of patients who developed PTLD, representing a sevenfold increased risk compared with patients with ischemic or congenital heart disease. Increased surveillance and individualized immunosuppression may therefore be indicated for patients transplanted for cardiomyopathy.

The incidence of PTLD increases with the degree of immunosuppression. However, considerable interest exists in the possible antineoplastic activity of the TOR inhibitors, everolimus and sirolimus.

Hypertension and renal insufficiency

Hypertension induced by CNIs usually requires antihypertensive medication as well as salt restriction. Diuretics alone are rarely sufficient. ACE inhibitors and angiotensin receptor-blocking agents are effective antihypertensive agents, but hyperkalemia can be problematic and exacerbated by the CNIs. Diltiazem is associated with a lower incidence of allograft vasculopathy early after transplantation, but cyclosporine and tacrolimus levels are increased by diltiazem and need close monitoring. β Blockers should be used cautiously, particularly early after transplantation, because the denervated heart may rely on catecholamines to augment ventricular performance. Nephrotoxicity is associated with CNIs, so the lowest possible dose should be used to minimize renal dysfunction. Dehydration should be avoided because it potentiates renal toxicity.

Prevention and treatment of osteoporosis

About 50% of advanced heart failure patients have low bone mineral density due to a combination of vitamin D deficiency, low dietary calcium intake, loop diuretics, prerenal azotemia, immobilization, hepatic congestion, and hypogonadism. After transplantation, bone loss is accelerated by steroids and CNIs. Bone loss and fractures are highest in the first 3–12 months, ranging from 8% to 65%. Therefore, prevention of post-transplant osteoporosis begins before transplantation. All patients awaiting heart transplantation should be evaluated for bone mineral metabolism disorders and osteoporosis with bone densitometry, spine radiographs, and blood tests for calcium, vitamin D, PTH, thyroid function, and testosterone (males). All transplant candidates should receive 400–800 IU vitamin D and 1000–1500 mg elemental calcium daily. Patients with osteoporosis or osteopenia should also receive bisphosphonates. In patients with normal bone mineral density, pretransplant bisphosphonates should be considered immediately after transplantation. Bisphosphonates are renally excreted and cannot be used in patients with a serum creatinine >3.0 mg/dL or a creatinine clearance <30 mL/min.

Dyslipidemia

The adverse metabolic effects of immunosuppressive drugs, coupled with a genetic predisposition to hyperlipidemia and obesity, make dyslipidemia problematic after heart transplantation. Studies using HMG-CoA reductase inhibitors (statins) confirm the efficacy of pravastatin, simvastatin, and lovastatin in lowering cholesterol by 18–42%. In the Canadian Study of Cardiac Transplantation Atherosclerosis (CASCADE), patients receiving a statin had less allograft coronary disease and greater 5-year survival than patients on no statin therapy.

Statins have immunomodulatory effects independent of cholesterol lowering. These agents inhibit growth factor-induced cellular proliferation and cytokine activity. Statin use has been associated with a decreased risk of death from allograft failure in the first post-heart transplantation year, a decreased incidence of severe cellular rejection, and a reduction in ischemic events due to plaque rupture, possibly due to modulation of platelet thromboxane A_2 biosynthesis.

Aspirin

There are few data on aspirin use after heart transplantation, but most centers prescribe aspirin for primary and secondary prevention of cardiac allograft vasculopathy in doses ranging from 81 mg to 325 mg daily. Although allograft vasculopathy is primarily immunologically mediated, ischemic injury at the time of transplantation causes platelet activation, aggregation, and degranulation. After transplantation patients continue to exhibit marked platelet hyperaggregation. Evidence of platelet resistance to the inhibitory effects of aspirin in heart transplant recipients may explain the failure of antiplatelet agents to prevent myocardial infarction after heart transplantation.

Cardiac surgery, including re-transplantation, in heart transplant recipients

As the number of heart transplant recipients accumulates, the need for cardiac reoperations, including cardiac re-transplantation, has emerged. Cardiac allograft vasculopathy and tricuspid regurgitation are the two major indications for cardiac surgery after cardiac transplantation.

Tricuspid regurgitation may result from endocarditis or biopsy-induced valve injury. Investigators at the Deutsches Herrzzentrum Berlin, Germany, investigated 647 cardiac transplant recipients at their institution and identified tricuspid regurgitation in 20.1% (mild in 14.5%, moderate in 3.1%, and severe in 2.5%). Seventeen patients underwent valve repair or replacement. Tricuspid valve pathology revealed biopsy-induced rupture of the chordae tendineae at various valve segments, mostly the anterior and posterior leaflets. Ten patients (62.5%) were alive at 29.9 months (range 4–81 months) follow-up with nine survivors in NYHA classes I–II and one in class III. In their series, mild-to-moderate tricuspid regurgitation responded to medical therapy and was non-progressive without having a detrimental effect on right ventricular performance. Therefore, the need for tricuspid valve surgery must be carefully assessed.

As discussed under "Cardiac allograft vasculopathy," the diffuse and distal nature of allograft vasculopathy precludes bypass surgery in many cases. In addition, mortality after bypass surgery for allograft vasculopathy is high, so its use in the treatment of allograft vasculopathy is palliative at best.

Early re-transplantation, especially within 6 months of primary cardiac transplantation, is associated with poor results and is not recommended. As donor organ shortage remains a major issue in cardiac transplantation, and outcomes after re-transplantation are inferior to those after primary transplantation, indications for re-transplantation need to be carefully evaluated.

Most published data about cardiac re-transplantation are single center experiences. However, Srivastava et al. retrospectively analyzed 514 patients from the Joint ISHLT/UNOS Thoracic Registry who underwent cardiac re-transplantation between 1987 and 1998 (see Further reading). The predominant indications for re-transplantation were cardiac allograft vasculopathy (56%), primary graft failure (18%), and acute rejection (9%). Time from primary transplant to re-transplant ranged from 1 day to 15.5 years. One-year survival after re-transplantation as a function of time between first and re-transplantation is shown in Figure 8.11. Multivariate analysis determined that risk factors for mortality at 1 month after re-transplantation were center volume less than nine transplants/year, older recipient age, and the requirement for life support (VAD, ventilator, and /or inotropic therapy) and ICU care before re-transplantation. Recipient age and pretransplant mechanical ventilation continued to predict poor outcomes at 1 year. Re-transplantation performed more recently (1995 and after versus 1987–1994) positively affected outcome.

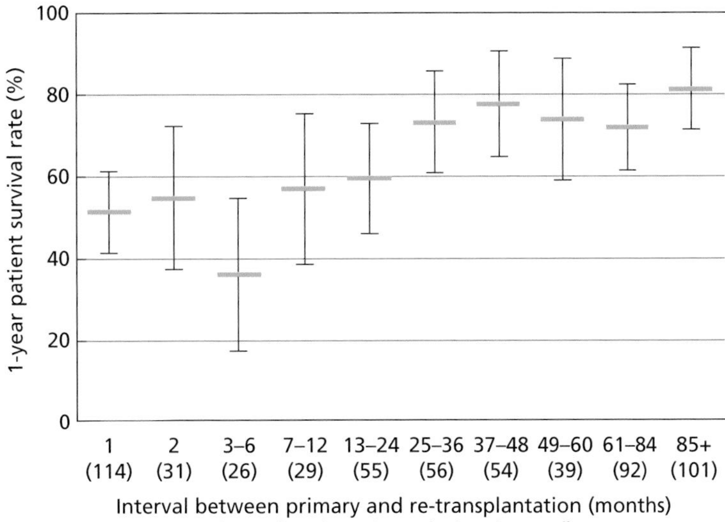

Figure 8.11 One-year survival after re-transplantation as a function of time between first transplant and re-transplantation. (Reprinted with permission from Srivastava R, Keck BM, Bennett LE, Hosenpud JD. The results of cardiac retransplantation: an analysis of the Joint International Society for Heart and Lung Transplantation/United Network for Organ Sharing Thoracic Registry. *Transplantation* 2000;70:606–12.)

Data from the ISHLT Registry show that, in 2003 and 2004, approximately 80 cardiac re-transplants were performed annually in North America, comprising 3–4% of all cardiac transplants. The 1-year survival rate in these patients reached 82.4% and the 3-year survival rate 71.6%, likely reflecting improved patient selection for re-transplantation.

Based on the above, selection criteria for re-transplantation at our institution (in addition to those defined for primary transplant) are as follows:

Indications

1. Diffuse cardiac allograft vasculopathy not amenable to angioplasty/stenting or bypass surgery, especially with associated LV dysfunction.
2. Graft failure from suboptimal donor or acute or chronic rejection, with symptomatic, progressive heart failure.

Contraindications

1. Graft failure for any reason within 2 weeks of transplantation
2. Graft failure within 6 months of transplantation if associated with acute rejection and hemodynamic compromise
3. Patient age >55 years
4. PTLD, if disease free for less than 5 years
5. Patient non-compliance.

Case: re-transplantation

A 48-year-old man is now 15 years after heart transplantation for non-ischemic cardiomyopathy. He had two rejection episodes that were successfully treated in the first postoperative year but otherwise did well. Three years ago at his annual cardiac catheterization, he was noted to have an 80% lesion in his LAD, which was successfully stented. Over the next 2 years, catheterizations have shown that his LAD stent remains patent but he has developed diffuse, progressive, allograft vasculopathy with a gradual decline in his LVEF to 25% and he now has symptomatic heart failure. He has been very compliant with his medical regimen, his creatinine is 1.5 mg/dL, and he has no contraindications to re-transplantation. What would you do?

The future of cardiac transplantation

Outcomes after cardiac transplantation have improved considerably since Dr Barnard performed the first heart transplantation in 1967. However, survival is still limited by deaths due to rejection, cardiac allograft vasculopathy, and complications of immunosuppression. The donor shortage also limits the number of heart transplantations performed. Improved outcomes after heart transplantation are critically dependent on more specific/targeted methods of immunosuppression, which can further decrease immunologic deaths without increasing morbidity and mortality due to complications of immunosuppression. Better utilization of available donor hearts, facilitated by improved donor management, is also critical.

Further reading

Anand IS, Fisher LD, Chiang YT, et al. Changes in brain natriuretic peptide and norepinephrine over time and mortality and morbidity in the Valsartan Heart Failure Trial (Val-HeFT). *Circulation* 2003;**107**:1278–83.

Argenziano M, Chen JM, Cullinane S, et al. Arginine vasopressin in the management of vasodilatory hypotension after cardiac transplantation. *J Heart Lung Transplant* 1999;**18**:814–17.

Ashton RC, Jr., Goldstein DJ, Rose EA, Weinberg AD, Levin HR, Oz MC. Duration of left ventricular assist device support affects transplant survival. *J Heart Lung Transplant* 1996;**15**:1151–7.

Aull MJ, Buell JF, Trofe J, et al. Experience with 274 cardiac transplant recipients with posttransplant lymphoproliferative disorder: a report from the Israel Penn International Transplant Tumor Registry. *Transplantation* 2004;**78**: 1676–82.

Aziz TM, Burgess MI, El-Gamel A, et al. Orthotopic cardiac transplantation technique: a survey of current practice. *Ann Thorac Surg* 1999;**68**:1242–6.

Aziz T, Burgess M, Khafagy R, et al. Bicaval and standard techniques in orthotopic heart transplantation: medium-term experience in cardiac performance and survival. *J Thorac Cardiovasc Surg* 1999;**118**:115–22.

Bardy GH, Lee KL, Mark DB, et al. Amiodarone or an implantable cardioverter-defibrillator for congestive heart failure. *N Engl J Med* 2005;**352**:225–37.

Barr ML, Sanchez JA, Seche LA, Schulman LL, Smith CR, Rose EA. Anti-CD3 monoclonal antibody induction therapy: immunological equivalency with triple-drug therapy in heart transplantation. *Circulation* 1990;**82**(suppl 5):IV-291–4.

Bengel FM, Ueberfuhr P, Schiepel N, Nekolla SG, Reichart B, Schwaiger M. Effect of sympathetic reinnervation on cardiac performance after heart transplantation. *N Engl J Med* 2001;**345**:731–8.

Benza RL, Zoghbi GJ, Tallaj J, et al. Palliation of allograft vasculopathy with transluminal angioplasty: a decade of experience. *J Am Coll Cardiol* 2004;**43**:1973–81.

Brandt M, Harringer W, Hirt SW, et al. Influence of bicaval anastomoses on late occurrence of atrial arrhythmia after heart transplantation. *Ann Thorac Surg* 1997;**64**:70–2.

Carrier M, Rivard M, Kostuk W, et al. The Canadian Study of Cardiac Transplantation Atherosclerosis. Investigators of the CASCADE Study. *Can J Cardiol* 1999;**15**:1337–44.

Chan BB, Fleischer KJ, Bergin JD, et al. Weight is not an accurate criterion for adult cardiac transplant size matching. *Ann Thorac Surg* 1991;**52**:1230–5.

Chen JM, Edwards NM. Donor selection and management of the high-risk donor. In: Edwards NM, Chen JM, Mazzeo PA (eds), *Cardiac Transplantation*. Totowa, NJ: Humana Press, 2004: 19–36.

Cleland JG, Daubert JC, Erdmann E, et al. The effect of cardiac resynchronization on morbidity and mortality in heart failure. *N Engl J Med* 2005;**352**:1539–49.

Copeland JG, Smith RG, Arabia FA. et al Cardiac replacement with a total artificial heart as a bridge to transplantation. *N Engl J Med* 2004;**351**:859–67.

Costanzo MR, Naftel DC, Pritzker MR, et al. Heart transplant coronary artery disease detected by coronary angiography: a multiinstitutional study of preoperative donor and recipient risk factors. Cardiac Transplant Research Database. *J Heart Lung Transplant* 1998;**17**:744–53.

Costanzo-Nordin MR, Grusk BB, Silver MA, et al. Reversal of recalcitrant cardiac allograft rejection with methotrexate. *Circulation* 1988;**78**(suppl III):47–57.

Costard-Jackle A, Fowler MB. Influence of preoperative pulmonary artery pressure on mortality after heart transplantation: testing of potential reversibility of pulmonary hypertension with nitroprusside is useful in defining a high risk group. *J Am Coll Cardiol* 1992;**19**:48–54.

de Boer J, Cohen B, Thorogood J, Zantvoort FA, D'Amaro J, Persijn GG. Results of acute heart retransplantation. *Lancet* 1991;**337**:1158.

Deleuze PH, Benvenuti C, Mazzucotelli JP, et al. Orthotopic cardiac transplantation with direct caval anastomosis: is it the optimal procedure? *J Thorac Cardiovasc Surg* 1995;**109**:731–7.

Deng MC, Edwards LB, Hertz MI, et al. Mechanical Circulatory Support Device Database of the International Society for Heart and Lung Transplantation: third annual report–2005. *J Heart Lung Transplant* 2005;**24**:1182–7.

Deng MC, Eisen HJ, Mehra MR, et al. Noninvasive discrimination of rejection in cardiac allograft recipients using gene expression profiling. *Am J Transplant* 2006;**6**:150–60.

Deng MC, Loebe M, El-Banayosy A, et al. Mechanical circulatory support for advanced heart failure: effect of patient selection on outcome. *Circulation* 2001;**103**:231–7.

Eisen HJ, Kobashigawa J, Keogh A, et al. Three-year results of a randomized, double-blind, controlled trial of mycophenolate mofetil versus azathioprine in cardiac transplant recipients. *J Heart Lung Transplant* 2005;**24**:517–25.

Eisen HJ, Tuzcu EM, Dorent R, et al. RAD B253 Study Group. Everolimus for the prevention of allograft rejection and vasculopathy in cardiac-transplant recipients. *N Engl J Med* 2003;**349**:847–58.

el Gamel A, Yonan NA, Grant S, et al. Orthotopic cardiac transplantation: a comparison of standard and bicaval Wythenshawe techniques. *J Thorac Cardiovasc Surg* 1995;**109**:721–9.

el-Gamel A, Deiraniya AK, Rahman AN, Campbell CS, Yonan NA. Orthotopic heart transplantation hemodynamics: does atrial preservation improve cardiac output after transplantation? *J Heart Lung Transplant* 1996;**15**:564–71.

Ensley RD, Hunt S, Taylor DO, et al. Predictors of survival after repeat heart transplantation. The Registry of the International Society for Heart and Lung Transplantation, and Contributing Investigators. *J Heart Lung Transplant* 1992;**11**(suppl V):142–58.

Fang JC, Kinlay S, Beltrame J, et al. Effect of vitamins C and E on progression of transplant-associated arteriosclerosis: a randomised trial. *Lancet* 2002;**359**:1108–13.

Felkel TO, Smith AL, Reichenspurner HC, et al. Survival and incidence of acute rejection in heart transplant recipients undergoing successful withdrawal from steroid therapy. *J Heart Lung Transplant* 2002;**21**:530–9.

Forni A, Faggian G, Luciani GB, et al. Reduced incidence of cardiac arrhythmias after orthotopic heart transplantation with direct bicaval anastomosis. *Transplant Proc* 1996;**28**:289–92.

Grande AM, Rinaldi M, D'Armini AM, et al. Orthotopic heart transplantation: standard versus bicaval technique. *Am J Cardiol* 2000;**85**:1329–33.

Griepp RB, Stinson EB, Clark DA, Dong E Jr, Shumway NE. The cardiac donor. *Surg Gynecol Obstet* 1971;**133**:792–8.

Gronda E, Bourge RC, Costanzo MR, et al. Heart rhythm considerations in heart transplant candidates and considerations for ventricular assist devices: International Society for Heart and Lung Transplantation guidelines for the care of cardiac transplant candidates-2006. *J Heart Lung Transplant* 2006;**25**:1043–56.

Halle AA III, DiSciascio G, Massin EK, et al. Coronary angioplasty, atherectomy and bypass surgery in cardiac transplant recipients. *J Am Coll Cardiol* 1995;**26**:120–8.

Hershberger RE, Starling RC, Eisen HJ, et al. Daclizumab to prevent rejection after cardiac transplantation. *N Engl J Med* 2005;**352**:2705–13.

Higgins R, Kirklin JK, Brown RN, et al. To induce or not to induce: do patients at greatest risk for fatal rejection benefit from cytolytic induction therapy? *J Heart Lung Transplant* 2005;**24**:392–400.

Ibrahim M, Masters RG, Hendry PJ, et al. Determinants of hospital survival after cardiac transplantation. *Ann Thorac Surg* 1995;**59**:604–8.

Jessup M, Banner N, Brozena S, et al. Optimal pharmacologic and nonpharmacologic management of cardiac transplant candidates: approaches to be considered prior to transplant evaluation: International Society for Heart and Lung Transplantation guidelines for the care of cardiac transplant candidates-2006. *J Heart Lung Transplant* 2006;**25**:1003–23.

Johnson MR. Transplant coronary disease: nonimmunologic risk factors. *J Heart Lung Transplant* 1992;**11**(suppl): 124–32.

Johnson MR, Mullen GM, O'Sullivan EJ, et al Risk/benefit ratio of perioperative OKT3 in cardiac transplantation. *Am J Cardiol* 1994;**74**:261–6.

Johnson MR, Aaronson KD, Canter CE, et al. Heart retransplantation. *Am J Transplant* 2007;**7**:2075–81.

Keogh A, MacDonald P, Mundy J, et al. Five-year follow-up of a randomized double-drug versus triple-drug therapy immunosuppressive trial after heart transplantation. *J Heart Lung Transplant* 1992;**11**:550–6.

Keogh A, Richardson M, Ruygrok P, et al. Sirolimus in de novo heart transplant recipients reduces acute rejection and prevents coronary artery disease at 2 years: a randomized clinical trial. *Circulation* 2004;**110**:2694–700.

Kirklin JK, Young JB, McGiffin DC. The heart transplant operation. In: Kirklin JK, Young JB, McGiffin DC (eds), *Heart Transplantation*. New York: Churchill Livingstone, 2002: 339–52.

Kobashigawa JA, Kirklin JK, Naftel DC, et al. Pretransplantation risk factors for acute rejection after heart transplantation: a multiinstitutional study. The Transplant Cardiologists Research Database Group. *J Heart Lung Transplant* 1993;**12**:355–66.

Kobashigawa J, Miller L, Renlund D, et al. A randomized active-controlled trial of mycophenolate mofetil in heart transplant recipients. Mycophenolate Mofetil Investigators. *Transplantation* 1998;**66**:507–15.

Kobashigawa JA, Moriguchi JD, Laks H, et al. Ten-year follow-up of a randomized trial of pravastatin in heart transplant patients. *J Heart Lung Transplant* 2005;**24**: 1736–40.

Kobashigawa JA, Miller LW, Russell SD, et al. Tacrolimus with mycophenolate mofetil (MMF) or sirolimus vs. cyclosporine with MMF in cardiac transplant patients: 1-year report. *Am J Transplant* 2006;**6**:1377–86.

Koelling TM, Joseph S, Aaronson KD. Heart failure survival score continues to predict clinical outcomes in patients with heart failure receiving β-blockers. *J Heart Lung Transplant* 2004;**23**:1414–22.

Kubo SH, Naftel DC, Mills RM Jr, et al. Risk factors for late recurrent rejection after heart transplantation: a multiinstitutional, multivariable analysis. Cardiac Transplant Research Database Group. *J Heart Lung Transplant* 1995;**14**:409–18.

Leyh RG, Jahnke AW, Kraatz EG, Sievers HH. Cardiovascular dynamics and dimensions after bicaval and standard cardiac transplantation. *Ann Thorac Surg* 1995;**59**: 1495–500.

Lietz K, Miller LW. Improved survival of patients with end-stage heart failure listed for heart transplantation. *J Am Coll Cardiol* 2007;**50**:1282–90.

McCarthy PM, Smith JA, Siegel LC, et al. Cardiac transplant admission, anesthesia, and operative procedures. In: Smith JA, McCarthy PM, Sarris GE, et al. (eds), *The Stanford Manual of Cardiopulmonary Transplantation*. Armonk, NY: Futura Publishing Co., Inc., 1996: 61–62.

Mancini DM, Eisen H, Kussmaul W, Mull R, Edmunds LH Jr, Wilson JR. Value of peak exercise oxygen consumption for optimal timing of cardiac transplantation in ambulatory patients with heart failure. *Circulation* 1991;**83**:778–86.

Mancini D, Pinney S, Burkhoff D, et al. Use of rapamycin slows progression of cardiac transplantation vasculopathy. *Circulation* 2003;**108**:48–53.

Massad MG, Cook DJ, Schmitt SK, et al. Factors influencing HLA sensitization in implantable LVAD recipients. *Ann Thorac Surg* 1997;**64**:1120–5.

Mather PJ, Jeevanandam V, Eisen HJ, et al. Functional and morphologic adaptation of undersized donor hearts after heart transplantation. *J Am Coll Cardiol* 1995;**26**: 737–42.

Mehra MR, Kobashigawa J, Starling R, et al. Listing criteria for heart transplantation: International Society for Heart and Lung Transplantation guidelines for the care of cardiac transplant candidates-2006. *J Heart Lung Transplant* 2006;**25**:1024–42.

Mehra MR, Uber PA, Park MH, Ventura HO, Scott RL. Corticosteroid weaning in the tacrolimus and mycophenolate era in heart transplantation: clinical and neurohormonal benefits. *Transplant Proc* 2004;**36**:3152–5.

Menkis AH, Novick RJ, Kostuk WJ, et al. Successful use of the "unacceptable" heart donor. *J Heart Lung Transplant* 1991;**10**:28–32.

Milano CA, Shah AS, Van Trigt P, et al. Evaluation of early postoperative results after bicaval versus standard cardiac transplantation and review of the literature. *Am Heart J* 2000;**140**:717–21.

Mills RM, Naftel DC, Kirklin JK, et al. Heart transplant rejection with hemodynamic compromise: a multiinstitutional study of the role of endomyocardial cellular infiltrate. Cardiac Transplant Research Database. *J Heart Lung Transplant* 1997;**16**:813–21.

Morgan JA, Edwards NM. Techniques of cardiac transplantation in adults. In: Edwards NM, Chen JM, Mazzeo PA (eds.) *Cardiac Transplantation*. Totowa, NJ: Humana Press, 2004: 63–77.

Musci M, Loebe M, Wellnhofer E, et al. Coronary angioplasty, bypass surgery, and retransplantation in cardiac transplant patients with graft coronary disease. *Thorac Cardiovasc Surg* 1998;**46**:268–74.

O'Neill JO, Young JB, Pothier CE, Lauer MS. Peak oxygen consumption as a predictor of death in patients with heart failure receiving beta-blockers. *Circulation* 2005;**111**: 2313–18.

Ojo AO, Held PJ, Port FK, et al. Chronic renal failure after transplantation of a nonrenal organ. *N Engl J Med* 2003;**349**:931–40.

Opelz G, Dohler B, Laux G. Long-term prospective study of steroid withdrawal in kidney and heart transplant recipients. *Am J Transplant* 2005;**5**:720–8.

Ott GY, Herschberger RE, Ratkovec RR, Norman D, Hosenpud JD, Cobanoglu A. Cardiac allografts from high-risk donors: excellent clinical results. *Ann Thorac Surg* 1994;**57**:76–81; discussion 81–2.

Owen VJ, Burton PB, Michel MC, et al. Myocardial dysfunction in donor hearts. A possible etiology. *Circulation* 1999;**99**:2565–70.

Packer M, Colucci WS, Sackner-Bernstein JD, et al. Double-blind, placebo-controlled study of the effects of carvedilol in patients with moderate to severe heart failure. The PRECISE Trial. Prospective Randomized Evaluation of Carvedilol on Symptoms and Exercise. *Circulation* 1996; **94**:2793–9.

Piccione W Jr. Bridge to transplant with the HeartMate device. *J Card Surg* 2001;**16**:272–9.

Prieto M, Lake KD, Pritzker MR, et al. OKT3 induction and steroid-free maintenance immunosuppression for treatment of high-risk heart transplant recipients. *J Heart Lung Transplant* 1991;**10**:901–11.

Radio SJ, McManus BM, Winters GL, et al. Preferential endocardial residence of B-cells in the "Quilty effect" of human heart allografts: immunohistochemical distinction from rejection. *Mod Pathol* 1991;**4**:654–60.

Radovancevic B, McGiffin DC, Kobashigawa JA, et al. Retransplantation in 7,290 primary transplant patients: a 10-year multi-institutional study. *J Heart Lung Transplant* 2003;**22**:862–8.

Reichart B, Meiser B, Vigano M, et al. European multicenter tacrolimus heart pilot study: Three year follow-up. *J Heart Lung Transplant* 2001;**20**:249–250.

Renlund DG, O'Connell JB, Gilbert EM, Watson FS, Bristow MR. Feasibility of discontinuation of corticosteroid maintenance therapy in heart transplantation. *J Heart Lung Transplant* 1987;**6**:71–8.

RESOLVD Investigators. Effects of metoprolol CR in patients with ischemic and dilated cardiomyopathy: the randomized evaluation of strategies for left ventricular dysfunction pilot study. *Circulation* 2000;**101**:378–84.

Rodino MA, Shane E. Osteoporosis after organ transplantation. *Am J Med* 1998;**104**:459–69.

Rosengard BR, Feng S, Alfrey EJ, et al. Report of the Crystal City meeting to maximize the use of organs recovered from the cadaver donor. *Am J Transplant* 2002;**2**: 701–11.

Rothenburger M, Hulsken G, Stypmann J, et al. Cardiothoracic surgery after heart and heart-lung transplantation. *Thorac Cardiovasc Surg* 2005;**53**:85–92.

Sarsam MA, Campbell CS, Yonan NA, Deiraniya AK, Rahman AN. An alternative surgical technique in orthotopic cardiac transplantation. *J Cardiovasc Surg* 1993;**8**: 344–9.

Shumway SJ. Operative techniques in heart transplantation. In: Shumway SJ, Shumway NE (eds), *Thoracic Transplantation*. Oxford: Blackwell Science, 1995: 163–73.

Sievers HH, Leyh R, Jahnke A, et al. Bicaval versus atrial anastomoses in cardiac transplantation. Right atrial dimension and tricuspid valve function at rest and during exercise up to thirty-six months after transplantation. *J Thorac Cardiovasc Surg* 1994;**108**:780–4.

Sievers HH, Weyand M, Kraatz EG, Bernhard A. An alternative technique for orthotopic cardiac transplantation, with preservation of the normal anatomy of the right atrium. *Thorac Cardiovasc Surg* 1991;**39**:70–2.

Srivastava R, Keck BM, Bennett LE, Hosenpud JD. The results of cardiac retransplantation: an analysis of the Joint International Society for Heart and Lung Transplantation/United Network for Organ Sharing Thoracic Registry. *Transplantation* 2000;**70**:606–12.

Stark RP, McGinn AL, Wilson RF. Chest pain in cardiac-transplant recipients. Evidence of sensory reinnervation after cardiac transplantation. *N Engl J Med* 1991;**324**: 1791–4.

Stewart S, Winters GL, Fishbein MC, et al. Revision of the 1990 working formulation for the standardization of nomenclature in the diagnosis of heart rejection. *J Heart Lung Transplant* 2005;**24**:1710–20.

Swinnen LJ, Costanzo-Nordin MR, Fisher SG, et al. Increased incidence of lymphoproliferative disorders after immunosuppression with the monoclonal antibody OKT3 in cardiac-transplant recipients. *N Engl J Med* 1990;**323**: 1723–8.

Taylor DO, Barr ML, Radovancevic B, et al. A randomized, multicenter comparison of tacrolimus and cyclosporine immunosuppressive regimens in cardiac transplantation: decreased hyperlipidemia and hypertension with tacrolimus. *J Heart Lung Transplant* 1999;**18**:336–45.

Taylor DO, Bristow MR, O'Connell JB, et al. Improved long-term survival after heart transplantation predicted by successful early withdrawal from maintenance corticosteroid therapy. *J Heart Lung Transplant* 1996;**15**: 1039–46.

Taylor DO, Edwards LB, Boucek MM, et al. Registry of the International Society for Heart and Lung Transplantation: twenty-fourth official adult heart transplant report – 2007. *J Heart Lung Transplant* 2007;**26**:769–81.

Topkara VK, Dang NC, John R, et al. A decade experience of cardiac retransplantation in adult recipients. *J Heart Lung Transplant* 2005;**24**:1745–50.

Traversi E, Pozzoli M, Grande A, et al. The bicaval anastomosis technique for orthotopic heart transplantation yields better atrial function than the standard technique: an echocardiographic automatic boundary detection study. *J Heart Lung Transplant* 1998;**17**:1065–74.

Trento A, Czer LS, Blanche C. Surgical techniques for cardiac transplantation. *Semin Thorac Cardiovasc Surg* 1996;**8**:126–32.

Wenke K, Meiser B, Thiery J, et al. Simvastatin initiated early after heart transplantation: 8-year prospective experience. *Circulation* 2003;**107**:93–7.

Wilson RF, Christensen BV, Olivari MT, Simon A, White CW, Laxson DD. Evidence for structural sympathetic reinnervation after orthotopic cardiac transplantation in humans. *Circulation* 1991;**83**:1210–20.

Wilson RF, Johnson TH, Haidet GC, Kubo SH, Mianuelli M. Sympathetic reinnervation of the sinus node and exercise hemodynamics after cardiac transplantation. *Circulation* 2000;**101**:2727–33.

Wood KE, Becker BN, McCartney JG, D'Alessandro AM, Coursin DB. Care of the potential organ donor. *N Engl J Med* 2004;**351**:2730–39.

Yacoub M, Alivizatos P, Khaghani A, Mitchel A. The use of cyclosporine, azathioprine and antithymocyte globulin with or without low-dose steroids for immunosuppression of cardiac transplant patients. *Transplant Proc* 1985; **XVII**:221–2.

Yankah AC, Musci M, Weng Y, et al. Tricuspid valve dysfunction and surgery after orthotopic cardiac transplantation. *Eur J Cardiothorac Surg* 2000;**17**:343–8.

9 Lung transplantation

Jonathan E Spahr[1] *and Keith C Meyer*[2]

[1]Children's Hospital of Pittsburgh and the University of Pittsburgh School of Medicine, Pittsburgh, Pennsylvania, USA

[2]University of Wisconsin School of Medicine and Public Health, Madison, Wisconsin, USA

Allotransplantation of the human lung was first performed in 1963 by Dr James Hardy at the University of Mississippi. It did not become successful enough to achieve acceptance as a treatment for end-stage lung disease (ESLD) until the mid-1980s to the early 1990s when improved surgical techniques, advances in organ preservation, and the development and clinical implementation of novel immunosuppressive drugs allowed long-term survival of lung allograft recipients. Lung transplantation has evolved considerably over the past two decades and is now a definitive treatment for ESLDs that do not respond to other therapeutic interventions. As lung transplantation has become accepted as a life-prolonging therapy for ESLD and performed at various centers world-wide, many complications have been identified, and methods for monitoring and treating those complications have arisen. Despite considerable progress in preventing and treating complications, only half of recipients survive more than 5 years after receiving a lung transplant. The risks and benefits of lung transplantation must be carefully weighed for each patient. In addition, the timing of the procedure is of critical importance. Thus, a great deal of attention has been focused on appropriate referral criteria and timing for this procedure in order to maximize its benefit. Improvements in surgical technique and immunosuppressive regimens combined with a growing awareness of common complications and the measures to prevent them have extended survival and provided most recipients with an improved quality of life after lung transplantation.

This chapter focuses on the three main aspects of optimizing the outcome of lung transplantation: first, patient selection and appropriate timing and criteria for lung transplantation is reviewed; the focus then turns to the technical aspects of the procedure; finally, attention focuses on perioperative and postoperative complications and strategies to prevent or treat such complications.

Selection of patients for lung transplantation

Indications and contraindications

Indications for lung transplantation include the broad categories of obstructive, restrictive, suppurative, and vascular pulmonary diseases. Older adults undergo transplantation much more frequently for chronic obstructive pulmonary disease (COPD) and interstitial lung disease (ILD) than children and young adults, who undergo lung transplantation predominantly for suppurative lung diseases, of which cystic fibrosis (CF) is the most common.

The task of determining eligibility for lung transplantation should be the responsibility of a multidisciplinary team that evaluates both the physiologic and psychosocial characteristics of individuals referred for transplantation. This team typically consists of physicians (medical and surgical), nurses, pharmacists, mental health specialists, and social workers. Patients and families should be informed of the rigors inherent

Primer on Transplantation, 3rd edition.
Edited by Donald Hricik.

in undergoing lung transplantation. Candidates for lung transplantation must have the ability to deal with these challenges physically, psychologically, and financially.

In 1998, the American Thoracic Society (ATS) and the European Respiratory Society (ERS) developed a consensus statement for the selection of candidates for lung transplantation. This statement, updated in 2006, considers both general and disease-specific factors, which include age, expected survival without lung transplantation, and quality of life. In general, most transplant centers would agree that the upper age limit is 65 years for single lung transplantation (SLT) and 60 years for bilateral lung transplantation (BLT). At the other end of the age spectrum, children are limited by the size of their thorax and the size of available donor lungs.

Of particular importance in deciding whether a patient with ESLD is a candidate for lung transplantation is the status of native lung function. As lung transplantation candidates generally wait an average of 18–24 months before they can be transplanted, the referring physician is charged with the difficult task of predicting 2-year mortality for their patients with ESLD so that the effectiveness of this potentially life-prolonging procedure can be optimized. Table 9.1

Table 9.1 Indications for disease-specific patient referral and transplantation

Recipient indication	Referral	Transplantation
Obstructive lung disease • COPD • Obliterative/constrictive bronchiolitis	• BODE index >5 (BODE is a composite score based on BMI, FEV_1, dyspnea index, and exercise capacity) • Criteria used before the creation of the BODE index: • Post-bronchodilator FEV_1 < 25% of predicted normal value • $PaCO_2$ > 7.3 kPa (55 mmHg) • Associated pulmonary arterial hypertension/cor pulmonale	Patients with a BODE index of 7–10 or at least one of: • history of hospitalization for exacerbation associated with acute hypercapnia (PCO_2 >50 mmHg) • pulmonary hypertension or cor pulmonale (or both) despite supplemental oxygen therapy • FEV_1 < 20% predicted and either *D*LCO < 20% predicted or homogeneous distribution of emphysema
Pulmonary fibrosis • IPF • Fibrotic NSIP • Sarcoidosis • Other ILD	Histologic or radiologic evidence of UIP irrespective of VC Histologic evidence of fibrotic NSIP Other characteristic with predictive value (IPF): • VC < 60–70% predicted • DL_{CO} < 50–60% predicted • Resting hypoxemia (PaO_2 < 7.3 kPa [55 mmHg]) • Hypercapnia ($PaCO_2$ >6 kPa [45 mmHg]) • Desaturation during 6-MWT to <88% • Secondary pulmonary arterial hypertension • NYHA functional class III/IV for other ILD (sarcoidosis, LAM, PLCH)	IPF or fibrotic NSIP: *D*LCO < 39% predicted (IPF) or <35% (fibrotic NSIP) ≥10% decline in FVC during 6-month follow-up (IPF, NSIP) Decrease in oxyhemoglobin saturation to <88% during 6MWT Honeycomb change on HRCT (fibrosis score >2) Sarcoidosis: NYHA class III/IV and any of: • resting hypoxemia • pulmonary hypertension • right atrial pressure >15 mmHg • LAM or PLCH: severe impairment in lung function and exercise capacity and/or resting hypoxemia

Table 9.1 (*Continued*)

Recipient indication	Referral	Transplantation
Septic obstructive lung disease • Cystic fibrosis • Non-CF bronchiectasis	Post-bronchodilator $FEV_1 < 30\%$ (especially young females) Exacerbation of pulmonary disease requiring ICU stay Increasing frequency of exacerbations requiring intravenous antibiotics Refractory and/or recurrent pneumothorax Recurrent hemoptysis not controlled by embolization Other factors with predictive value for CF: • hypercapnia ($PaCO_2$ >6 kPa [45 mmHg]) • rapidly progressive decline in lung function • resting hypoxemia ($PaO_2 < 7.3$ kPa [55 mmHg])	• Oxygen-dependent respiratory failure • Hypercapnia • Pulmonary hypertension
Pulmonary vascular disease • Primary pulmonary hypertension (PPH) • Chronic thromboembolic disease	• NYHA class III/IV regardless of ongoing therapy • Rapidly progressive disease (e.g. worsening functional capacity despite escalating doses of vasodilator therapy) • Not a surgical candidate if indication is chronic thromboembolic disease	• Persistent NYHA class III/IV on maximal medical therapy • Low (<350 m) or declining 6MWT • Failing therapy with intravenous epoprostenol or equivalent (PPH) • Cardiac index <2 L/min per m^2 • Right atrial pressure > 15 mmHg
Heart and lung disease[a] • Eisenmenger's syndrome • Other cardiopulmonary disease	• NYHA class III/IV despite optimal therapy • Progressive symptoms • Other factors to consider: cor pulmonale, declining cardiac output, presence of cyanosis	• Persistent NYHA class III/IV on maximal medical therapy • Low (<350 m) or declining 6MWT distance

6MWT, 6-minute walk test; BODE, body mass index, airflow obstruction, dyspnea, and exercise capacity index in COPD; CF, cystic fibrosis; COPD, chronic obstructive pulmonary disease; *D*LCO, diffusion capacity of the lung for carbon monoxide; FVC, forced vital capacity; FEV_1, forced expiratory volume in 1 s; HRCT, high-resolution computed tomography of the thorax; ILD, interstitial lung disease; IPF, idiopathic pulmonary fibrosis; LAM, lymphangioleiomyomatosis; NSIP, non-specific interstitial pneumonia; NYHA, New York Heart Association; PLCH, pulmonary Langerhans' cell histiocytosis; PPH, primary pulmonary hypertension; VC, vital capacity; UIP, usual interstitial pneumonia.
[a]Heart–lung transplant usually required.See Orens, et al. *J Heart Lung Transplant* 2006;25:745–55.

summarizes referral criteria and ideal timing of transplantation according to specific indications for the procedure. For each indication, guidelines for listing are discussed separately below.

As the primary goal of lung transplantation is to prolong life rather than to permanently cure an ESLD, consideration of how the patient will benefit from lung transplantation must be made. There is ongoing debate about the survival benefit of lung transplantation based on the underlying disease. For the most part, individuals with CF, ILD, and pulmonary hypertension appear to derive a survival benefit from lung transplantation. However, studies evaluating survival benefit for patients with COPD have yielded mixed results. For many patients with an otherwise untreatable form of ESLD, lung transplantation can provide palliation of symptoms and improved quality of life even when long-term survival is not extended. For example, in patients with Eisenmenger's syndrome, a clear survival benefit of lung transplantation has not been identified. However, most patients with this disorder experience improvement in exercise tolerance and are able to improve their daily function after lung transplantation.

The absolute and relative contraindications to lung transplantation vary from center to center (see Key points 9.1). In general, absolute contraindications include severe extrapulmonary disease, use of tobacco or alcohol, impaired functional status, and refractory psychosocial problems. Examples of severe extrapulmonary disease that would preclude lung transplantation are infection with human immunodeficiency virus (HIV), active tuberculosis, hepatitis B, significant left ventricular dysfunction, active malignancy within 5 years, renal insufficiency, hepatic dysfunction, portal hypertension, diabetes mellitus with end-organ damage, and osteoporosis with vertebral compression fractures.

Key points 9.1 Absolute and relative contraindications to lung transplantation[a]

- **Absolute contraindications**
  Malignancy within 2 years, with the exception of cutaneous squamous and basal cell tumors[b]
  Untreatable, advanced dysfunction of another major organ system
  Non-curable chronic extrapulmonary infection
  Significant chest wall and/or spinal deformity
  Documented non-adherence or inability to follow through with medical therapy and monitoring
  Untreatable psychiatric or psychologic condition that will impair compliance with medical therapy
  No reliable social support system
  Substance addiction within past 6 months
- **Relative contraindications**
  Critical or unstable condition
  Severely limited functional status with poor rehabilitation potential
  Colonization with highly resistant or highly virulent microorganisms
  Severe obesity (BMI >30 kg/m^2)
  Severe or symptomatic osteoporosis
  Mechanical ventilation
  Suboptimally treated serious medical condition

[a]See Orens et al. *J Heart Lung Transplant* 2006;**25**:745–55.
[b]In general, a 5-year disease-free interval is prudent.

The need for mechanical ventilation at the time of transplantation is an absolute contraindication for some centers but a relative contraindication at others, depending on the underlying ESLD. Adults with CF should not be excluded from undergoing lung transplantation if they are mechanically ventilated, because mortality rates are not influenced by the need for ventilation at the time of transplantation. In contrast, the need for mechanical ventilation in children with CF is associated with poor short- and long-term outcomes. Many individuals require supplemental oxygen and even non-invasive ventilation in the form of bi-level positive airway pressure (BiPAP) as a "bridge" to transplantation. Currently available data suggest that post-transplant outcomes are improved for recipients with CF who use BiPAP before lung transplantation.

There are some factors that may make lung transplantation more challenging and place the patient at considerable risk for suboptimal outcome. Patients who have had previous chest surgery or pleurodesis (chemical or surgical) may have significant pleural fibrosis and adhesion of the visceral and parietal pleura. This makes explantation of the native lungs extremely difficult and prone to hemorrhagic complications. Nevertheless, prior surgery or pleurodesis is not considered an absolute contraindication to future lung transplantation. Oral corticosteroids are known to impair wound healing, and many centers consider a daily dose of prednisone >20 mg to be a contraindication, although this is not universal.

Pretransplant evaluation

As there are contraindications to lung transplantation, a comprehensive pretransplant evaluation is required to identify potential comorbidities that present potentially insurmountable problems in the perioperative and postoperative periods and that may significantly decrease the likelihood of long-term survival. Table 9.2 lists both medical and psychosocial evaluations that are helpful in assessing risk in a lung transplantation candidate. This list, although extensive, is not absolute and may not cover all situations. Subsequent sections will address specific disease states and/or comorbidities that may require additional evaluation.

COPD and α_1-antitrypsin deficiency-associated emphysema

COPD, including the obstructive disease resulting from α_1-antitrypsin deficiency, is the most common

Table 9.2 Evaluation of potential candidates for lung transplantation

- Psychosocial evaluation
  - ? Tobacco use within 6 months
  - ? Illicit drug use, drug-seeking behavior
  - Compliance with medical therapies
  - ? Significant psychiatric illness
  - Adequate social support
- Cardiopulmonary
  - Full pulmonary function tests
  - Standardized exercise test (e.g., 6-minute walk test)
  - Electrocardiogram
  - Stress echocardiogram (plus coronary catheterization as appropriate)
  - High-resolution CT scan of thorax
  - Lipid profile
- Other
  - Peripheral blood cell survey
  - Glucose and hemoglobin A1C
  - 24-hour creatinine clearance
  - Bone mineral density scan
- Infection specific
  - Quarterly respiratory tract cultures (for suppurative lung disease)
  - Gram-negative bacilli
  - Meticillin-resistant *Staphylococcus aureus*
  - Mycobacteria
  - Fungi
  - Serology
  - HIV
  - Hepatitis B and C
  - Varicella
  - Cytomegalovirus
  - Toxoplasmosis
  - Vaccinations
  - PPD skin test
  - Evaluation and treatment of paranasal sinus disease

indication for lung transplantation in adults. As the surgical risks are lower for SLT versus BLT in patients with COPD, SLT is commonly performed for this lung transplantation indication, which helps to expand the donor pool when a single donor can be used for two recipients. Although there may be an advantage to BLT with regard to outcome and lung function, exercise capacity is comparable for SLT versus BLT recipients with COPD.

Certain criteria must be met to list candidates with COPD for lung transplantation, and these include a demonstrated ability to abstain from smoking. Most transplant centers require abstinence from cigarette smoking anywhere from 6 months to 12 months. Physiologic parameter thresholds for lung transplantation in COPD have included forced expiratory volume at 1 s (FEV_1) <25% predicted without reversibility and/or $PaCO_2 \geq 7.3$ kPa (55 mmHg) with or without elevated pulmonary artery pressures and progressive deterioration. The most recent recommendations from the International Society for Heart and Lung Transplantation (ISHLT), however, advocate use of the BODE index (body mass index, airflow obstruction, dyspnea, and exercise capacity index in COPD) for decision-making (see Table 9.1) The American Thoracic Society and European Respiratory Society (ATS/ERS) have also made the recommendation that priority for lung transplantation be given to patients who require oxygen supplementation and who exhibit progressive deterioration and elevated $PaCO_2$ because mortality is increased for such patients.

Interstitial lung disease

Idiopathic pulmonary fibrosis (IPF) is the most common form of ILD for which lung transplantation is performed. Indications for referral include symptomatic and progressive disease recalcitrant to therapy, significantly impaired lung function with decrease in forced vital capacity (FVC) to <60–70% of the predicted normal value and/or diffusion capacity for carbon monoxide (DLCO) <50–60% predicted. As the median survival after diagnosis of IPF is approximately 2–3 years, current ISHLT guidelines recommend referral to a lung transplantation center at the time of diagnosis due to the progressive nature of the disease. Hemoglobin oxygen desaturation during a 6-minute walk test (6MWT) may be helpful in determining the degree of lung function decline. Specifically, desaturation to 88% or less predicts a survival rate of approximately 35% at 4 years.

The progression of other ILDs is quite variable. In the case of non-specific interstitial lung disease (NSIP) and sarcoidosis, progression tends to be less rapid (compared with IPF) and more likely to respond to immunomodulatory medications. However, the fibrotic variant of NSIP, if accompanied by oxyhemoglobin desaturation to ≤88% during a 6MWT, carries a prognosis that is fairly similar to that for IPF. Therefore, recommendations to refer patients with NSIP are based on the aggressiveness of the disease and whether it is characterized by a cellular and/or fibrotic histopathology. Likewise, sarcoidosis may progress to extensive pulmonary fibrosis, and wait-listed patients with severe impairment of lung function have a projected survival that is very similar to that for wait-listed patients with IPF.

In the case of ILD, SLT is more commonly performed than BLT. However, BLT should be considered if there is significant bronchiectasis in the native lungs that would predispose the lungs to a chronic suppurative process.

Bronchiectasis/Cystic fibrosis

BLT is the recommended procedure for severe suppurative lung disease due to bronchiectasis (sometimes the result of advanced CF), which is typically widespread throughout both lungs. Conventional wisdom dictates that, if only one lung is transplanted, residual infection in the native lung can spread to the transplanted lung and cause unacceptable complications in the immunocompromised recipient. The suppurative and fluctuating nature of CF lung disease presents a significant and often vexing challenge to physicians in determining the appropriate and optimal time for referral as well as preparing the patient for referral to a lung transplantation center.

The presence of multidrug-resistant *Pseudomonas aeruginosa* is not a contraindication for transplantation, but persistent carriage of pan-resistant *P. aeruginosa* is considered to be a contraindication at some centers. However, several studies have shown no difference in post-lung transplantation survival for patients infected with pan-resistant *P. aeruginosa* and those with antibiotic-sensitive strains. Additionally in vitro sensitivities of *P. aeruginosa* may not accurately reflect in vivo sensitivity and should be interpreted with caution because some individuals have been shown to improve clinically despite the use of anti-pseudomonal antibiotics that would not be considered effective according to in vitro susceptibility testing. In some cases, the use of aerosolized colistin has been reported to cause a re-emergence of sensitive *P. aeruginosa* in CF patients awaiting lung transplantation.

Chronic infection with *Burkholderia cepacia* in patients with CF is viewed by some centers to be a contraindication to lung transplantation. One retrospective study of patients with cystic fibrosis showed that 6-month mortality was significantly increased only in cases where genomovar III strains of *B. cepacia* caused the chronic infection. These data suggest that determining the specific *B. cepacia* genomovar may be useful in weighing the risk of lung transplantation for patients who harbor *B. cepacia* in their respiratory secretions before transplantation.

Aspergillus fumigatus is commonly isolated from respiratory secretions of patients with CF. Surprisingly, this fungus is rarely a serious pathogen in the post-transplant patient with CF. When aspergillosis occurs in lung transplant recipients with CF, it is usually in the form of tracheobronchial aspergillosis in the allograft bronchi adjacent to the anastomoses (the injured epithelium at the anastomosis is susceptible to aspergillus infection as it heals after reperfusion).

Severe malnutrition with very low body mass index (BMI), which frequently occurs in patients with CF and ESLD, may place the patient in a risk category that is too high to safely perform lung transplantation. Supplemental nutrition via enterostomy tube may be required before transplantation to improve a low BMI. Another consideration in patients with CF is the presence of significant hepatobiliary disease. As survival into adulthood progressively increases, advanced liver disease is becoming more prevalent and may pose a problem after otherwise successful lung transplantation. Although combined lung and liver transplantation can be considered, relatively few centers are willing to perform a combined lung–liver transplantation during the same operation.

The timing of referral for patients with advanced CF lung disease presents a significant challenge to referring physicians. The recommended physiologic parameters that predict respiratory failure within 2 years and, thus, the basis for referral include post-bronchodilator $FEV_1 < 30\%$ predicted, $PaO_2 < 7.3$ kPa (55 mmHg), and $PaCO_2 > 6$ kPa (45 mmHg). Other criteria or complex scoring systems that utilize multiple parameters have not shown significantly better predictive value. Determining the optimal time for referral and transplantation for children is particularly difficult. Although FEV_1, PaO_2, and $PaCO_2$ continue to be important factors in deciding when to refer the child with CF for lung transplantation, most centers continue to evaluate on a case-by-case basis. Pneumothorax and hemoptysis are associated with a significant increase in 2-year mortality, even when FEV_1 is not severely impaired, and their occurrence may indicate a need to consider early referral. In addition, a rapid and sustained decline in lung function, especially when occurring in young females, may indicate a need to refer for lung transplantation. Lastly, frequent, recurrent exacerbations that require hospitalizations and/or antibiotic treatment also may herald a rapid decline in lung function and impending need for lung transplantation referral.

Pulmonary hypertension

Patients with primary pulmonary hypertension who meet criteria for New York Heart Association (NHYA) class III or IV, and who have progressive disease despite medical therapy, meet the criteria for lung transplantation. Right heart catheterization measurements that show mean pulmonary artery pressure >55 mmHg, mean right atrial pressure >15 mmHg, and cardiac index <2.0 L/min per m^2 support the decision to refer for lung transplantation. An important decision when evaluating patients with pulmonary hypertension for lung transplantation is whether SLT or BLT should be performed. Although a well-functioning single lung should have adequate capacitance to prevent right heart strain or failure, published data do not provide clear guidelines, and the decision to perform SLT versus BLT should be made on a case-by-case basis. Heart and lung transplantation is necessary when left ventricular function is irreversibly compromised.

Patients with Eisenmenger's complex may tolerate mean pulmonary artery pressures >55 mmHg and mean right atrial pressures >15 mmHg, making their risk of mortality and clinical course more difficult to predict. For these patients, heart–lung transplantation appears to confer a better outcome in regard to mortality.

With the advent of new medications (e.g., bosentan, prostaglandin infusion, and sildenafil) to treat pulmonary hypertension, patients are able to live longer without the need for lung transplantation. In contrast to other indications for lung transplantation, the need for donor lungs for this indication has decreased with the advent of medical therapies that successfully lower pulmonary arterial pressures and improve cardiac output.

UNOS allocation (old and new systems)

The United Network for Organ Sharing (UNOS) recently made a significant change to the allocation system for lung donation in the USA, and implemented the new system in 2005. Before this change, recipient rank on the lung transplantation wait-list was based on waiting time, blood group compatibility, and size matching. In contrast to policies for heart and liver transplantation, severity of disease was not a factor in the old system, with the exception of patients with IPF, who were automatically credited 90 days of accrued wait-list time due to the relatively severe and progressive nature of their disease.

The new UNOS allocation system does take into account severity of disease and assigns each potential recipient a lung allocation score based on medical information. The medical parameters taken into account by the new lung allocation system (LAS) are listed in Table 9.3. Specific types of ESLD are prioritized according to the inherent degree of severity and expected progression of the disease. However, the LAS scoring system applies only to individuals aged >12 years. For those aged <12 years, waiting time is still the most significant factor in determining lung allocation priority.

Once the potential recipient is determined to be a candidate for lung transplantation, they are registered into the UNet secure internet-based system for organ allocation and data collection, and the data are used to compile a score ranging from 0 to100, with higher scores corresponding to higher priority. This score, along with the ABO blood group compatibility, size matching, and the patient's distance from the hospital, will determine the order of patient eligibility when an offer for a donor lung is received by the lung transplantation center where the patient is listed. In the case of a tie score, time spent on the list is used to break the tie. Information must be updated every 6 months, but data may be updated at any time to reflect changes in the patient's status. If lung transplantation center physicians believe that certain patients have exceptional circumstances and their LAS does not accurately reflect the patient's situation and urgency for transplantation, they may petition the Lung Review Board to determine if an adjustment can be made.

In the case of pediatric lung allocation, lung size needs to be taken into account and recipient priority is based on donor age. Those under the age of 12 continue to have their recipient priority determined

Table 9.3 Lung allocation scoring (LAS) system in the USA

LAS score determinants
• Specific disease indication for lung transplant
• Forced vital capacity (percent predicted)
• Pulmonary arterial systolic pressure
• Supplemental oxygen requirement (L/min)
• Age
• Height and weight
• Functional status (I, II, III)
• 6MWT distance
• Ventilator use
• Pulmonary capillary wedge pressure
• Serum creatinine
• PCO_2
Calculation of the LAS score
• Waiting list survival probability during next year is calculated
• Calculate wait-list urgency
• Calculate post-transplant survival probability during first post-transplantation year
• Calculate post-transplant survival measure
• Calculate raw allocation score
• Raw allocation score is then normalized (0–100; organ offers go to candidate with highest score within specific blood group and thoracic dimension category)

by the time spent on the waiting list. Key points 9.2 also reflects how children receive priority over adult patients for donor lungs.

Key points 9.2 Pediatric transplantation: matching and prioritization

• Donor age (years)	<12	12–17	18+
• First priority recipient	Age <12	Age 12–17	Age ≥12
• Second priority recipient	Age 12–17	Age <12	Age <12
• Third priority recipient	Age 18+	Age 18+	

Policies for listing and delisting in other countries do not use a LAS scoring system as is done in the USA. The Eurotransplant organization, a supranational consortium of numerous European countries, still uses time on the wait-list combined with donor–recipient suitability to match recipients with donor organs. However, patients who display imminent need for invasive mechanical ventilation or other evidence of rapid decompensation can be granted a high urgency status and be given the highest transplant priority.

Before the change in the US allocation system, time spent on the waiting list ranged from a median of 18 months to 24 months and the number of wait-listed lung transplant candidates continued to rise as the donor pool remained static. The goal of the new system is to decrease the number of patients dying while awaiting lung transplantation by allocating lungs to those individuals most in need. The new LAS system takes into account the anticipated benefit linked to the underlying cause of ESLD, as well as the anticipated mortality without a transplant. However, the ability to predict mortality from ESLD continues to be limited due to marked variability across different patient cohorts and disease processes. Early results indicate that the new allocation system has shifted recipient diagnoses toward pulmonary fibrosis while reducing the overall mortality rate for those on lung transplantation wait-lists. One concern is that this shift will tend to select patients who will have a decreased post-transplant survival due to the severity of their illness at the time of transplantation.

Technical considerations

The donor

Careful selection of an organ donor and optimized donor management are crucial determinants of post-lung transplant outcome. Unfortunately, the rate of donor procurement for lungs remains <20% (17% in the USA and 12% in Europe) and represents the major limiting factor for the number of lung transplantations performed. Potential donors vary considerably in terms of clinical stability and organ function, and significant decline in pulmonary function all too frequently occurs during the critical management period when donors are managed in an intensive care setting. The lungs are particularly prone to injury, and maintaining optimal lung function in a potential donor requires tactics that are counterproductive to maintaining optimal function of other organs (e.g., providing high perfusion pressures to maintain adequate intravascular volume for procurement of optimally functioning kidneys). High central venous pressures may cause the lungs to develop hydrostatic edema, loss of compliance, and impaired gas exchange. The period of time from the inciting illness, such as a traumatic brain injury, to the point when brain death is declared poses significant risk for pulmonary complications that include aspiration, barotrauma, ventilator-associated pneumonia, diffuse lung injury, and non-cardiogenic pulmonary edema.

Brain death adversely affects cardiovascular function, and donor management includes measures to achieve optimal hemodynamics by maintaining normovolemia, blood pressure, and cardiac output to sustain adequate perfusion pressure and blood flow, and thereby preserve organ function while trying to limit vasoactive drug requirements. Supportive interventions required to stabilize and maintain optimal organ function in the donor may include infusion of fluids and red blood cells for hypovolemia and anemia, sodium bicarbonate for acidosis, hypotonic solutions for hypernatremia, insulin infusions for hyperglycemia, and vasoactive drug support for hypotension, (see Chapter 3).

Traditional ("standard") criteria that were initially used to define ideal donors included donor age <55 years, minimal tobacco exposure, normal chest radiograph, $PaO_2 : FiO_2$ ratio >300 during ventilation with 5 cmH_2O of positive end-expiratory pressure (PEEP) and FiO_2 100%, and the absence of aspiration, purulent secretions, or trauma (Table 9.4). However, adherence to these ideal criteria would exclude most potential donors, and adequate objective evidence to support their value has not been forthcoming. Therefore, most centers have judiciously relaxed these requirements to expand the donor pool. Atelectasis and excessive fluid resuscitation are correctable causes of hypoxemia, and aggressive management protocols that include ventilator manipulation to promote lung expansion, early bronchoscopy and aggressive secretion clearance, antibiotic administration, and judicious fluid management have allowed donors who were initially considered unsuitable by traditional criteria to become lung donors.

Table 9. 4 Criteria for acceptability of donor lungs

Traditional criteria
• Age <50 years
• Minimal tobacco exposure
• Normal chest radiograph
• PaO_2 > 39.9 kPa (300 mmHg) on 5 cmH_2O PEEP with FiO_2 = 100%
• No evidence of aspiration
Liberalized criteria (marginal/extended donor)
• Age up to 65
• Smoking up to 20 pack-years
• Severe chest trauma
• Mechanical ventilation >4 days
• Positive Gram stain on tracheobronchial washing and/or BAL
Interventions to improve donor lung function
• Frequent suctioning to remove secretions
• Ventilatory manipulation to promote lung expansion and reverse atelectasis (e.g. alveolar recruitment with inspiratory pressures at 25 cmH_2O and PEEP 15 cmH_20 for 2 h)
• Reverse fluid overload (diuresis and fluid restriction)
Absolute criteria required when donor lungs with extended criteria utilized
• PaO_2/FiO_2 > 300
• No persistent radiographic infiltrates
• No copious purulent secretions
• No bronchoscopic evidence of aspiration

BAL, bronchoalveolar lavage; PEEP, positive end-expiratory pressure.

Indeed, most centers have relaxed a number of the "standard" criteria (e.g., age up to 65 years, smoking history >20 years, $PaO_2/FiO_2 < 300$), and the acceptance of extended donor criteria coupled with improvements in donor management has contributed to an increase in lung transplantation procedures over the past decade. Outcomes using allografts with extended donor criteria have not been shown to be significantly different from outcomes when lungs were used from candidates who met ideal donor criteria. For certain disease states, however, use of lungs with extended donor criteria may lead to poor outcome. SLT for pulmonary hypertension and IPF with secondary hypertension presents situations in which the native lung would be unable to support a marginal donor lung. In addition, donor conditions that exclude use of a donor lung include uncontrolled sepsis, positive HIV status, viral hepatitis or encephalitis, active tuberculosis, Guillain–Barré syndrome, illicit drug use, malignancy, and significant chronic lung disease. Regardless of HIV antibody testing, potential donors with significant risk factors for HIV infection should be excluded from donation unless the risk to the recipient of not performing the transplantation is perceived to be greater than the risk of transmitting HIV infection and disease to the recipient. These risk factors include men who have had sex with another man within 5 years, use of non-medical drugs via injection within the preceding 5 years, engaging in sex for money or drugs within 5 years, inmates of a correctional institution, and people having contact with an HIV-infected individual within 12 months (sexual, shared needles, open wound contact, or mucous membrane contact).

In addition to the use of lungs with extended donor criteria, some centers have expanded the donor pool further by considering potential donors who do not meet criteria for brain death but have catastrophic, irreversible illness. Viable lungs can be procured and utilized after life support has been withdrawn and cardiac arrest has occurred in this setting, and the use of lungs from donation after cardiac death (DCD) donors represents one strategy to increase the donor pool. Another technique that can increase the donor pool in lung transplantation is the living lobar lung transplantation. Introduced in 1993, living lobar lung transplantation uses two donors who each provide one lobe (usually the lower lobe) to supply the recipient with adequate lung tissue for the transplant. The most common use of this technique is for patients with CF (usually children) with two parents serving as donors. A recent report of a 10-year experience with living lobar donation indicated that survival was similar to that of recipients transplanted with deceased donor grafts, except in cases of re-transplantation or when the recipient was intubated and mechanically ventilated.

The graft

Careful explantation of the lungs, which is done together with explantation of the heart, is crucial to achieving optimal post-transplant physiologic function. Careful attention to all aspects of excising the lung from the donor and preserving it ex vivo are crucial for preventing primary graft dysfunction (PGD), which accounts for a substantial number of all deaths in lung transplant recipients.

Just before cross-clamping the major vessels to free the lungs from the donor, the explant is typically flushed with epoprostadil followed by flushing with cold preservation fluid, and the explanted lungs are maintained at 4–10°C (on ice) until reimplantation is performed. Retrograde flushing (pulmonary vein to pulmonary artery) with preservation fluid can be done before implantation to try to free any clots that have embolized to the lung before explantation. When retrograde flush is performed through the pulmonary veins *in situ* while the lungs are still ventilated (following antegrade flush), lung preservation may be enhanced with better distribution of flush solution throughout the vasculature and less impairment of surfactant function. Retrograde flush may also be performed in vivo when the lung has been partially implanted (before construction of vascular anastomoses) in the recipient. Once *in situ* perfusion of the donor lungs has been cut off, minimization of ischemic time is of key importance in preventing graft injury. Older donor age and prolonged ischemic time have been shown to correlate with decreased 1-year survival, and early graft function is significantly affected by prolonged ischemic times with a threshold estimated at 330 min, although ischemic time may be extended to 8 h for young donors.

Optimal ex vivo preservation of the donor lung and minimization of ischemic time are critical to postimplantation allograft function. Poor initial graft function can have considerable adverse effects upon postimplantation recovery and prolong the need for invasive mechanical ventilation, thereby predisposing recipients to nosocomial infections and other complications of prolonged intensive care unit (ICU) stays. Furthermore, poor initial graft function may increase the risk of developing subsequent allograft rejection. The ideal preservation solution should prevent intracellular acidosis, calcium accumulation, and edema while suppressing the generation of oxyradicals and promoting the regeneration of intracellular energy metabolism. Although intracellular preservation solutions (e.g., Euro-Collins, University of Wisconsin [UW] Solution) have been used by many centers, experimental and clinical evidence now support the use of extracellular solutions, in particular the low-potassium dextran–glucose agent, Perfadex, as an optimal preservation fluid. Antegrade flush of the lungs is typically performed in concert with inflation of the lungs with an adequate tidal volume (10 mL/kg) and maintenance of airway pressures in the range of 20–25 cmH_2O before cross-clamping. Equilibration airway pressures should, however, be limited to 10–15 cmH_2O to avoid barotrauma during storage and air transport, and flushing pressures should be limited to 10–15 mmHg.

Other therapies may be administered to optimize the donor lung. Prostaglandins, which counteract ischemia-induced vasoconstriction, and corticosteroids, which prevent intense inflammatory responses, are used to prevent reperfusion injury. Newer interventions that seek to prevent or mitigate primary graft dysfunction (PGD) include the use of inhaled nitric oxide (NO), surfactant replacement, continuous infusion of prostaglandin E_1 into the recipient during early stages of reperfusion, preimplantation donor leukocyte depletion, administration of oxyradical scavengers, donor leukocyte infusion, and administering other anti-inflammatory therapies (inhibition of platelet-activating factor, chemokine receptor inhibition, complement antagonists). Although promising, these latter interventions have yet to be adopted in clinical lung transplantation protocols that attempt to improve early graft function and prevent PGD.

The match

Donor–recipient matching is primarily based on donor lung size, which must approximate the predicted lung size of the recipient, and ABO blood group match. With the exception of living donor lung transplantation, HLA matching is not feasible. Matching for cytomegalovirus (CMV) status is desirable but not mandatory with currently used antiviral prophylaxis.

Size matching is done by measuring dimensions on a standard chest radiograph or computed tomography (CT) of the thorax. Total lung capacity (TLC) of recipients with pulmonary fibrosis usually approximates that of the donor lung post-transplantation when SLT is performed. However, the donor lung may be restricted and TLC may be lower than expected due to increased compliance of the residual native lung when SLT is performed for COPD. TLC should approximate the recipient's predicted value after BLT. For children, size matching varies from institution to institution and even within institutions. Matching recipient and donor within 10 cm or 10% of the body length are two examples of estimations used for size matching in children. If there is a mismatch in the sizing where the donor lung is too large for the recipient thoracic cage, the donor lung can be down-sized via plication or lobectomy.

Case

A suitable donor was identified for a 56-year-old man with idiopathic pulmonary fibrosis. However, CT of the thorax revealed that the donor lung was 12 cm longer than the lung of the recipient. Lobectomy was performed to achieve adequate size matching and single lung transplantation was performed successfully.

The implantation procedure

A well-coordinated effort that minimizes ischemia time and allows the surgical team to create technically perfect vascular and bronchial anastomoses is extremely important in maximizing the likelihood of postoperative success. Inhaled NO and cardiac bypass should be available for every procedure. Intraoperative cardiopulmonary bypass (CPB) or extracorporeal membrane oxygenation (ECMO) may be needed to support the recipient during surgery and should be used as needed to support recipient gas exchange during the procedure. CPB, when performed intraoperatively in higher-risk patients, allows controlled initial reperfusion of the graft(s) while using lower inspired oxygen tensions, thus helping to limit reperfusion injury. In addition to surgical expertise, experienced anesthesiologists play a key role in surgical management. Decisions about the use of double-lumen intubation techniques, ventilation strategies, the need for cardiac bypass, the role of vasoactive medications such as NO, and hemodynamic support, must be addressed jointly by surgeons and anesthesiologists during removal of native lungs and implantation of donor organs.

Single lung transplantation

SLT can be performed for all recipient indications with the exception of suppurative lung diseases (CF and non-CF bronchiectasis). In the case of IPF and pulmonary hypertension, the graft should have optimal appearance and function because the native lung will have little to contribute to respiratory function. Also, although some centers find SLT acceptable for patients with pulmonary hypertension, there may be specific circumstances for which a BLT would be more advantageous. In cases of pulmonary hypertension with left ventricular dysfunction, heart–lung transplantation is indicated.

Ventilation–perfusion (V/Q) scanning in the potential recipient plays an important role in determining which lung should be transplanted. It can demonstrate areas of poor ventilation and perfusion and can estimate the relative contribution of each lung to respiratory function. The native lung with poorest function should be chosen for replacement.

Surgical pneumonectomy is typically performed through a posterolateral incision for SLT recipients. However, posterolateral thoracotomy for the left lung and anterolateral thoracotomy for the right lung will optimally expose the hilar structures. The procedure can be performed without the need for CPB if the non-transplanted native lung has residual function that is adequate to support the individual during the procedure. The non-transplanted lung is selectively ventilated as the contralateral lung is deflated and removed. If significant hypoxemia occurs due to shunting through the deflated lung, the pulmonary artery is clamped to promote better *V*/*Q* matching. If refractory hypoxemia or other manifestations of inadequate residual lung function occur, CPB should be used.

Once the recipient native lung has been explanted, the donor lung is positioned and anastomoses are made between donor and recipient bronchus, donor and recipient pulmonary artery, and donor pulmonary veins to recipient left atrium. Precautions must be taken not to disrupt the phrenic and vagus nerves and, in the case of left SLT, the recurrent laryngeal nerve. Bronchial anastomoses are often performed by telescoping the donor and recipient bronchi because end-to-end anastomoses tend to require a tissue patch and are more prone to healing complications. As the bronchial circulation provides blood flow to the airways, anastomosis of the donor and recipient bronchial arteries may theoretically prevent airway mucosal ischemia and anastomotic complications. However, outcomes when the bronchial arteries are anastomosed are not significantly different from outcomes without bronchial artery anastomosis, and perfusion of the bronchi via retrograde flow through the bronchial artery from the pulmonary circulation appears to be adequate to promote healing and to maintain viability of the bronchial mucosa.

Bilateral lung transplantation

Originally performed as an en bloc procedure (double lung transplantation) whereby both lungs were transplanted at once via a single airway anastomosis at the trachea, BLT is now most often performed by bilateral sequential transplantation of the lungs via an anterior clam-shell incision. The advantage to sequential transplantation is that the patient may not need to undergo CPB, and the bilateral bronchial anastomoses are more stable than a single tracheal anastomosis. In addition, the transverse thoracosternotomy incision used in the sequential technique allows for better exposure of the pleura when compared with the median sternotomy incision used in the en bloc double lung transplant procedure. The contralateral lung is selectively ventilated during the transplantation, and CPB can be utilized in the event of refractory hypoxemia or when transplantation is being performed for pulmonary hypertension. Hypoxemia or hemodynamic instability may occur during cross-clamping of the first pulmonary artery, after perfusion of the first transplanted lung, or after clamping of the second pulmonary artery.

Living lobar transplantation

As previously stated, the living lobar lung transplantation represents a technique established to expedite transplantation and relieve some of the stress on the UNOS donor pool. The donors must be larger than the recipient to allow adequate matching of the donor lobe to the dimensions of the recipient thoracic cage. Inadequate donor graft size may result in pleural complications and the development of bullae. Blood group matching must be performed, but donor–recipient HLA mismatches appear to have no significant influence on survival. The operation is performed similarly to SLT or sequential BLT. Donor morbidity generally consists of a prolonged need for thoracotomy tubes or a need for additional thoracotomy tubes, and donor mortality is quite low. Recipient survival has been reported to be comparable to cadaveric lung transplant survival at 1, 3 and 5 years post-transplantation.

The postoperative period

The perioperative period

Initial postoperative management is directed by the hemodynamic status of the patient and initiation of appropriate immunosuppressive and prophylactic therapies. Upon completion of the surgical procedure, intensive supportive care should start, including hemodynamic monitoring, close attention to allograft function, use of vasoactive medications as needed to maintain appropriate perfusion, assessment of renal function, appropriate prophylaxis for peptic ulcer disease and deep vein thrombosis, and strict glucose control and nutritional supplementation. Hemodynamic support during the early postoperative period should focus on avoiding pulmonary edema while maintaining adequate perfusion pressure. Pulmonary capillary occlusion pressure should be kept as low as possible while maintaining adequate urine output and systemic blood pressure. Vasoactive agents, fluid restriction, and diuretics should be used as needed to achieve this goal.

The goals of mechanical ventilation include avoiding any additional damage to the reperfused allograft and using low tidal volume ventilation strategies as needed to avoid barotrauma. Inspired oxygen should be weaned as rapidly as possible to avoid tissue injury due to hyperoxia. The ultimate goal is to liberate the patient from mechanical ventilation as soon as possible and thereby avoid complications related to prolonged ventilatory support. In the case of SLT for COPD, PEEP and high airway pressures should be minimized to avoid overdistension of the native lung. In extenuating circumstances such as severe early graft failure, individual lung ventilation may be needed to provide appropriate airway pressures for each lung and avoid ventilator-induced lung injury. Most recipients are weaned from mechanical ventilation within 48–72 h. In the case of lung transplantation for pulmonary hypertension, the patients may need to be sedated for a slightly longer period of time to prevent the occurrence of hemodynamic compromise due to the relative instability of the pulmonary vascular bed combined with a heart that has been chronically conditioned to high pulmonary artery pressures.

Protocols should be in place to begin immunosuppressive therapies and prophylactic antimicrobial agents to prevent rejection and post-lung transplant infectious complications. Immunosuppressive regimens are discussed below. Monitoring for hyperacute rejection (a rare occurrence) and acute rejection (AR) is extremely important and is discussed below.

Complications in the perioperative period

Perioperative lung transplantation complications include, but are not limited to, pulmonary edema, immediate graft failure, acute bacterial infection, bleeding, diaphragmatic paresis or paralysis, anastomotic stenosis or dehiscence, renal failure, and stroke (Table 9.5). Size matching is a key issue in transferring lungs from one thoracic cavity to another, and problems may arise from size discrepancy. Undersized lungs may over-inflate, leading to possible graft dysfunction, and pleural effusions may form. Lungs that are too large for the recipient are prone to the development of atelectasis and pneumonia, and oversized lungs may compromise hemodynamic parameters. Although size matching is important, surgical lung volume reduction can be done to allow a better fit for oversized lungs and has no apparent ill-effects on graft survival or mortality.

Pulmonary edema is almost always present in the immediate postoperative period. Although usually mild, severe pulmonary edema may occur as a consequence of multiple complications that include fluid overload, reperfusion injury, massive transfusions, and acute renal failure. Disruption of lymphatic vessels or vascular anastomoses also may cause pulmonary edema.

Reperfusion lung injury (Figure 9.1) caused by damage of endothelial–alveolar interfaces is a major contributor to early respiratory failure and mortality in patients receiving lung transplantation and is now termed PGD and graded on the basis of severity of gas exchange impairment (see Key points 9.3). PGD occurs in 13–25% of lung transplant recipients and typically has an overwhelmingly negative effect on recovery, causing prolonged hospitalization and increased mortality. One group has suggested that an even higher incidence of primary graft failure (50%) can be detected using criteria of radiographic infiltrate in the first 3 days after transplantation with $PaO_2 : FiO_2$ ratios <300. A higher incidence of ICU mortality occurs in those with PGD versus those without (29% vs 10.9%, respectively). Four variables predict higher mortality in the setting of PGD: age, degree of impaired gas exchange, graft ischemia time, and severe early hemodynamic failure.

Key points 9.3 Classification of primary graft dysfunction

PGD grade	Infiltrates on chest radiography	PaO2/FiO2 ratio
0	None	≥300
1	Present	≥300
2	Present	200–300
3	Present	<200

Bronchial anastomoses may develop ischemia, dehiscence, ulcerations, malacia, or stenosis. Implantation of grafts with smaller airways, particularly lung transplantation performed on children, are more prone to develop significant airway

Table 9.5 Post-transplant complications

Allograft rejection
- hyperacute (humoral)
- acute cellular
- lymphocytic bronchitis/bronchiolitis
- chronic rejection (bronchiolitis obliterans)

Primary graft dysfunction
Bronchial anastomosis complications (dehiscence, malacia, stenosis)
Infection
- bacterial (pneumonia, bacterial tracheobronchitis, empyema)
- fungal infection (e.g. *Aspergillus, Candida* spp., tracheobronchial aspergillosis)
- viral (e.g. CMV, RSV, influenza)
- mycobacterial
- *Pneumocystis* spp.
- Coagulation/thrombotic events
- hemorrhage
- hypercoagulability
- thrombosis of venous anastomoses
- venous thromboembolism
- axillary vein thrombosis
- heparin-induced thrombocytopenia with thrombosis
- Multisystem failure

Neurological complications (usually drug induced)
- central nervous system dysfunction
- tremor

Pleural effusion
Phrenic nerve injury
Vocal fold paralysis
Renal dysfunction/insufficiency
Native lung complications (single lung transplantation)
- hyper-inflation (emphysema)
- infection
- pneumothorax

Cardiovascular
- systemic hypertension
- cardiac rhythm disturbances
- hyperlipidemia

Hemolytic–uremic syndrome
Diabetes mellitus
- new onset
- worsened control of established disease

Gastrointestinal complications
- impaired motility (diarrhea, bezoar)
- colonic (diverticulitis, perforation, colitis)
- hepatobiliary dysfunction

Musculoskeletal complications
- Impaired bone metabolism:
  - osteoporosis
  - compression fractures
  - avascular necrosis
- Myopathy

Myelosuppression
Malignancies/lymphoproliferative disease (PTLD, primary lung cancer, other)
Menstrual irregularities

CMV, cytomegalovirus; PTLD, post-transplantation lymphoproliferative disease; RSV, respiratory syncytial virus.

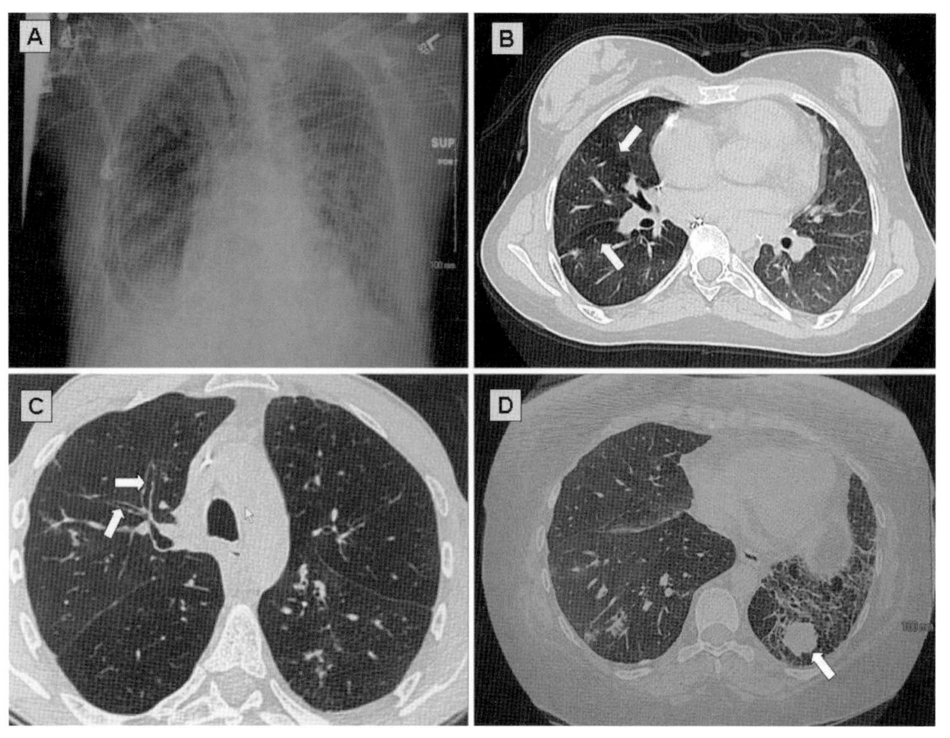

Figure 9.1 Thoracic imaging of lung transplant recipients. (a) Anteroposterior chest radiograph of a recipient with grade 3 primary graft dysfunction (PGD). (b) High-resolution CT (HRCT) scan showing air trapping in a bilateral lung transplant recipient with bronchiolitis obliterans syndrome. (c) HRCT scan showing allograft bronchiectasis (arrows). (d) HRCT scan showing a new small cell carcinoma in the fibrotic native lung of a single lung transplant recipient with idiopathic pulmonary fibrosis.

complications. Preoperative steroid use, CPB, reperfusion injury, acute rejection, airway infection, and administration of postoperative cytolytic drugs have all been linked to anastomotic dysfunction. Anastomotic complications arising in the first year after lung transplantation may be increased in recipients who are tall or in those receiving organs from donors who had prolonged mechanical ventilation. Aspergillus infection of tracheobronchial anastomoses may occur, especially in CF patients. Risk factors for anastomotic complications in children include prolonged mechanical ventilation and infection with *B. cepacia* or fungus.

Infection is a constant concern in the perioperative period and can arise from aspiration, surgical sites, or nosocomial infections. Pediatric recipients appear to have a higher incidence of pneumonia than adults. Infection in the perioperative period is largely caused by bacterial organisms, although viral and fungal infections should not be overlooked. Broad-spectrum antibiotics should be given until organisms can be identified, and it is important to consider infections that may have existed in the donor before transplantation. Infectious complications are discussed in more detail under "Postoperative period".

Phrenic nerve injury or diaphragmatic dysfunction can occur due to the transplant procedure. Diaphragmatic dysfunction can have significant effects on weaning from the ventilator and, thus, tends to prolong hospitalization. Fortunately, this complication does not seem to have a significant impact on long-term outcome.

Pulmonary embolism can be a devastating complication that may occur during the perioperative period, especially during the first postoperative month, with an incidence that ranges up to 30%. As with all postoperative patients, lung transplant recipients are at high risk for developing deep venous thrombosis (DVT) and subsequent pulmonary emboli (PEs). In addition, clot can form at sites of vascular anastomoses. As a result of the potentially devastating effects of DVT/PE, patients should receive adequate DVT prophylaxis. In some situations, it may be prudent to place an inferior vena cava filter to prevent fatal PEs.

Hyperacute, antibody-mediated rejection may occur in the immediate postoperative period, although very few cases have been reported. Hyperacute rejection is characterized by the development of diffuse infiltrates within a few hours of lung transplantation. These recipients test positively for panel-reactive antibodies and retrospective tissue cross-match studies. Clinical features of this aggressive clinical syndrome include sudden, rapid increases in airway pressure, copious amounts of blood-tinged fluid emanating from the airways, a precipitous decline in $PaO_2 : FiO_2$, and coagulopathy. Treatment includes escalation of immunosuppressive therapy combined with plasmapheresis to attenuate the production and the presence of pre-formed antibodies.

The postoperative period

Patients who survive the perioperative period and leave the hospital usually experience a significant improvement in lung function over the next few months. It is imperative that the patient and the healthcare team work to ensure the vitality of the transplanted lung to achieve and maintain this improvement in lung function over time. Although there is no consensus for various aspects of postoperative surveillance, lung transplantation programs are more likely to succeed if frequent and reasonably intense surveillance is employed to prevent or recognize complications. The rigorous post-transplant surveillance program and the complex medical regimen that lung transplant recipients must adhere to as outpatients underscores one reason why patients must be carefully screened before listing for lung transplantation. Nevertheless, even with rigorous surveillance protocols in place, multiple complications may occur.

As the recipient recovers from the transplant procedure and management shifts to long-term ambulatory care, complications associated with long-term immunosuppressive agents emerge as major issues. The combinations of immunosuppressive drugs required to prevent graft rejection pose a risk of side effects and toxicities that include renal dysfunction, central nervous system complications, osteoporosis, hyperlipidemia, and increased risk of malignancy. Other potential complications include pulmonary disorders that can affect the transplanted lung, such as acute rejection, allograft infection, recurrence of disease in the transplanted lung (e.g., pulmonary Langerhans' cell histiocytosis, lymphangioleiomyomatosis, sarcoidosis), problems with the native lung that may affect allograft function in recipients of SLT (e.g., hyperinflation of an emphysematous native lung, infection, pneumothorax), post-transplant lymphoproliferative disorder (PTLD), and bronchiolitis obliterans (BO).

Immunosuppression

The goal of immunosuppressive therapy is to promote immune tolerance of the lung allograft. Despite seemingly adequate immunosuppressive regimens, a high proportion of lung transplant recipients will develop acute rejection, which tends to occur more frequently in lung transplantation than in other solid organ transplantations. Immunosuppression of the lung transplant recipient must be intense and sustained to suppress the numerous factors that promote and drive allograft rejection. Immune system components that mediate a rejection cascade include innate immunity, adaptive immunity, humoral immunity, and autoimmune responses. As a result of the complexity and overlap in these components of the immune system, there is no simple physiologic "switch" that can be shut off to control rejection. The post-transplant immunosuppressive regimen usually consists of a calcineurin inhibitor (CNI), a purine synthesis inhibitor, and a corticosteroid. In addition, almost 45% of lung transplantation centers report that they utilize induction therapy with either anti-thymocyte globulins (ATGs), monoclonal anti-CD3 antibody (OKT3), or anti-interleukin (IL)-2-receptor antibodies. The rationale for use of induction antibody therapy in lung transplantation includes the high risk of acute rejection and the beneficial effect of providing time to achieve therapeutic levels of maintenance agents. Recent data from the International Society for Heart and Lung Transplantation (ISHLT) database show a small but statistically significant survival advantage associated with the use of induction antibodies in the early postoperative period. Unfortunately, adequately powered, prospective, randomized controlled trials are lacking to support or refute the use of any specific induction/maintenance immunosuppressive regimen to optimize long-term allograft survival after lung transplantation.

Adequate maintenance immunosuppressive therapy, which is started immediately postoperatively, is of key importance in preventing AR. Currently, the CNIs (cyclosporine and tacrolimus) provide the "backbone" for maintenance regimens administered to lung transplant recipients. Although tacrolimus may have greater efficacy for refractory AR, and switching from cyclosporine to tacrolimus has been reported to stabilize or slow declining allograft function due to "chronic rejection," it remains unclear whether tacrolimus is truly better than cyclosporine in preventing AR. The purine synthesis inhibitors, azathioprine or mycophenolate (mycophenolate mofetil or mycophenolate sodium) are generally used in combination with a CNI. Although smaller studies have suggested that mycophenolate may have superior efficacy over azathioprine in preventing AR, results from larger prospective, randomized, multicenter trials have not demonstrated any convincing difference between the two agents in suppressing AR. Finally, prednisone is the corticosteroid of choice in most centers and is helpful for preventing as well as treating AR. As a result of its adverse effects, especially on blood sugar control and bone mineral density, some centers significantly decrease or discontinue prednisone dosing over the first year after lung transplantation. Large doses of intravenously administered methylprednisolone followed by a gradual taper of oral prednisone are typically used to treat episodes of AR.

Strategies to avoid toxicity (e.g., monitoring CNI levels in peripheral blood) yet maintain adequate immunosuppression and avoid opportunistic infection must be followed. Trough levels (C_0) of cyclosporine and tacrolimus have traditionally been used for monitoring CNIs. However, in the case of cyclosporine, some centers use C_2 levels that may better reflect area-under-the-curve (AUC) pharmacokinetics. Although C_2 monitoring has been linked to enhanced clinical benefit in heart, liver, and kidney transplant recipients, data that support improved outcomes in association with its use in lung transplantation remain limited.

Data from the 2007 report of the ISHLT indicate that lung transplantation centers prefer tacrolimus over cyclosporine and mycophenolate over azathioprine. Target of rapamycin (TOR) inhibitors (sirolimus and everolimus) have been touted as CNI-sparing agents. However, sirolimus therapy has been sporadically linked to adverse pulmonary reactions and must be monitored carefully. Moreover, new use of these agents has been associated with impaired wound healing and, in lung transplant recipients, with dehiscence of the tracheal anastomosis. Novel approaches to preventing or treating AR include the administration of inhaled cyclosporine. One single-center, randomized, placebo-controlled trial of inhaled cyclosporine demonstrated improvement in overall allograft survival and chronic rejection-free survival, although a significant effect on preventing AR was not demonstrated.

AR can be treated with high-dose intravenous corticosteroids and, when applicable, conversion from cyclosporine to tacrolimus. If this is unsuccessful, cytolytic therapy with ATG or OKT3 may be used. If further treatment is needed, high-dose intravenous immunoglobulin (IVIG) provides another option. Chronic rejection should be treated by switching from cyclosporine to tacrolimus for at least 3–6 months, and high-dose corticosteroids and ATG can also tried if refractory. Finally, other modalities such as total lung irradiation, photopheresis, or chronic use of azithromycin may be helpful in stabilizing lung function in recipients with progressive loss of lung function due to chronic rejection.

Complications in the postoperative period

The major complications that occur beyond the perioperative period are predominantly linked to rejection and infection. Successful transplant programs must have systems in place to identify and treat these complications early and effectively, and various measures should be taken to minimize complications and optimize post-transplant outcomes (Table 9.6).

Acute rejection Malaise, cough, fever, and/or leukocytosis, decrease in FEV_1, changes on chest radiograph, and gastrointestinal complaints should signal the possibility of AR. It is graded histologically based on a commonly accepted scale that was most recently revised in 2005 (Table 9.7). Perivascular mononuclear infiltrates with or without lymphocytic

Table 9.6 Measures to optimize post-transplant outcomes

Experienced and multidisciplinary transplant team in place (thoracic surgeons, pulmonologists, consultants, coordinators/nursing, pharmacists, nutritionists, health psychologists, social workers)
Adequate yearly transplant volume to keep team skills at a high level
Careful selection of transplant candidates
Optimized pretransplant management
• Adequate pharmacologic therapies
• Avoidance of debilitation/deconditioning (optimal nutrition, pulmonary rehabilitation)
Donor management
• Careful selection
• Optimal supportive care
Use of strategies to avoid/minimize ex vivo allograft preservation injury
Aggressive postoperative ICU management
• Avoid ventilator-induced injury
• Consider early extracorporeal membrane oxygenation for severe, refractory graft dysfunction
• Judicious fluid restriction
• Closely monitor graft function
Prophylactic/pre-emptive therapies
• Adequate immune suppression
• Cytomegalovirus
• *Aspergillus* spp.
• *Pneumocystis* spp.
Surveillance
• Lung allograft
– spirometry
– radiologic imaging
– bronchoscopy (BAL and transbronchial biopsy)
• Immunosuppressant monitoring
– CNI peripheral blood levels
– bone marrow function
• Intermittent assessment of non-pulmonary issues
– renal function
– gastrointestinal function (GER, etc.)
– cardiac function
– lipid profile
– systemic blood pressure
– nutrition
– bone metabolism
– glucose metabolism
– malignancy risk

BAL, bronchoalveolar lavage; CNI, calcineurin inhibitor; GER, gastroesophageal reflux; ICU, intensive care unit.

Table 9.7 Grading of acute rejection and bronchiolitis obliterans syndrome

Disorder	Grade	Findings/Severity	Comments
Acute rejection (perivascular and interstitial inflammation)	A0 A1 A2 A3 A4	None Minimal Mild Moderate Severe	Adequate specimen requires five or more pieces of alveolated parenchyma Routine H&E processing at three levels required Special stains for microorganisms (GMS, AFB) required Connective tissue stain (e.g. elastic) recommended
Lymphocytic bronchiolitis (airway inflammation)	B0 B1 B2 BX	None Low grade High grade Ungradable	Lymphocytic bronchitis/bronchiolitis (LBB) is also a form of acute rejection
Bronchiolitis obliterans syndrome	BOS 0 BOS 1 BOS 2 BOS 3	$FEV_1 \geq 80\%$ of baseline[a] FEV_1 66–80% of baseline FEV_1 51–65% of baseline $FEV_1 \leq 50\%$ of baseline	Other causes of lung function decline must be excluded: • acute rejection • infection • native lung problems (single lung transplant recipients) • excessive recipient weight gain • anastomotic dysfunction • respiratory muscle dysfunction • technical problems

[a]Baseline defined as the average of the two best FEV_1 determinations post-lung transplantation.
AFB, acid-fast bacilli; GMS, Gomori methenamine silver; H&E, hematoxylin and eosin.

bronchitis/brochiolitis in the absence of infection is the histologic hallmark of AR (Figure 9.2). Acute cellular rejection is by far the most common rejection response. Hyperacute rejection is rare. However, another form of AR, characterized by alveolar septal capillary injury that lacks the lymphocyte infiltration characterizing cellular AR, has been reported to be associated with anti-endothelial antibodies specific for non-major histocompatibility (MHC) antigens.

The grading for AR ranges from A0 to A4. Grade A2 or greater is generally considered to be clinically significant and requiring intervention. Grade A1 (minimal) is commonly seen on surveillance transbronchial lung biopsy (TBLB) and is of unclear significance. Although grade A1 rejection has generally been considered to be clinically insignificant, it has been associated with increased risk for developing BO. However, no clear benefit has been demonstrated with intensifying immunosuppression for recipients with A1 rejection detected via surveillance bronchoscopy (SB). AR of grade A2 or higher requires intensified immunosuppression because it is usually accompanied by worsening lung function and oxygenation. One of the main reasons why surveillance TBLB is performed is because some patients may have grade A2 or even A3 AR that is clinically occult without a perceptible decline in lung function or gas exchange. A follow-up TBLB should be performed after the intensification of immunosuppression and corticosteroid burst to verify that the rejection episode has been adequately treated and suppressed.

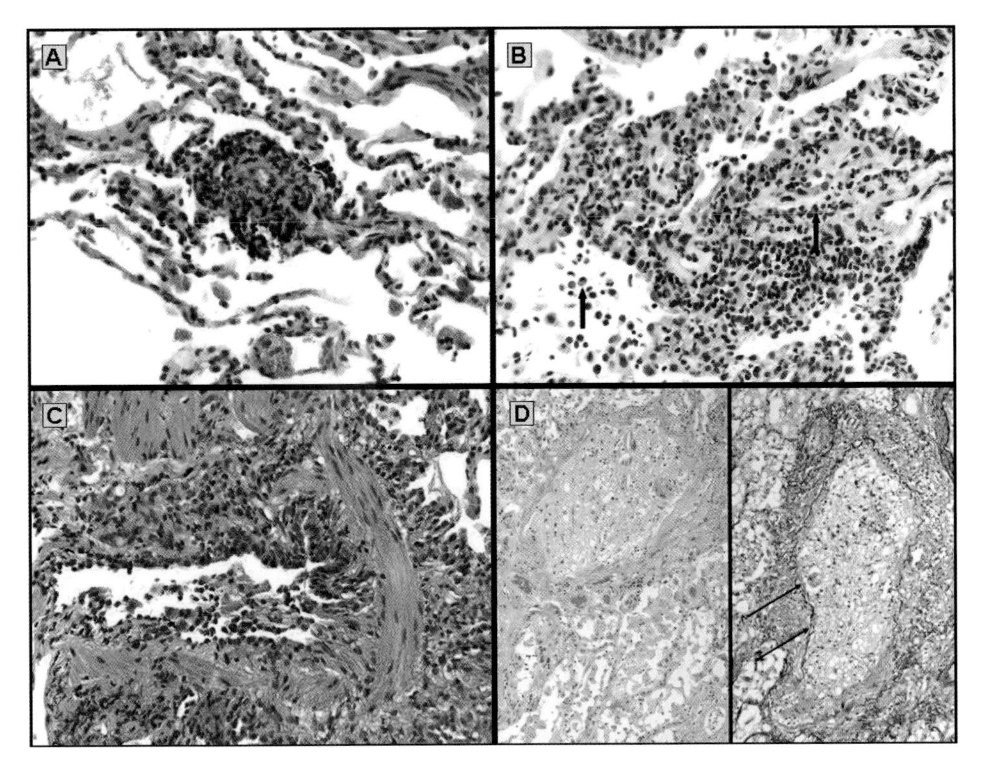

Figure 9.2 Histopathology of acute and chronic rejection. (Images provided courtesy of Henry Tazelaar, MD.) (a) International Society for Heart and Lung Transplantation (ISHLT) grade A2 acute rejection with one dense perivascular mononuclear infiltrate and no interstitial extension. (b) ISHLT grade A3 acute rejection; note the presence of eosinophils (arrows). (c) ISHLT grade B1 with mild bronchiolar lymphocytic infiltrate. (d) Chronic airway rejection (obliterative bronchiolitis), with complete airway scarring. The right panel shows an adjacent section stained with an elastic stain, highlighting the internal elastic lamina (arrows).

Case

A 23-year-old woman developed fever and leukocytosis 9 weeks after bilateral lung transplantation for cystic fibrosis. THE FEV_1 was 15% lower than a baseline value obtained 1 month earlier. Transbronchial lung biopsy revealed grade A2 acute rejection and no evidence of infection. She was treated with high doses of intravenous methylprednisolone. Cyclosporine was switched to tacrolimus. Fever and leukocytosis resolved. Repeat transbronchial biopsy 1 month later showed no evidence of acute rejection.

Infection Infection can occur at any time after lung transplantation. The incidence of bacterial pneumonia is approximately 16% in the first month after lung transplantation. Prolonged mechanical ventilation predisposes individuals to ventilator-associated bacterial pneumonia, and impaired cough reflexes and mucociliary clearance combined with immunosuppression sustain this risk after extubation. Undetected infection may be present in the lung allograft before donor explantation. Ischemic mucosa in the perianastomotic areas and impaired lymphatic drainage contribute to the risk of bacterial pneumonia. Fever, radiographic infiltrate, and culture-positive lower airway secretions can be diagnostic of pneumonia in the transplanted patient, but bronchoscopy with bronchoalveolar lavage (BAL) may be needed to make the diagnosis.

Gram-negative organisms, especially *P. aeruginosa*, are the predominant organisms followed by *Staphylococcus aureus*, which may be meticillin resistant. Empyema occasionally complicates lung transplantation and may be difficult to distinguish from postoperative pleural effusions which frequently occur as a consequence of disrupted lymphatic drainage. Although pneumonia usually occurs in the transplanted lung in single lung transplant recipients, pneumonia can occasionally occur in the residual native lung. Antimicrobial prophylaxis and aggressive treatment of infection in the early postoperative period can decrease the incidence or progression of lung infection and, ultimately, improve early graft function. In the case of recipients transplanted for suppurative lung disease (CF or non-CF bronchiectasis), pathogens isolated from pre-lung transplantation sputum cultures or pathogens typically isolated from these individuals are usually the causative pathogens when post-lung transplantation bacterial pneumonia occurs. In addition, the paranasal sinuses continue to harbor organisms that can infect the lower respiratory tract after lung transplantation. As a result of this possibility, paranasal sinus disease should be optimally managed in the pre- and perioperative period. Some centers perform endoscopic sinus surgery to enhance sinus drainage, although there are no convincing data that such intervention has a significant impact on post-lung transplantation outcome.

CMV can cause serious infection that can be life threatening, and patients are at greatest risk during the first 3 months post-transplantation. Although most patients have been exposed before transplantation, recipients with negative CMV serology at the time of transplantation are particularly at risk, especially if they receive a graft from a CMV-positive donor. Other risk factors for CMV disease include blood transfusions, immunosuppressive induction regimens that deplete lymphocytes, co-infection with human herpesviruses 6 or 7, and bronchiolitis obliterans syndrome (BOS).

Infection with CMV may manifest as a pulmonary syndrome, with increased shortness of breath and decreased graft function mimicking AR. In addition, CMV may involve other organ systems and cause extrapulmonary disease including pancytopenia, gastrointestinal dysfunction, or dermatologic reactions. As pulmonary CMV infection may be difficult to distinguish from AR (and both may be present simultaneously), bronchoscopy with TBLB is usually required to make a definitive diagnosis. The advent of rapid shell-vial culture techniques and polymerase chain reaction (PCR) methodologies has greatly enhanced the ability to rapidly detect CMV in BAL fluid, but CMV infection must be distinguished from CMV disease, which is characterized by a cytopathologic process in the lung allograft. The demonstration of inclusion bodies in cytomegalic cells on TBLB specimens is diagnostic of CMV pneumonitis. However, obtaining diagnostic TBLB may be difficult, and a presumptive diagnosis of CMV disease can be made on the basis of clinical features and positive culture or PCR results.

There is no consensus as to the timing, duration, or optimal dose of prophylactic agents for CMV. Some centers employ universal prophylaxis with either ganciclovir or valganciclovir, whereas others utilize pre-emptive treatment that is based on screening and early identification of CMV infection. Disadvantages of universal prophylaxis include cost, toxicity, and the possible emergence of resistant organisms, while disadvantages of the pre-emptive method are the cost of screening and the possibility of failure to identify individuals with CMV infection before they develop a serious form of CMV disease. Nevertheless, significant CMV infection during the early post-lung transplantation period is now rare, and most centers continue prophylactic therapy for the first year after lung transplantation. Although the appearance of drug-resistant CMV is a concern and has been estimated to range in frequency from 3% to 16% in solid organ transplant recipients, such approaches appear to have significantly decreased the morbidity and mortality of CMV infection in lung transplant recipients. When CMV pneumonitis or CMV affecting other organ systems occurs, treatment with ganciclovir or valganciclovir is usually effective. In addition, CMV-specific or polyvalent immune globulin may be used to augment the treatment regimen in recipients with CMV disease.

Most opportunistic fungal infections are caused by *Candida* and *Aspergillus* spp. Pneumonia caused by *Candida* spp. is rare, but surgical site infection and dissemination can occur. Aspergillosis is a common post-transplantation opportunistic infection that can cause pulmonary and/or extrapulmonary disease, and invasive disease occurs in approximately 5% of recipients. *Aspergillus* spp. can cause infection at the anastomotic site and may cause dehiscence in the early post-transplant time period. In addition, aspergillosis can affect the lung parenchyma and cause angioinvasive disease with cavitating lesions, and sometimes involves other organ systems. Prophylactic regimens, especially when used for patients with known pre-transplant colonization, may decrease the risk of post-transplant aspergillosis. A confident diagnosis of aspergillosis is made by obtaining biopsy specimens that show tissue invasion. However, *Aspergillus* spp. growing in culture, combined with the appropriate clinical picture, may be sufficient to make a presumptive diagnosis and commence therapy.

Aspergillus spp. can produce devastating, life-threatening illness if not identified rapidly and treated appropriately. When aspergillosis is suspected, immediate evaluation of the patient for the extent of organ system involvement, combined with the administration of intense, multiagent, appropriate antifungal therapy, is required. Treatment has traditionally consisted of intravenous amphotericin B, but newer approaches include the administration of voriconazole and caspofungin, depending on the site and severity of disease. Many programs administer antifungal agents (e.g., inhaled, nebulized amphotericin B, oral itraconazole, oral voriconazole) for prophylaxis, especially to patients known to be colonized with *Aspergillus* spp. pretransplantation.

Many other infectious complications can occur in the lung transplant recipient. Possible viral infections include herpes simplex virus, adenovirus, respiratory syncytial virus (RSV), influenza, and parainfluenza. Other fungal infections include *Cryptococcus* and *Coccidioides* spp. Mycobacterial infections with both *Mycobacterium tuberculosis* and non-tuberculous mycobacteria may also occur. Finally, other agents such as *Pneumocystis jiroveci* can cause life-threatening illness in the intensely immunosuppressed lung transplant recipient. Trimethoprim–sulfamethoxazole (or other agent if true allergy exists) is used routinely as prophylaxis for *Pneumocystis* spp.

Case

A 55-year-old man with a history of end-stage lung disease from COPD developed fever and exertional dyspnea 8 months after a single lung transplantation. Chest radiograph revealed new bilateral interstitial infiltrates. Hybrid capture DNA for CMV was previously negative, but CMV prophylaxis had been discontinued 6 months post-transplantation. Transbronchial biopsy revealed inclusion bodies consistent with CMV. The patient completed a 4-week course of therapy (intravenous ganciclovir for 1 week, oral valganciclovir for 3 weeks) and the syndrome resolved.

Bronchiolitis obliterans The development of BO, which is widely perceived to occur as a consequence of chronic rejection, continues to be the major factor that limits long-term survival and quality of life after lung transplantation. Despite improvements in immunosuppression and other elements of patient management, BO still occurs in more than half of all lung transplant recipients who survive to 5 years after lung transplantation. As BO is difficult to diagnose by radiologic imaging or transbronchial biopsy, the surrogate marker of FEV_1 (see Table 9.7) is used to detect and grade BO, which is then termed BO syndrome. However, when this diagnosis is made, other potentially reversible causes of a decline in lung function (e.g., AR, infection, native lung problems for single lung transplant recipients, excessive recipient weight gain that impairs lung function) must be ruled out as causes of chronic allograft dysfunction. BOS rarely occurs in the first 6 months post-lung transplantation, and median time to diagnosis is 16–20 months. Some patients may not display symptoms at all and may be identified only by screening lung function tests.

Risk factors that have been linked to the development of BOS include episodes of AR, HLA mismatching, and an autoimmune reaction to the lung matrix component, collagen V. However, alloimmune-independent factors such as inhaled irritants, airway ischemia, viral infections (e.g., CMV and respiratory viruses including influenza virus, RSV, parainfluenza virus, adenovirus, and rhinovirus), gastroesophageal reflux (GER), and donor factors (underlying asthma, smoking, and head injury as the cause of death) may also cause or contribute to the pathogenesis of BOS. Recipients who have three or more episodes of acute rejection in the first 6–12 months have a three- to fourfold increased risk of developing BO. However, some recipients do not develop BO despite multiple episodes of AR, and recipients who have never had AR may develop BO. In the pediatric lung transplant population, GER appears to be quite prevalent, and most pediatric lung transplant centers are very aggressive about identifying and treating GER. Finally, one must consider non-adherence to the medical regimen when evaluating rejection in the lung transplant recipient.

Although the pathogenesis of BO is not completely understood, both animal and human data suggest that there is an initial injury to airway epithelium that leads to a significant recruitment of inflammatory cells. Prominent among these inflammatory cells are neutrophils which accumulate in airspace secretions and may orchestrate the activation of the immune system. Proinflammatory cytokines and chemokines mediate and potentiate this inflammatory response, eventually leading to progressive airway damage, fibrosis, and airway smooth muscle proliferation with bronchiolar scarring and obliteration – all culminating in irreversible airflow obstruction. However, it should be emphasized that BO is a heterogeneous disorder with causes and immune/inflammatory responses that may vary from one lung transplant recipient to another.

One of the first clues to the presence of BO is a decrease in small airway function (forced expiratory flow at 25–75% – $FEF_{25-75\%}$), which may precede symptoms of cough, mucus production and dyspnea. Transbronchial lung biopsy has a disappointingly low sensitivity (17%) for detecting BO, necessitating adoption of the FEV_1 as a surrogate marker for BOS, with a sustained decline in FEV_1 to <80% of the best value post-transplantation indicating the onset of BOS. Revision in the BOS staging system in 2002 included a decline in $FEF_{25-75\%}$ to <75% of the best post-lung transplantation value as indicating the probable onset of BOS, because this parameter may identify airway obliteration earlier in the disease process. As AR (especially if it occurs early, is high grade, and recurrent) is thought to be a major risk for developing BOS, most lung transplantation centers use frequent monitoring to identify and treat AR early and hopefully prevent the development of BOS. Existing data support the use of intensive induction immunosuppression post-lung transplantation, combined with aggressive treatment of AR detected via frequent surveillance bronchoscopy (SB), with TBLB as a way of decreasing the risk of developing chronic rejection precipitated by episodes of AR. In addition, as GER is highly prevalent in patients with advanced lung disease and has been linked to chronic allograft dysfunction and BOS, some investigators have taken a more aggressive approach to its management. Fundoplication performed early after lung transplantation has been reported to be associated with both improved lung function and survival in comparison to control groups and appears to have relatively little morbidity. Laparoscopic fundoplication can also be performed safely on patients with ESLD before lung transplantation.

BO has a devastating effect on long-term survival with only 30–40% of recipients with BOS surviving 5 years after its onset, and management of BOS is difficult and usually ineffective. Treatment of BOS must take into consideration the delicate balance of immunosuppression and risk of opportunistic infection. Although increasing immunosuppressive therapy would be beneficial to control the immune/inflammatory response, it also places the patient at increased risk of infection. Nevertheless, both infection and inflammation must be aggressively treated in an attempt to prevent the progression of BOS. Patients with BOS after transplantation may have increased sputum production, grow *P. aeruginosa* on sputum culture, and show signs of bronchiectasis and end-expiratory air trapping on chest CT. Chronic azithromycin administration has been associated with stabilization or improvement in lung function in some recipients. Use of HMG-CoA (hydroxymethylglutaryl coenzyme A) reductase inhibitors ("statins") also has been associated with a decreased risk of developing BOS. Total lymphoid irradiation (TLI), initiated early in the course of chronic rejection that is refractory to conventional medical management, has been associated with an attenuation of the rate of decline in lung function, and extracorporeal photopheresis may also help stabilize declining graft function in recipients with early BOS. Newer approaches that can prevent or effectively treat BOS are desperately needed. Re-transplantation may be considered, but survival statistics for re-transplantation are significantly worse than that for recipients of primary lung transplantation. Candidates for re-transplantation due to progressive, refractory BOS must be evaluated with intense scrutiny.

Other complications

Gastrointestinal A number of gastrointestinal complications can occur at any time after lung transplantation and affect approximately 50% of lung transplant recipients. GER is highly prevalent in patients with advanced lung disease and has been linked to declines in lung function and the development of BO. Reflux can occur for a variety of reasons that include postoperative changes to the lower esophageal sphincter and diaphragmatic crura, dysmotility associated with diabetes mellitus, and changes in body habitus (e.g., from corticosteroid-associated weight gain). Non-acid GER occurs in many patients and must be detected via impedance/pH monitoring. Ideally, all candidates and recipients should be screened (pH and impedance measurements) for GER and receive appropriate medical or surgical therapies as needed to prevent significant reflux. Recipients with CF are particularly predisposed to gastrointestinal complications due to disease-related intestinal tract dysfunction. Patients with CF can develop bezoars that often form in the early post-transplant period and that can inhibit absorption of orally administered drugs. Recipients with CF are also at risk for distal intestinal obstruction, biliary tract complications (cholecystitis, significant biliary stasis, ascending cholangitis), and intestinal neoplasm (especially colon cancer).

Renal dysfunction Recipients are at a major risk for developing renal dysfunction after lung transplantation, and renal function should be checked frequently in the first post-transplant months and then at regular intervals thereafter. Blood levels of CNIs need to be monitored closely and doses adjusted to ensure an adequate (but not excessive) level that will give the desired degree of immunosuppression. Other electrolytes that can affect renal function (e.g., magnesium) or rise to dangerous levels (e.g., potassium) also need to be frequently monitored. When serum creatinine rises irreversibly >1.5 g/dL (or estimated glomerular filtration rate [GF]R <50 mL/min), or if significant proteinuria is detected on urinalysis, referral to a nephrologist who is familiar with transplant issues should be considered.

Cardiovascular Common cardiovascular complications include systemic hypertension, rhythm disturbances (e.g., atrial fibrillation), and hyperlipidemia. Systemic hypertension has been linked to corticosteroids, CNI administration, and weight gain. Hyperlipidemia is also linked to immunosuppressive agents, and the administration of statins for hyperlipidemia has been linked to improved survival and decreased risk of developing BO. Systemic hypertension and hyperlipidemia will eventually develop in most lung transplant recipients, and systemic blood pressure and peripheral blood lipid profiles should be monitored frequently to facilitate the detection and treatment of these complications.

Bone metabolism There is a very high prevalence of osteopenia and osteoporosis in patients with advanced lung disease, and lung transplantation can accelerate bone loss. All recipients should have bone mineral density checked frequently (e.g., 6–12 months post-transplantation and then yearly) via bone mineral density scanning and receive appropriate therapies if *T*-scores indicate the presence of osteopenia.

Glucose intolerance Corticosteroids and other transplant medications often disrupt glucose metabolism. Patients with CF are particularly at risk and have a relatively high pretransplant prevalence of diabetes mellitus that increases significantly post-transplantation. Frequent monitoring should be performed to assess glycemic control and to detect new onset of glucose intolerance.

Malignancy The profound immunosuppression required for lung transplant recipients places them at increased risk for developing dermatologic malignancies and PTLD. The latter occurs in approximately 5% of lung transplant recipients, and nearly all cases of PTLD are associated with the Epstein–Barr virus (EBV). Recipients who are EBV seronegative seem to be at highest risk for developing PTLD in the postoperative period. Peripheral blood semi-quantitative EBV PCR may identify recipients at increased risk for PTLD and may warrant cautious reduction of immunosuppression and continued prophylactic antiviral agents to prevent CMV as a cofactor in the pathogenesis of PTLD. Treatment consists of decreasing the level of immunosuppression to attempt to restore immunity against EBV. Other modalities, such as rituximab, have been used with some success. Overall, the mortality rate attributed to PTLD for recipients who develop this complication after lung transplantation is 37–50%.

Primary lung neoplasms may arise in the native lung of single lung transplant recipients, and other neoplasms such as bladder and colon cancer have been reported. Patients and their care providers need to maintain vigilance for any skin changes that may herald the development of a cutaneous malignancy, and internal malignancy must be considered when unexplained symptoms or signs arise in the post-transplant setting. Cancer screening, including routine skin examinations, mammography, cervical cancer screening and colonoscopy, must be maintained in the post-transplant setting.

Long-term surveillance

The goal of a surveillance program is to identify any acute or evolving issue that is related to an infectious process, acute rejection, or other potential complications, and to intervene before graft function is irreversibly affected or other complications occur. A typical surveillance program should include monitoring of allograft function, evaluation for infectious complications, intermittent laboratory testing and drug monitoring, monitoring of other organ system function (renal, cardiovascular function, and gastrointestinal function), intermittent assessment of bone and glucose metabolism, and attention to risk for malignancy. Most centers require frequent performance of home spirometry to detect declining FEV_1 values once the recipient has been discharged from the hospital, and patients should be educated to recognize changing symptoms including increased shortness of breath, fever, chills, or decline in exertional capacity.

Lung transplant recipients require close and frequent evaluation in the postoperative period to detect allograft dysfunction, particularly rejection and infection. As a result of their high prevalence in lung transplant recipients, there are a number of significant complications (hyperlipidemia, diabetes mellitus, osteoporosis, renal insufficiency, GER, and systemic hypertension) for which screening should be performed. Most of these complications are linked to the intense immunosuppressive regimens initiated at the time of lung transplantation, and frequent monitoring of immunosuppression, especially blood levels of cyclosporine and tacrolimus, should be performed to guide treatment and avoid toxicities.

Heart rate, blood pressure, temperature, and spirometry should be measured on a regular basis to detect complications. Most lung transplantation centers provide their patients with home spirometers and monitor lung function on a daily or even twice-daily basis. Fever and significant decline in lung function (decrease in FEV_1 >10% over 48h) require immediate evaluation, and bronchoscopy with transbronchial biopsy is usually performed to establish an accurate diagnosis of rejection and/or infection. For recipients with CF, extrapulmonary problems such as CF-related diabetes mellitus, CF liver disease, various other gastrointestinal complications, and paranasal sinus disease must be managed intensively. Frequent clinic visits at a CF center allow the patient to be evaluated for nutritional status, pulmonary status, and identification of early complications including medical and psychosocial problems.

Bronchoscopy with TBLB and BAL is an important tool for the detection of rejection and infection and is performed when clinically indicated. Examination of BAL fluid is particularly helpful in identifying bacterial, viral, and fungal infections, whereas TBLB is especially useful for identifying AR and/or CMV pneumonia. Quantitative bacterial cultures and stains, cultures for fungi and mycobacteria, and viral studies are typically obtained on BAL fluid, and transbronchial biopsies are obtained to evaluate allograft tissue for evidence of rejection and/or infection. The sensitivity and specificity of TBLB in identifying AR are approximately 72% and 90–100%, respectively. Sensitivity and specificity for the detection of CMV pneumonitis are approximately 91% and 70%, respectively. Follow-up bronchoscopy with TBLB is typically performed 4 weeks after the detection and treatment of significant acute rejection to ensure that enhanced immunosuppression has effectively eliminated the process.

Scheduled SB can detect occult infection or AR in patients who appear to be stable and lack radiographic or physiologic manifestations of rejection. However, the routine use of SB is controversial, and SB is routinely performed in only two-thirds of lung transplantation centers in the USA. For those institutions that perform SB, schedules differ from center to center and are usually determined by the lung transplantation center's previous experience. Nevertheless, SB is an important tool that allows inspection of airways and anastomoses, and retrieval of diagnostic specimens via TBLB and BAL for the detection of occult rejection and/or infection. Occult infection and AR are often detected when SB is performed, especially during the first 6 months post-transplantation, and the benefit of detecting and treating AR are thought to be improved survival and decreased risk of developing BO. A significant limitation of SB is the very limited ability to diagnose chronic rejection because of the limited ability to sample tissue that demonstrates histologic changes consistent with BO.

Thoracic CT scanning can be a useful tool to evaluate the lung allograft. By using end-expiratory, thin-section CT scanning (high-resolution CT [HRCT]) in the postoperative period, changes consistent with BOS may be detected relatively early (see Figure 9.1). When using air trapping as a marker for detecting BOS, studies have shown a sensitivity ranging from 74% to 91% and a specificity ranging from 67% to 94%. Although HRCT with inspiratory and expiratory views may be useful in detecting and assessing the severity of BOS in recipients who are suspected of having developed it, HRCT is not recommended as a routine surveillance test. It can, however, detect changes in addition to air trapping (e.g., small nodules, bronchiectasis) in the lung allograft as well as complications in the native lung of single lung transplant recipients (e.g., opportunistic infection or malignancy) that cannot be detected on routine chest radiographic imaging (see Figure 9.1).

Outcomes

The 5-year survival rate (Kaplan–Meier) is approximately 50% for both adults and children and remains significantly lower than survival for other solid organ transplantations. A steep, early decline in survival that levels off at 1–3 months post-lung transplantation reflects the impact of early events such as surgical complications, PGD, and thromboembolism. BO and infection appear to have the greatest impact on long-term survival, and constant exposure to ambient air as well as aspiration of upper airway and/or refluxed gastroesophageal secretions are likely the major contributors to graft failure and death. As a result of its significant prevalence and tendency to relentlessly progress, BO claims the lives of most individuals who survive the early postoperative period.

Fortunately, most lung transplant recipients experience significant improvements in lung function, exercise tolerance and quality of life (QoL). Average values for vital capacity increase from 43% predicted pre-lung transplantation to 65% and 69% predicted at 3 months and 1 year, respectively, for patients receiving a SLT for IPF. The greatest improvement in lung function usually occurs in the first 3 months after lung transplantation and slowly reaches a plateau at about 1 year, barring any significant complications that affect lung function. For patients receiving SLT for COPD, FEV_1 increases from 20% pre-lung transplantation to 45–60% 1 year after transplantation. Patients with COPD who receive a BLT can expect normal or near-normal lung function 1 year postoperatively. Patients with CF who receive BLT display an increase in FEV_1 from a mean of 20% predicted before lung transplantation to 70–80% predicted at 1 year post-lung transplantation. Finally, normalization of pulmonary pressures, right ventricular function, and cardiac output is expected for patients who receive a BLT for pulmonary hypertension, although single lung transplant recipients should also experience normalization of hemodynamic parameters. Exercise tolerance improves greatly and allows most recipients to perform activities of daily living without limitation or need for supplemental oxygen. However, cardiopulmonary exercise testing reveals that maximum oxygen consumption is limited to 50–60% predicted at peak exercise. Deconditioning, and a possible myopathy that is linked to the immunosuppressant regimen or other factors, likely accounts for this limited exercise capacity, because cardiopulmonary reserve appears to be maintained. Recipients of heart, liver and kidney transplants have similar limitations on cardiopulmonary exercise, suggesting that factors other than organ function may account for the subnormal maximum oxygen consumption at peak exercise.

Quality of life and cost-effectiveness have been scrutinized as important outcome factors in lung transplantation. Recently, a plethora of research has been published on QoL in lung transplant recipients. Most patients who have undergone lung transplantation have been found to be happy with their decision to undergo the procedure. The recipient approval rating of their lung transplantation is approximately 75%, and over 90% of those who have had the procedure would elect to have it again. Over 80% of survivors at 1, 3, and 5 years post-transplantation have no activity limitations. However, only 20% of recipients are working full-time at 1 year post-transplantation despite their lack of activity limitation. Improvements in QoL appear to have a lasting effect even at 7 years post-transplantation, and there does not seem to be a difference in QoL when comparing single with bilateral lung transplant recipients. Cost-effectiveness data are relatively scarce, and results inconclusive.

Recurrence of lung disease is very unusual. Sarcoidosis and lymphangioleiomyomatosis are diseases that may recur after lung transplantation. In addition, there have been case reports of recurrence in recipients transplanted for Langerhans' cell histiocytosis, giant cell interstitial pneumonitis, pulmonary alveolar proteinosis, and diffuse panbronchioloitis.

Re-transplantation

PGD, severe airway complications, refractory acute rejection, and progressive BOS can lead to irreversible allograft dysfunction and respiratory failure after lung transplantation. Re-transplantation can be performed to treat these complications if refractory to all other interventions, but outcomes after re-transplantation have been significantly worse than outcomes after primary lung transplantation. Due to ethical concerns about proper organ distribution when an overall organ scarcity prevents successful transplantation of many wait-listed candidates and various reports of poor outcome after re-transplantation, the value of re-transplantation has been open to question. More recent data suggest that survival after re-transplantation for certain recipient groups approaches that for primary lung transplantation, and outcomes after lung re-transplantation have generally improved. Early re-transplantation (within 30 days) and re-transplantation for PGD have the worst outcomes, whereas re-transplantation for BOS appears to provide survival rates that are similar to long-term survival rates for primary lung transplantation. Re-transplantation should be considered on a case-by-case basis for recipients of primary lung transplantation whose allografts have developed severe dysfunction that is refractory to non-surgical interventions.

Further reading

Aboyoun CL, Tamm M, Chhajed PN, et al. Diagnostic value of follow-up transbronchial lung biopsy after lung rejection. *Am J Respir Crit Care Med* 2001;**164**:460–3.

Aigner C, Jaksch P, Taghavi S, et al. Pulmonary retransplantation: is it worth the effort? A long-term analysis of 46 cases. *J Heart Lung Transplant* 2008;**27**:60–5.

Amital A, Shitrit D, Raviv Y, et al. Development of malignancy following lung transplantation. *Transplantation* 2006;**81**:547–551.

Angel LF, Levine DJ, Restrepo MI, et al. Impact of lung transplantation donor-management protocol on lung donation and recipient outcomes. *Am J Respir Crit Care Med* 2006;**174**:710–16.

Anonymous. *Lung Allocation Score System for Transplant Professionals*. United Network for Organ Sharing, 2005. Available at: www.unos.org.

Arcasoy SM, Hersh C, Christie JD, et al. Bronchogenic carcinoma complicating lung transplantation. *J Heart Lung Transplant* 2001;**20**:1044–53.

Aris RM, Gilligan PH, Neuringer IP, Gott KK, Rea J, Yankaskas JR. The effects of panresistant bacteria in cystic fibrosis patients on lung transplant outcome. *Am J Respir Crit Care Med* 1997;**155**:1699–1704.

Aris RM, Neuringer IP, Weiner MA, et al. Severe osteoporosis before and after lung transplantation. *Chest* 1996; **109**:1176–83.

Aris RM, Routh JC, LiPuma JJ, Heath DG, Gilligan PH. Lung transplantation for cystic fibrosis patients with Burkholderia cepacia complex. Survival linked to genomovar type. *Am J Respir Crit Care Med* 2001;**164**:2102–6.

Bando, K, Armitage, JM, Paradis, IL, et al. Indications for and results of single, bilateral, and heart-lung transplantation for pulmonary hypertension. *J Thorac Cardiovasc Surg* 1994;**108**:1056–65.

Bankier AA, Muylem AV, Knoop C, Estenne M, Gevenois PA. BOS in heart-lung transplant recipients: diagnosis with expiratory CT. *Radiology* 2001;**218**:533–9.

Barraclough K, Menahem SA, Bailey M, Thomson NM. Predictors of decline in renal function after lung transplantation. *J Heart Lung Transplant* 2006;**25**:1431–5.

Bartz R, Will L, Welter D, Love R, Meyer K. Outcome following lung transplantation for mechanically ventilated patients with cystic fibrosis. *Am J Respir Crit Care Med* 2001;**163**:A335.

Benden C, Aurora P, Curry J, Whitmore P, Priestley L, Elliott MJ. High prevalence of gastroesophageal reflux in children after lung transplantation. *Pediatr Pulmonol* 2005;**40**:68–71.

Blondeau K, Mertens V, Vanaudenaerde BA, et al. Acid, non-acid GER and gastric aspiration in lung transplant patients with or without chronic rejection. *Eur Respir J* 2007;**37**:625–30.

Boehler A, Estenne. Post-transplant bronchiolitis obliterans. *Eur Respir J* 2003;**22**:1007–18.

Botha P, Fisher AJ, Dark JH. Marginal lung donors: a diminishing margin of safety? *Transplantation* 2006;**82**: 1273–9.

Bowdish ME, Arcasoy SM, Wilt JS, et al. Surrogate markers and risk factors for chronic lung allograft dysfunction. *Am J Transplant* 2004;**4**:1171–8.

Braith RW, Conner JA, Fulton MN, et al. Comparison of alendronate vs alendronate plus mechanical loading as prophylaxis for osteoporosis in lung transplant recipients: a pilot study. *J Heart Lung Transplant* 2007;**26**:32–137.

Canales M, Youssef P, Spong R, et al. Predictors of chronic kidney disease in long-term survivors of lung and heart-lung transplantation. *Am J Transplant* 2006;**6**:2157–63.

Caplan-Shaw CE, Arcasoy SM, Shane E, et al. Osteoporosis in diffuse parenchymal lung disease. *Chest* 2006;**129**: 140–6.

Chakinala MM, Ritter J, Gage BF, et al. Yield of surveillance bronchoscopy for acute rejection and lymphocytic bronchitis/bronchiolitis after lung transplantation. *J Heart Lung Transplant* 2004;**23**:1396–404.

Chamberlain D, Maurer J, Chaparro C, Idolor L. Evaluation of transbronchial lung biopsy specimens in the diagnosis of bronchiolitis obliterans after lung transplantation. *J Heart Lung Transplant* 1994;**13**:963–71.

Chatila WM, Furukawa S, Gaughan JP, Criner, GJ. Respiratory failure after lung transplantation. *Chest* 2003;**123**:165–73.

Choong CK, Meyers BF. Quality of life after lung transplantation. *Thorac Surg Clin* 2004;**14**:385–407.

Christie JD, Bavaria JE, Palevsky HI, et al. Primary graft failure following lung transplantation. *Chest* 1998;**114**: 51–60.

Christie JD, Kotloff RM, Ahya VN, et al. The effect of primary graft dysfunction on survival after lung transplantation. *Am J Respir Crit Care Med* 2005;**171**: 1312–16.

Cooper JD, Billingham M, Egan T, et al. A working formulation for the standardization of nomenclature and for clinical staging of chronic dysfunction in lung allografts. *J Heart Lung Transplant* 1993;**12**:713–16.

Corris P, Glanville A, McNeil K, et al. One year analysis of an ongoing international randomized study of mycophenolate mofetil (MMF) vs azathioprine (AZA) in lung transplantation. *J Heart Lung Transplant* 2001;**20**:149–50.

Daud SA, Yusen RD, Meyers BF, et al. Impact of immediate primary lung allograft dysfunction on bronchiolitis obliterans syndrome. *Am J Respir Crit Care Med* 2007;**175**: 507–13.

deJong PA, Dodd JD, Coxson HO, et al. Bronchiolitis obliterans following lung transplantation: early detection using computed tomographic scanning. *Thorax* 2006;**61**:799–804.

Dellon ES, Morgan DR, Mohanty SP, Davis K, Aris RM. High incidence of gastric bezoars in cystic fibrosis patients after lung transplantation. *Transplantation* 2006;**81**: 1141–6.

DeMeo DL, Ginns LC. Clinical status of lung transplantation. *Transplantation* 2001;**72**:1713–24.

Efrati O, Kremer MR, Barak A, et al. Improved survival following lung transplantation with long-term use of bilevel positive pressure ventilation in cystic fibrosis. *Lung* 2007;**185**:73–9.

Egan TM. Non-heart-beating donors in thoracic transplantation. *J Heart Lung Transplant* 2004;**23**:3–10.

Egan TM, Edwards LB, Coke MA, et al. Lung allocation in the United States. In: Lynch JP III, Ross DJ (eds), *Lung Biology in Health and Disease*, Vol **217**. Lung and Heart-Lung Transplantation New York, Taylor & Francis, 2006: 285–300.

Elizur A, Sweet SC, Huddleston CB, et al. Pre-transplantation mechanical ventilation increases short-term morbidity and mortality in pediatric patients with cystic fibrosis. *J Heart Lung Transplant* 2007;**26**:127–31.

Estenne M, Maurer JR, Boehler A, et al. Bronchiolitis obliterans syndrome 2001: an update of the diagnostic criteria. *J Heart Lung Transplant* 2002;**21**:297–310.

Ettinger NA, Bailey TC, Trulock EP, et al. Cytomegalovirus infection and pneumonitis: impact after isolated lung transplantation. *Am Rev Respir Dis* 1993;**147**:1017–23.

Fischer S, Bohn D, Rycus P, et al. Extracorporeal membrane oxygenation for primary graft dysfunction at lung transplantation: analysis of the Extracorporeal Life Support Organization (ELSO) registry. *J Heart Lung Transplant* 2007;**26**:472–7.

Flume PA, Egan TM, Paradowski LJ, Detterbeck FC, Thompson JT, Yankaskas JR. Infectious complications of lung transplantation: impact of cystic fibrosis. *Am J Respir Crit Care Med* 1994;**149**:1601–7.

Gammie JS, Keenan RJ, Pham SM, et al. Single- versus double-lung transplantation for pulmonary hypertension. *J Thorac Cardiovasc Surg* 1998;**115**:397.

George I, Xydas S, Topkara VK, et al. Clinical indication for use and outcomes after inhaled nitric oxide therapy. *Ann Thorac Surg* 2006;**82**:2161–9.

Gerbase MW, Spiliopoulos A, Rochat T, Archinard M, Nicod LP. Health-related quality of life following single or bilateral lung transplantation: a 7-year comparison to functional outcome. *Chest* 2005;**128**:1371–8.

Glanville AR. The role of bronchoscopic surveillance monitoring in the care of lung transplant recipients. *Semin Respir Crit Care Med* 2006;**27**:480–91.

Glanville AR, Estenne M. Indications, patient selection and timing of referral for lung transplantation. *Eur Respir J* 2003;**22**:845–52.

Glanville AR, Aboyoun CL, Morton JM, et al. Cyclosporine C2 target levels and acute cellular rejection after lung transplantation. *J Heart Lung Transplant* 2006;**25**:928–34.

Groetzner J, Kur F, Spelsberg F, et al., Munich Lung Transplant Group. Airway anastomosis complications in de novo lung transplantation with sirolimus-based immunosuppression. *J Heart Lung Transplant* 2004;**23**: 632–8.

Hadijiliadis D, Madill J, Chaparro C, et al. Incidence and prevalence of diabetes mellitus in patients with cystic fibrosis undergoing lung transplantation before and after lung transplantation. *Clin Transplant* 2005;**19**:773–8.

Hadjiliadis D, Angel LF. Controversies in lung transplantation: Are two lungs better than one? *Semin Respir Crit Care Med* 2007;**27**:561–6.

Hardy JD, Webb WR, Dalton ML, Walker GR. Lung homotransplantation in man: report of the initial case. *JAMA* 1963;**186**:1065–74.

Helmi M, Welter D, Cornwell RD, Love RB, Meyer KC. Tracheobronchial aspergillosis in lung transplant recipients with cystic fibrosis; risk factors and outcome comparison to other transplant recipients. *Chest* 2003;**123**: 800–8.

Horning NR, Lynch JP, Sundaresan SR, Patterson GA, Trulock EP. Tacrolimus therapy for persistent or recurrent acute rejection after lung transplantation. *J Heart Lung Transplant* 1998;**17**:761–7.

Husain S, Paterson DL, Studer S, et al. Voriconazole prophylaxis in lung transplant recipients. *Am J Transplant* 2006;**6**:3008–16.

Iacono AT, Johnson BA, Grgurich B, et al. A randomized trial of inhaled cyclosporine in lung-transplant recipients. *N Engl J Med* 2006;**354**:141–50.

Ishani A, Erturk S, Hertz MI, Matas AJ, Savik K, Rosenberg ME. Predictors of renal function following lung or heart-lung transplantation. *Kidney Int* 2002;**61**:2228–34.

Kahan ES, Petersen G, Gaughan JP, Criner GJ. High incidence of venous thromboembolic events in lung transplant recipients. *J Heart Lung Transplant* 2007;**26**:339–44.

Kaneda H, Waddell TK, de Perrot M, et al. Pre-implantation multiple cytokine mRNA expression analysis of donor lung grafts predicts survival after lung transplantation in humans. *Am J Transplant* 2006;**6**:544–51.

Kawut SM, Lederer DJ, Keshavjee S, et al. Outcomes after lung retransplantation in the modern era. *Am J Respir Crit Care Med* 2008;**177**:114–20.

Kerem E, Reisman J, Corey M, Canny GJ, Levison H. Prediction of mortality in patients with cystic fibrosis. *New Engl J Med* 1992;**326**:1187–91.

Knoop C, Thiry P, Saint-Marcoux F, Rousseau A, Marquet P, Estenne M. Tacrolimus pharmacokinetics and dose monitoring after lung transplantation for cystic fibrosis and other conditions. *Am J Transplant* 2005;**5**:1477–82.

Knoop C, Vervier I, Thiry P, et al. Cyclosporine pharmacokinetics and dose monitoring after lung transplantation: comparison between cystic fibrosis and other conditions. *Transplantation* 2003;**76**:683–8.

Kotloff RM, Ahya VN. Medical complications of lung transplantation. *Eur Respir J* 2004; **23**:334–42.

Kroshus TJ, Kshettry VR, Savik K, John R, Hertz MI, Bolman RM III. Risk factors for the development of bronchiolitis obliterans syndrome after lung transplantation. *J Thorac Cardiovasc Surg* 1997;**114**:195–202.

Lama VN, Flaherty KR, Toews GB, et al. Prognostic value of desaturation during 6-minute walk test in idiopathic interstitial pneumonia. *Am J Respir Crit Care Med* 2003; **168**:1084–90.

Leblond V, Sutton L, Dorent R, et al. Lymphoproliferative disorders after organ transplantation: A report of 24 cases observed at a single center. *J Clin Oncol* 1995;**13**:961–8.

Lee E-S, Gotway MB, Reddy GP, Golden JA, Keith FM, Webb WR. Early bronchiolitis obliterans following lung transplantation: accuracy of expiratory thin-section CT for diagnosis. *Radiology* 2000;**216**:472–7.

Levy G, Thervet E, Lake J, et al. Patient management by Neoral C2 monitoring: an international consensus statement. *Transplantation* 2002;**73**:S12–18.

Levy RD, Ernst P, Levine SM, et al. Exercise performance after lung transplantation. *J Heart Lung Transplant* 1993; **12**:27–33.

Lu BS, Garrity ER Jr, Bhorade SM. Immunosuppressive drugs: cyclosporine, tacrolimus, sirolimus, azathioprine, mycophenolate mofetil, and corticosteroids. In: Lynch JP III, Ross DJ (eds), *Lung Biology in Health and Disease*, Vol **217**. Lung and Heart-Lung Transplantation. New York: Taylor & Francis, 2006: 363–99.

McAnally KJ, Valentine VG, LaPlace SG, McFadden PM, Seoane L, Taylor DE. Effect of pre-transplantation prednisone on survival after lung transplantation. *J Heart Lung Transplant* 2006;**25**:67–74.

Martinez, FJ, Safrin S, Weycker D, et al. The clinical course of patients with idiopathic pulmonary fibrosis. *Ann Intern Med* 2004;**142**:963–7.

Maurer JR, Frost AE, Estenne M, et al. International Guidelines for the Selection of Lung Transplant Candidates. *J Heart Lung Transplant* 1998;**17**:703–9.

Maurer JR. Metabolic bone disease in lung transplant recipients. In: Lynch JP III, Ross DJ (eds), *Lung Biology in Health and Disease*, Vol **217**. Lung and Heart-Lung Transplantation. New York: Taylor & Francis, 2006: 895–9.

Mayer-Hamblett N, Rosenfeld M, Emerson J, et al. Developing cystic fibrosis lung transplant referral criteria using predictors of 2-year mortality. *Am J Respir Crit Care Med* 2002;**166**:1550–5.

Meade MO, Granton JT, Matte-Martyn A, et al. A randomized trial of inhaled nitric oxide to prevent ischemia-reperfusion injury after lung transplantation. *Am J Respir Crit Care Med* 2003;**167**:1483–9.

Meyer K. Allogeneic recognition and immune tolerance in lung transplantation. In: Lynch JP III, Ross DJ (eds), *Lung Biology in Health and Disease*, Vol **217**. Lung and Heart-Lung Transplantation. New York: Taylor & Francis, 2006: 47–60.

Moro J, Almenar L, Martinez-Dolz L, et al. mTOR inhibitors: do they help preserve renal function? *Transplant Proc* 2007;**39**:2135–7.

Orens JB, Boehler A, de Perrot M, et al. A review of lung transplant donor acceptability criteria. *J Heart Lung Transplant* 2003;**22**:1183–200.

Orens JB, Estenne M, Arcasoy S, et al. International guidelines for the selection of lung transplant candidates: 2006 update – a consensus report from the Pulmonary Scientific Council of the International Society for Heart and Lung Transplantation. *J Heart Lung Transplant* 2006;**25**:745–55.

Palmer SM, Miralles AP, Howell DN, et al. Gastroesophageal reflux as a reversible cause of allograft dysfunction after lung transplantation. *Chest* 2000;**118**:1214–7.

Patterson GA. Historical development of pulmonary transplantation. *Semin Respir Crit Care Med* 1996;**17**:103–7.

Pierre F, Keshavjee S. Lung transplantation: donor and recipient critical care aspects. *Curr Opin Crit Care* 2005;**11**:339–44.

Pilcher DV, Scheinkestel CD, Snell GI, et al. A high central venous pressure is associated with prolonged mechanical ventilation and increased mortality following lung transplantation. *J Thoracic Cardiovasc Surg* 2005;**129**:912–8.

Ramalingam P, Rybicki L, Smith MD, et al. Posttransplant lymphoproliferative disorders in lung transplant patients: the Cleveland Clinic experience. *Mod Pathol* 2002;**15**:647–56.

Reams BD, McAdams HP, Howell DN, et al. Posttransplant lymphoproliferative disorder: incidence, presentation, and response to treatment in lung transplant recipients. *Chest* 2003;**124**:1242–9.

Ross DJ, Waters PF, Levine M, Kramer M, Ruzevich S, Kass RM. Mycophenolate mofetil versus azathioprine immunosuppressive regimens after lung transplantation: preliminary experience. *J Heart Lung Transplant* 1998;**17**:768–74.

Shumway, SJ, Hertz, MI, Petty, MG, Bolman, RM. Liberalization of donor criteria in lung and heart-lung transplantation. *Ann Thorac Surg* 1994;**57**:92–5.

Smeritschnig B, Jaksch P, Kocher A, et al. Quality of life after lung transplantation: a cross-sectional study. *J Heart Lung Transplant* 2005;**24**:474–80.

Snyder LD, Palmer SM. Immune mechanisms of lung allograft rejection. *Semin Respir Crit Care Med* 2006;**27**:534–43.

Starnes VA, Barr ML, Cohen RG. Lobar transplantation: indications, technique and outcome. *J Thorac Cardiovasc Surg* 1994;**108**:403–10.

Starnes VA, Bowdish ME, Woo MS, et al. A decade of living lobar lung transplantation: recipient outcomes. *J Thorac Cardiovasc Surg* 2004;**127**:114–22.

Studer SM, Levy RD, McNeil K, Orens JB. Lung transplant outcomes: a review of survival, graft function, physiology, health-related quality of life and cost-effectiveness. *Eur Respir J* 2004;**24**:674–85.

Swanson SJ, Mentzer SJ, Reilly JJ, et al. Surveillance transbronchial lung biopsies: implication for survival after lung transplantation. *J Thorac Cardiovasc Surg* 2000;**119**:27–37.

Thabut G, Mal H, Cerrina J, Dartevelle P, et al. Graft ischemic time and outcome of lung transplantation. *Am J Respir Crit Care Med* 2005;**171**:786–91.

Thabut G, Vinatier I, Stern JB, et al. Primary graft failure following lung transplantation: Predictive factors of mortality. *Chest* 2002;**121**:1876–82.

Trulock EP, Ettinger NA, Brunt EM, Pasque MK, Kaiser LR, Cooper JD. The role of transbronchial lung biopsy in the treatment of lung transplant recipients. An analysis of 200 consecutive procedures. *Chest* 1992;**102**:1049–54.

Trulock, EP. Lung Transplantation. *Am J Respir Crit Care Med* 1997;**155**:789–815.

Van De Wauwer C, Van Raemdonck D, Verleden GM, et al. Risk factors for airway complications within the first year after lung transplantation. *Eur J Cardiothorac Surg* 2007;**31**:703–10.

Venuta F, De Giacomo T, Rendina EA, et al. Recovery of chronic renal impairment with sirolimus after lung transplantation. *Ann Thorac Surg* 2004;**78**:1940–3.

Verleden GM, Dupont LJ. Azithromycin therapy for patients with bronchiolitis obliterans syndrome after lung transplantation. *Transplantation* 2004;**77**:1465–7.

Verschuuren EA, Stevens S, Pronk I, et al. Frequent monitoring of Epstein–Barr virus DNA load in unfractionated whole blood is essential for early detection of post-transplant lymphoproliferative disease in lung transplant patients. *J Heart Lung Transplant* 2001;**20**:199–200.

Weigt SS, Lynch JP III, Langer LR, et al. Lymphoproliferative disorders complicating solid organ transplantation. In: Lynch JP III, Ross DJ (eds), *Lung Biology in Health and Disease*, Vol **217**. Lung and Heart-Lung Transplantation. New York: Taylor & Francis, 2006: 901–34.

Wigfield CH, Lindsey JD, Steffens TG, et al. Early institution of extracorporeal membrane oxygenation for primary graft dysfunction after lung transplantation improved outcome. *J Heart Lung Transplant* 2007;**26**:331–8.

Williams TJ, Patterson GA, McClean PA, Zamel N, Maurer JR. Maximal exercise testing in single and double lung transplant recipients. *Am Rev Respir Dis* 1992;**145**:101–5.

Wood KE, Becker BN, McCartney JG, et al. Care of the potential organ donor. *N Engl J Med* 2004;**351**:2730–9.

Yates B, Murphy DM, Forrest IA, et al. Azithromycin reverses airflow obstruction in established bronchiolitis

obliterans syndrome. *Am J Respir Crit Care Med* 2005; **172**:772–5.
Young LR, Hadjiliadis D, David D, et al. Lung transplantation exacerbates gastroesophageal reflux disease. *Chest* 2003;**124**:1689–93.
Yousem SA, Berry GJ, Cagle PT, et al Revision of the 1990 working formulation for the classification of pulmonary allograft rejection: Lung Rejection Study Group. *J Heart Lung Transplant* 1996;**15**:1–15.
Zamora MR, Davis RD, Leonard C, et al. Management of cytomegalovirus infection in lung transplant recipients: evidence-based recommendations. *Transplantation* 2005; **80**:157–63.
Zuckermann A, Klepetko W, Birsan T, et al. Comparison between mycophenolate mofetil- and azathioprine-based immunosuppressions in clinical lung transplantation. *J Heart Lung Transplant* 1999;**18**:432–40.

Addendum: glossary

α_1-Antitrypsin deficiency: a deficiency of a protein produced in the liver that blocks the destructive effects of certain enzymes.This inherited condition can be associated with emphysema and/or liver disease.

Atelectasis: absence of gas from a part or the whole of the lungs, due to failure of expansion or resorption of gas from the alveoli.

ARDS: acute respiratory distress syndrome – a malfunction of the lung resulting from injury to the small air sacs and the capillaries of the lungs. Upon injury, blood and fluid leak into the air sacs, making breathing difficult. The condition can be fatal.

BAL: Bronchoalveolar lavage – a technique that allows the recovery of both cellular and noncellular components from the epithelial surface of the lower respiratory tract and differs from bronchial washings, which refer to the aspiration of either secretions or small amounts of instilled saline from the large airways.

BiPAP: bilevel positive airway pressure – a noninvasive means to deliver both inspiratory and expiratory pressure for ventilatory support.

BO/BOS: bronchiolitis obliterans/bronchiolitis obliterans syndrome – irreversible scarring of the terminal and respiratory bronchioles which may either partially or totally obliterate the lumen of the airway.

Bronchiectasis: chronic dilation of bronchi. It can be the result of inflammation, infection, and/or lung tissue fibrosis (traction bronchiectasis).

Bronchoscopy: the direct visualization of the trachea and bronchi through a rigid or flexible tube (bronchoscope).

CPB: cardiopulmonary bypass – to surgically insert a shunt to bypass a chamber of the heart to carry blood directly to the aorta.

COPD: Chronic obstructive pulmonary disease – a progressive lung disease process characterized by difficulty breathing, wheezing, and a chronic cough. Airflow obstruction usually does not improve after inhaled bronchodilator medications.

CF: cystic fibrosis – an inherited disease (autosomal recessive) that affects the lungs, exocrine pancreas and gastrointestinal system resulting in chronic lung disease.

DVT: deep venous thrombosis – blockage of the deep veins; particularly common in the leg.

Diffuse panbronchiolitis: an idiopathic chronic obstructive airway disease more commonly affecting Japanese individuals. Lymphocytic and plasma cell infiltration of bronchial walls occurs.

DIOS: distal intestinal obstructive syndrome – inspissation of intestinal contents in the terminal ileum, cecum, and proximal colon in patients with CF.

ECMO: extracorporeal membrane oxygenation – a technique that is used to oxygenate blood by passing it through an external membrane.

Eisenmenger's syndrome: the process in which a left-to-right shunt in the heart causes increased flow through the pulmonary vasculature, resulting in pulmonary hypertension, which causes increased pressures in the right side of the heart and reversal of the shunt into a right-to-left shunt.

Empyema: the presence of pus in a body cavity, especially the pleural cavity.

FEV_1: forced expiratory volume in 1 s – the volume of air that can be exhaled during the first second of a forced exhalation.

FVC/VC: forced vital capacity/vital capacity – the maximum volume of air that can be (forcibly) expired from the lungs.

ILD: interstitial lung disease – a disorder resulting in scarring of lung tissue or the lining of the air sacs (alveolus); often results in poor oxygen diffusion from the alveolus into the bloodstream.

IVC filter: inferior vena cava filter – a device placed in the inferior vena cava intended to disrupt the flow of a blood clot from the lower extremities to the lungs.

IPF: idiopathic pulmonary fibrosis – scarring or thickening of lung parenchyma of unknown etiology.

NO: nitric oxide – a free radical gas synthesized from arginine by nitric oxide synthase. It is one of the endothelium-dependent relaxing factors released by the vascular endothelium and mediates vasodilation. It also inhibits platelet aggregation, induces disaggregation of aggregated platelets, and inhibits platelet adhesion to the vascular endothelium.

PCR: polymerase chain reaction – a technique for amplifying DNA sequences in vitro by separating the DNA into two strands and incubating it with nucleotide triphosphates.

Pleuredesis: the surgical or medical creation of a fibrous adhesion between the visceral and parietal layers of the pleura, thus obliterating the pleural cavity.

PE: pulmonary embolism – lodging of a blood clot in the lumen of a pulmonary artery, causing dysfunction in respiratory function. PEs often originate in the deep leg veins and travel to the lungs through the blood circulation. Symptoms include sudden shortness of breath, chest pain, and rapid heart and respiratory rates.

PGD primary graft dysfunction: reperfusion injury that occurs after implantation and causes parenchymal infiltrates and impaired gas exchange.

Pulmonary hypertension: elevated blood pressure in the pulmonary circulation. Primary pulmonary hypertension indicates that the etiology is not secondary to diseases of the heart or lungs.

Sarcoidosis: a multisystem disorder characterized in affected organs by a type of granulomatous inflammation. The etiology is unknown.

Six-minute walk test: 6MWT – a test that measures the distance that a patient can quickly walk on a flat, hard surface in a period of 6 min. It evaluates the global and integrated responses of all the systems involved during exercise, including the pulmonary and cardiovascular systems, systemic circulation, peripheral circulation, blood, neuromuscular units, and muscle metabolism.

TBLB: transbronchial lung biopsy – a lung biopsy obtained during bronchoscopy in which tiny forceps are passed to the distal bronchi and air sacs to obtain tissue.

10 Liver transplantation

Kimberly Brown, Mary Ann Huang, Marwan Kazimi, and Dilip Moonka

Henry Ford Hospital, Detroit, Michigan, USA

Orthotopic liver transplantation (OLT) is the mainstay of treatment of end-stage liver disease in the USA and much of the world. The first transplantation with extended survival was performed by Thomas Starzl in 1967. The recipient was an 18-month-old girl with hepatocellular carcinoma. Additional historical landmarks include the development of cyclosporine as an effective and tolerated immunosuppressant agent, and a 1983 National Institutes of Health consensus conference which concluded that liver transplantation was no longer an experimental procedure, but a "therapeutic modality" for advanced liver disease. Over 6500 deceased and living donor liver transplant procedures are now performed in the USA annually.

One of the most far-reaching changes in liver transplantation in the past decade centered on the implementation of the model for end-stage liver disease (MELD) system for organ allocation in 2002. Before implementation of the MELD system, organs were allocated using a "status" system that relied on a combination of disease severity and recipient waiting time. The MELD system, using a score that incorporates serum bilirubin, serum creatinine and the international normalized ratio (INR), prioritizes patients for transplantation based on their calculated 90-day mortality rate without a liver transplant. The implementation of the MELD system, along with a steady growth in the number of deceased donor livers between 2000 and 2007, has led to shorter waiting lists, a shorter median time to transplantation, and reduced death rates for patients awaiting liver transplantation. Moreover, the transparent and quantitative nature of the MELD system allows an on-going rational and statistical evaluation of the efficacy of organ allocation. This has facilitated additional changes in the allocation system, including the "share 15 rule" (see below) and changes in priority accorded to patients with "MELD exceptions," including the exception allotted to the growing number of patients transplanted for hepatocellular carcinoma (HCC).

The 5-year patient survival rate after liver transplantation is currently about 73%, and the 5-year graft survival rate is 68%. However, major challenges remain in the care of liver transplant recipients before graft and patient survival rates can improve further. This chapter focuses on several of these obstacles, including optimization of patient and graft selection, management of recurrent underlying liver disease with a focus on hepatitis C, and the care of complications of long-term immunosuppressive therapy, including nephrotoxicity.

Patient and allograft outcomes

Patient and graft survival after liver transplantation have continued to improve over the last decade. From 1987 to 1997, the 1-year patient survival rate increased from 64% to 86% with the 10-year survival rate increasing from 42% to 60%. During the same time period, the graft survival rate at 1 year increased from 55% to 79% and the 10-year graft survival rate from 34% to 52%. In 2008, the 1-year patient and

Primer on Transplantation, 3rd edition.
Edited by Donald Hricik.

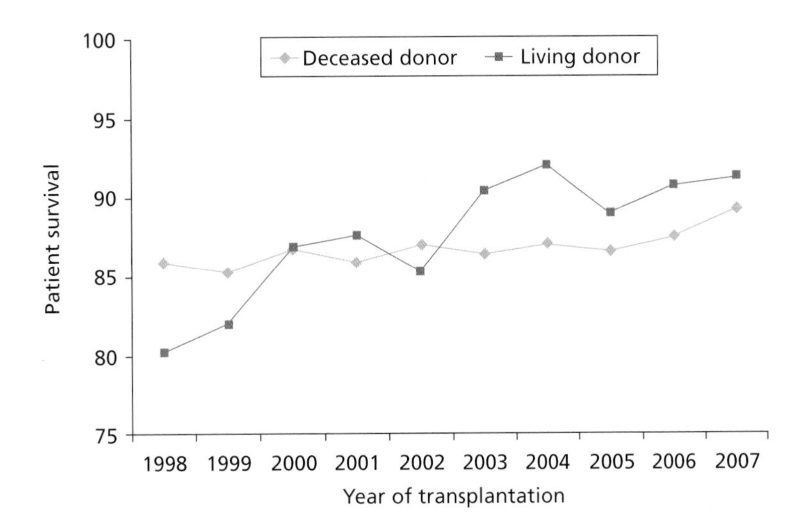

Figure 10.1 Changes in patient survival rates over time in liver transplantation in the USA.

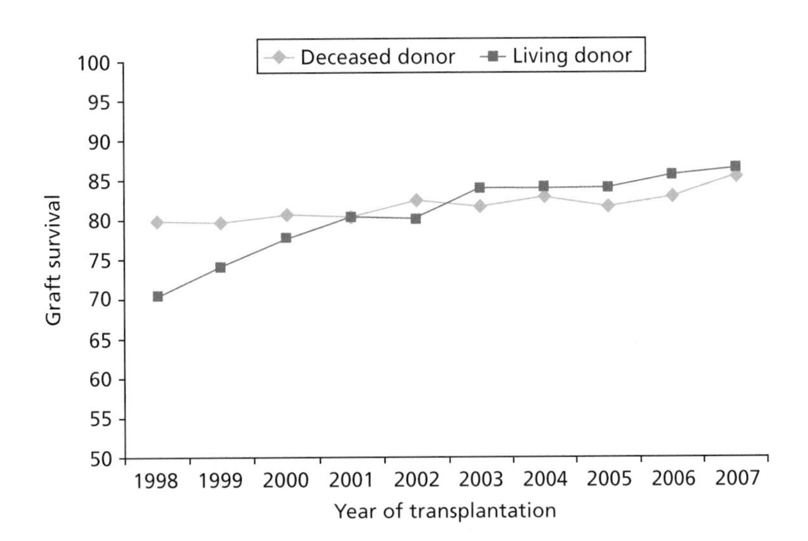

Figure 10.2 Changes in graft survival rates over time in liver transplantation in the USA.

graft survival rates nationally were 88% and 84%, respectively (Figures 10.1 and 10.2).

One of the biggest challenges facing patients awaiting liver transplantation is the increasing discrepancy between the number of transplantations performed yearly and the number of patients on the waiting list. In general, this has led to more ill patients receiving transplants while at the same time changing donor selection as transplant centers become more aggressive in attempting to match donor availability with recipient needs. Over the last 20 years, the number of new registrants on the waiting list has far exceeded transplantations performed and subsequently has resulted in increased wait-list mortality. From 2002 to 2008, the number of patients waiting for liver transplantation has remained high, approximately 16 000 each year. Over this time, approximately 6000 liver transplantations were performed annually in the USA with approximately 2000 deaths per year during the same time period (Figure 10.3).

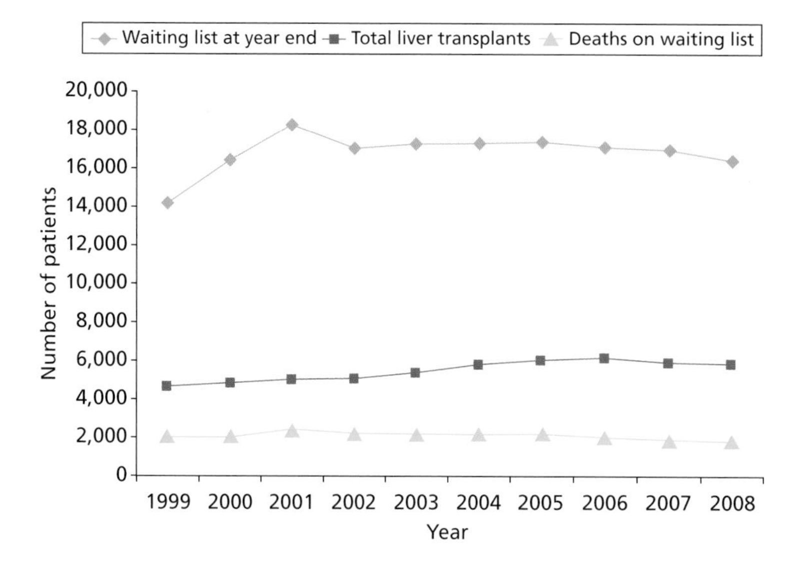

Figure 10.3 Changes in the size of the liver transplant waiting list, number of transplants performed, and deaths on the waiting list over time in the USA.

As noted above MELD was implemented in 2002 as a way to prioritize patients on the wait-list. MELD takes into account only severity of illness, and minimizes waiting time as a variable, and has been shown to effectively predict 3-month mortality from liver disease. Utilizing the MELD system for allocation of livers in the USA has resulted in a reduction in wait-list mortality by 15%, with the median wait time reduced from 656 days to approximately 300 days. Transplantation in patients with MELD scores ≤14 has been associated with higher mortality than for patients with the same MELD score who did not undergo transplantation. This finding led to the "share 15" policy which indicates that, if an organ is available and the highest MELD score of local patients is <15, the organ should be offered to a larger region first before it can be used locally. Several studies have shown that patients transplanted with MELD scores >25 have a lower survival than patients transplanted for lower MELD scores. However, the survival benefit remains high among patients with such scores. As a result, there is currently no MELD score for which removal from the list is mandated. It is important to note that MELD was designed to predict mortality risk from liver disease while waiting for liver transplantation and is less useful in predicting duration of survival *after* transplantation.

Key points 10.1 The MELD (model for end-stage liver disease) score

MELD calculators, requiring only an INR, serum creatinine, and serum bilirubin concentration, are widely available on the internet and on hand-held computers. The actual formula for calculating MELD is as follows:

$$\begin{aligned}\text{MELD score} &= 0.957 \times \log_e(\text{creatinine, mg/dL})^* \\ &+ 0.378 \times \log_e(\text{bilirubin, mg/dL}) \\ &+ 1.120 \times \log_e(\text{INR}) \\ &+ 0.643\end{aligned}$$

Multiply the score by 10 and round to the nearest whole number. Laboratory values <1.0 are set to 1.0.

*The maximum serum creatinine considered within the MELD score equation is 4.0 mg/dL. For candidates on dialysis, defined as having two or more dialysis treatments within the prior week or 24 h of continuous venovenous hemodialysis (CVVH) within the prior week, the serum creatinine entered in the MELD equation is automatically entered as 4.0 mg/dL.

Liver re-transplantation is associated with relatively poor survival rates, as has been established by many investigators. Multiple prognostic factors have been evaluated, including interval to re-transplantation, age, gender, and diagnosis of primary non-function (PNF) versus non-PNF. In addition, higher MELD scores have been shown to result in poorer survival after re-transplantation. Graft survival is significantly reduced in patients undergoing re-transplantation compared with first transplantation. For patients undergoing re-transplantation, 1-, 5- and 10-year graft survival rates are 69%, 54, and 38% which are significantly lower than those reported (84%, 69%, and 55%) for patients undergoing a first transplantation.

Deceased donor transplantation

Multiple factors contribute to outcomes after primary OLT. These can be classified as donor, recipient, operative, and postoperative factors.

Donor characteristics associated with poor post-OLT outcomes can be divided into relative and absolute factors. Many of the studies attempting to identify donor factors that contribute to poor post-transplant outcome have been performed at single centers, and the results have been variable and often contradictory. However, a compilation of multiple studies has identified 15 donor factors that may be associated with poor outcomes. These include donor age, gender, ethnicity, weight, ABO compatibility status, cause of brain death, length of hospital stay, pulmonary insufficiency, pressor use, steatosis, cardiac arrest, prolonged cold ischemia time, serum sodium level, and blood chemistry. Severe macrosteatosis (>60%) and cold ischemia time >30 h are absolute risk factors associated with poor post-transplant outcomes. Relative risk factors include moderate steatosis (defined as steatosis 30–60%), cold ischemia time >12 h, and donor age >50 years.

Recipient outcomes do vary by recipient age, gender, race, and diagnosis. In general, recipient characteristics have also been extensively investigated, including etiology of liver disease, age, coagulopathy, impaired renal function, ventilator status, hepatic function, and MELD score. Of all these factors, renal function before transplantation appears to be most closely associated with post-transplant outcomes. Ultimately, only a few absolute contraindications for liver transplantation exist., including extrahepatic malignancy, uncontrolled sepsis, and irreversible multisystem organ failure.

Operative and postoperative factors associated with post-transplant survival are often difficult to identify, because many of these factors have never been assessed in survival models. In terms of operative risk factors, warm ischemia time has been the most extensively evaluated in pretransplant models. Postoperatively, it has been extremely difficult to identify when urgent re-transplantation should occur. Although factors, such as bilirubin, prothrombin time, and creatinine, have been identified to help predict graft failure, the models generated may not be applicable for daily use and, currently, the decision to re-transplant relies on clinical assessment rather than mathematical models.

MELD is effective in predicting pretransplant mortality. Unfortunately, MELD scores have not been as helpful in predicting post-transplant outcomes. The transplant community has discussed the need for identifying the "upper limit" of utility, i.e., the need for identifying patients who have become too ill to benefit from transplantation. Thus far, criteria for determining when a patient should be removed from the list have not been established, and the decision remains with the transplant center. This is still a major difficulty with liver organ allocation, because the patients most in need of transplantation may not be the patients who will reap the most long-term survival and benefit.

Living donor transplantation

Adult to adult living donor transplantation (LDLT) began to grow in the 1990s as a possible solution to the widespread organ shortage. Previous work in Asia and Europe had established the utility of LDLT using the right hepatic lobe of a living donor for transplantation into adults with liver failure. Early on, from 1997 to 2001, the number of LDLTs being performed in the USA increased to a peak of over 400 in 2001. At that time, this represented about 8% of liver transplantations being performed in the USA. However, since that time, there has been a plateau and subsequent decrease in the number of adult LDLTs performed, partly due to concerns over donor morbidity and mortality (Figure 10.4).

Several factors suggest that outcomes from LDLT would be better than for deceased donor transplantation. These include decreased waiting time for the

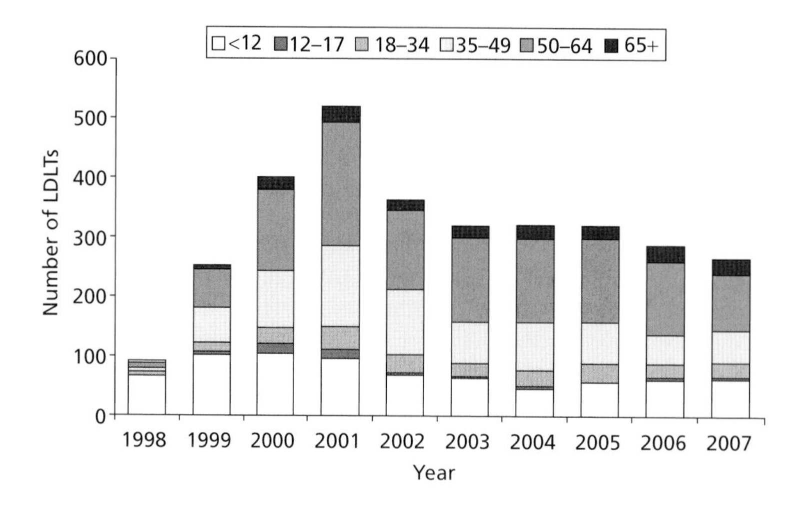

Figure 10.4 Number of living donor liver transplants (LDLTs) by recipient age, 1998–2007.

recipient, optimal evaluation of the donor organ before selection, and reduced cold ischemia time. In fact, both patient and graft survivals are improved in LDLT compared with deceased donor transplantation. The 1- and 3-year patient survival rates in LDLT are 91% and 82%, compared with 88% and 78% for deceased donor transplant recipients. The 1- and 3-year graft survival rates for LDLT are 86% and 76% compared with 84% and 73% for deceased donor liver transplantation. Overall, recipient outcomes have been shown to be comparable to those of deceased donor transplants. However, recipients of living donor livers are generally younger and have less severe liver disease.

Recipient selection and evaluation

There are several diagnostic indications for liver transplantation (Table 10.1). However, the need for transplantation is determined by weighing the natural history of the patient's liver disease against the likely outcome of transplantation. There are several basic questions that should be asked when evaluating patients referred for liver transplantation. First, is the liver disease severe enough to consider transplantation? In other words, is the patient at the point in the natural history of their disease at which no other alternate therapy is likely to improve their state of health other than transplantation? Second, is the patient an acceptable candidate? Are there recipient factors that would likely alter the expected outcome of transplantation, or are there factors that would interfere with the ability of the patient to benefit from transplantation? Finally, if patients appear to need a transplant and if they are found to be acceptable, are they willing and do they have the support to fully participate in the process?

With respect to the first question, the Childs–Turcotte–Pugh (CTP) score (Table 10.2) has been utilized to assess severity of cirrhosis, with minimal listing criteria considered a CTP score of ≥7 (Child's B cirrhosis). In these patients, the 1-year survival with a liver transplant would be expected to exceed the 1-year survival without a transplant. Obviously, other complications of cirrhosis, such as a diagnosis of HCC, hepatopulmonary syndrome, refractory ascites, or refractory encephalopathy, may make a candidate eligible for transplantation if the benefit outweighs the risk of surgery.

Case

A 43-year-old woman with autoimmune hepatitis is referred for possible liver transplantation. She has been taking prednisone for more than 1 year. On physical examination, she is alert and oriented and has no asterixis. She has a cushingoid appearance with centripetal obesity but no obvious ascites. An abdominal ultrasound scan does, however, show mild ascites. Laboratory evaluation shows a bilirubin of 1.4 mg/dL, albumin of 3.2 g/dL, and INR of 1.3. Based on her CPT score and her MELD score, you recommend that liver transplantation would likely not offer a survival advantage over medical therapy at this point in time. You also recommend close

Table 10.1 Indications for liver transplantation

Decompensated cirrhosis
Non-cholestatic
Viral hepatitis B or C
Alcohol
Non-alcoholic steatohepatitis
Autoimmune
Drug induced
Cryptogenic
Cholestatic
Primary biliary cirrhosis
Secondary biliary cirrhosis
Sclerosing cholangitis
Drug induced
Sarcoidosis
Cystic fibrosis
Biliary atresia
Alagille's syndrome
Progressive familial intrahepatic cholestasis
Metabolic/Inherited
α_1-Antitrypsin deficiency
Wilson's disease
Hereditary hemochromatosis
Glycogen storage disease
Tyrosinemia
Benign disorders
Polycystic liver disease
Budd–Chiari syndrome
Non-cirrhotic portal hypertension
Hemangioma (giant)
Malignant disorders
Hepatocellular carcinoma
Hepatoblastoma
Epithelioid hemangioendothelioma
Endocrine tumors
Other
Type 1 primary hyperoxaluria
Familial amyloidosis
Urea cycle or branched-chain amino acid disorders
Acute liver failure
Drugs
Toxins
Vascular
Immune
Metabolic (Wilson's disease)
Neonatal hemochromatosis
Acute graft loss
Primary non-function
Vascular
Humoral rejection
Late graft loss
Recurrent disease
Chronic rejection

Table 10.2 Child–Pugh classification of severity of liver disease

Parameter	Points		
	1	2	3
Ascites	Absent	Slight	Moderate
Bilirubin (mg/dL)	<2	2–3	>3
Albumin (g/dL)	>3.5	2.8–3.5	<2.8
International normalized ratio	<1.7	1.7–2.3	>2.3
Encephalopathy	None	Grade 1–2	Grade 3–4

follow-up with serial re-evaluations of the severity of her liver disease.

Medical evaluation

The answer to the second question involves the medical evaluation of the patient. Initial assessment should begin with a consultation with a hepatologist and a transplant surgeon as well as preliminary evaluation of financial coverage. Patients at this point may be deemed either too early or too ill for transplantation and no further evaluation may be necessary. However, in most patients it would be expected that further evaluation would be required to determine suitability for transplantation. The general evaluation consists of several consultations as well as laboratory and diagnostic testing (Table 10.3). The hepatologist evaluates the patient for disease diagnosis and assesses severity and considers whether alternate treatments may be appropriate. The surgeon's assessment should consider the technical aspects of the operation as well as donor selection and postoperative issues. Consultation with the "psychosocial team" may include evaluation by a social worker, clinical psychologist, chemical dependency specialist, or a combination of these consultants. Social support, risk of recidivism, and determination of patient ability to understand and cooperate with recommendations should be evaluated. A financial counselor should meet with the patient and family to assist them in understanding coverage and any out-of-pocket expenses. Consultation with a dietician or other specialists would be warranted based on specific patient issues or medical needs. In particular, clearance by cardiology would be warranted in patients aged >40 or those with a past medical history that dictates concern.

Laboratory testing is used to assess disease etiology, the degree of hepatic dysfunction and other comorbidities. Further evaluation of abnormal findings may warrant consultation with specific specialists such as infectious disease or nephrology. Basic laboratory testing includes a complete blood count, biochemical profile, and coagulation profile, blood group and cross-match, thyroid-stimulating hormone, and lipid profile. Further evaluation may vary from center to center, but should also include serologic work-up for viral hepatitis, testing for autoimmune and metabolic liver disease, screening for HCC with α-fetoprotein, urinalysis, and determination of the glomerular filtration rate (GFR) and arterial blood gas, a toxicology screen, and appropriate screening for extrahepatic malignancy (i.e. breast cancer screening in women aged >40 years, colon cancer screening). A patient may undergo more extensive testing if comorbid medical conditions or some positive test during the evaluation reveals a potential contraindication for transplantation.

Imaging is used to define the portal vasculature and to exclude malignancy. In patients with documented hepatocellular cancer, additional imaging of the chest with computed tomography (CT) is mandatory before listing. Cardiovascular testing with an echocardiogram is important to screen for increased pulmonary pressures. If evidence of increased pulmonary pressures is suspected, right heart catheterization and evaluation by both cardiology and pulmonary medicine is warranted. Cardiovascular testing should include some form of stress testing with either a dobutamine stress echo or nuclear stress testing to screen for ischemic disease.

In addition to the medical evaluation for transplantation, a psychosocial assessment is mandatory. Almost half of potential candidates for liver transplantation have at least one psychiatric disorder. A thoughtful and thorough assessment of each patient's psychiatric status will aid in assessing suitability for liver transplantation as well as in making recommendations for further evaluation or treatment before listing.

Patients with a history of substance abuse need further evaluation by a chemical dependency specialist. A generalized requirement of 6 months of abstinence has been accepted by most transplant centers. In addition, active participation in treatment may be recommended and required. Patients must participate in their abstinence. Poor prognostic factors include multiple prior episodes of relapses with substance abuse, limited insight into the consequences of substance abuse, and refusal or inability to participate in recovery.

Finally, evaluation of support and finances is mandatory. Patients must have adequate insurance to undergo transplantation and the resources to maintain health after transplantation. Evaluation of prescription coverage, patient and family resources, family and friend support, and individual barriers to success must be investigated by the social worker and other team members.

Selection of candidates

There are several absolute and relative contraindications for liver transplantation (Table 10.4). Uncontrolled sepsis or infection, extrahepatic malignancy, active substance abuse, and significant cardiopulmonary disease are absolute contraindications. Advanced age is a relative contraindication for transplantation, and the age cut-off varies from center to center. Patients aged >70 years may have poorer post-transplant outcomes compared with younger patients. Prior substance abuse, especially a history of

Table 10.3 Evaluation of the liver transplant recipient

Consultations
Hepatology
Transplant surgery
Cardiology
Social work
Financial
(Psychiatry, chemical dependency, nutritional, gynecology, other as necessary)
Laboratory
Complete blood count
Complete chemistry
International normalized ratio
Lipid profile
Blood group
Viral serology: HBsAg, HBcAb, HBsAb, HCV antibody, HAV antibody, HIV antibody, CMV, EBV
TSH
VDRL
α-Fetoprotein
Urinalysis
Measurement of GFR (calculated or 24 hours)
Toxicology screen
Arterial blood gas
(CEA, CA 19-9, PSA)
Imaging
Chest radiograph
EKG
Echocardiogram with/without stress
Cardiovascular stress testing
Dual-phase CT or MRI
Other
Colonoscopy (age >50, family or personal history, primary sclerosing cholangitis)
Mammography (age >40 or family or personal history)
Dental
Pap and pelvic

CEA, carcinoembryonic antigen; CMV, cytomegalovirus; EBV, Epstein–Barr virus; GFR, glomerular filtration rate; HBcAb, hepatitis B core antibody; HAV, hepatitis A virus; HBsAb, hepatitis B surface antibody; HBsAg, hepatitis B surface antigen; HCV, hepatitis C virus; PSA, prostate-specific antigen; TSH, thyroid-stimulating hormone; VDRL, Venereal Disease Reference Laboratory.

heavy alcohol use, may be a relative contraindication for transplantation. Data have shown that 20–50% of patients will consume some alcohol within the first 5 years after transplant, and 10–15% of those patients will have significant alcohol intake. Unfortunately, no reliable predictors exist to help determine which patients will be at highest risk of relapse after transplantation. Presence of significant pulmonary disease

Table 10.4 Absolute and relative contraindications to liver transplantation

Absolute
Severe uncontrolled sepsis
Extrahepatic malignancy
Active alcohol or substance abuse
Lack of adequate social support
Inability or unwillingness to comply with medical recommendations
Severe pulmonary hypertension
Severe cardiopulmonary disease
Relative
Advanced age
Hepatocellular carcinoma outside the Milan criteria
Previous history of malignancy
HIV
Intra-abdominal vascular thrombosis
Neuroendocrine malignancy

including pulmonary hypertension increases a patient's perioperative mortality and may become an absolute contraindication for transplantation due to anticipated worse post-transplant survivals. Finally, infection with HIV was once considered to be an absolute contraindication for liver transplantation. It is now felt to be a relative contraindication in the setting of well-controlled HIV disease because short-term outcomes appear to be reasonably good in these patients. Currently, only select centers in the USA have protocols for transplantation of HIV patients.

Once patients have completed their evaluation, they are reviewed individually by the multidisciplinary transplant team. The ideal candidate for listing is a patient with liver disease advanced to the point where the benefit of transplantation outweighs the risk (Child–Pugh score ≥7), in whom no obvious medical or social issues have been discovered that would interfere with a successful outcome. Once it is recommended that the patient undergo transplantation, if the patient and family agree, the patient is placed on the waiting list.

Table 10.5 American Association for the Study of Liver Disease guidelines for diagnosis and follow-up of varices

Screening esogastroduodenoscopy (EGD) for the diagnosis of esophageal and gastric varices when the diagnosis of cirrhosis is made
In patients with compensated cirrhosis and no varices on the initial EGD, repeat in 3 years
In patients with decompensated cirrhosis, EGD should be repeated annually
In patients with cirrhosis and small varices without prior bleeding but increased risk for hemorrhage (Child's B/C or red weal marks on varices); non-selective β blocker should be used for the prevention of first variceal hemorrhage
In patients with medium/large varices that have not bled but have high risk of hemorrhage (Child's B/C or red weal markings); non-selective β blockers or variceal ligation may be recommended for prevention of first variceal bleed

Management of patients listed for liver transplantation

The advent of MELD has changed the landscape of liver transplantation by allocating organs according to need rather than accumulated waiting time. The key for maintaining patients on the transplant list includes monitoring for complications of cirrhosis. Patients should be screened for HCC with an imaging study and α-fetoprotein every 6 months. Upper endoscopy should be performed to screen for varices. Both the treatment of varices and the timing of subsequent endoscopies depend on the presence and size of varices according to American Association for the Study of Liver Disease (AASLD) guidelines (Table 10.5). Yearly cardiac evaluation is mandated by most insurance carriers. In addition, other screening tests, such as mammograms and pap smears in women, should be updated.

Patients with cirrhosis related to hepatitis C may benefit from attempts to clear viremia, because such patients have better short- and long-term outcomes compared with patients with viremia. Unfortunately, most patients cannot tolerate therapy with pegylated interferon and ribavirin, and the presence of cirrhosis is associated with significantly decreased rates of a sustained virologic response (SVR). Thus, although attempts can be made to treat a patient for hepatitis C while they are waiting for transplantation, most patients will not be able to tolerate treatment.

In patients with hepatitis B and cirrhosis, those with active viral replication should be placed on oral antiviral treatment. Oral nucleoside and nucleotide reverse transcriptase inhibitors, such as lamivudine, adefovir, telbivudine, entecavir, and tenofovir, may be used for viral suppression. Current guidelines from the AASLD recommend use of an antiviral agent in patients diagnosed with cirrhosis. Avoidance of resistance is mandatory in this population to prevent both further decompensation before and viral resistance after transplantation. Most transplant centers choose either entecavir or tenofovir because these drugs have very potent viral suppression in addition to minimal documented resistance.

The MELD scores should be updated regularly. On average, recalculation of scores occurs every 90 days. However, patients with higher scores as well as those with clinical deterioration should have MELD scores updated more frequently. The interval in patients who are critically ill is defined by the United Network for Organ Sharing (UNOS). Finally, deterioration of clinical status may compromise a patient's candidacy for transplantation. Presence of active infection, multisystem organ failure, or other significant changes in clinical status should prompt the transplant team to re-evaluate the patient's candidacy, potentially resulting in either delisting or a change to "hold" status.

Patients should be screened for and immunized against both hepatitis A and hepatitis B if not already immune. Patients should receive the pneuomococcal vaccine, and be referred to infectious disease if childhood immunizations are not up to date.

Evaluation and selection of liver allograft donors

Major advances in the long-term success of liver transplantation have resulted in a broadening of the criteria used in the evaluation of potential liver allografts. A continued imbalance between the number of patients on the wait-list for liver transplant and the number of deceased donors highlights the need for optimizing the use of extended criteria donor (ECD), donation after cardiac death donor (DCD), and living donor liver allografts. Further advances in the technical aspects of the transplant procedure may continue, although more slowly than in the growth phase of liver transplantation. In contrast, donor management and the matching of donor allografts to appropriate recipients continue to evolve.

In selecting livers for transplantation, surgeons and hepatologists take a myriad of variables into account. Donor profiles include age, body mass index, social history including drug and alcohol use, medical and surgical history, liver function tests, serological testing, and, in some cases, pre-donation liver biopsies. These are balanced against the recipient's current medical condition, especially cardiac and renal function, history of a prior liver transplantation or other abdominal surgery, etiology of the liver disease, and known presence of HCC. A number of special considerations sometimes come in to play, e.g., although patients on the waiting list with the highest MELD scores are frequently the most sick, not all of them do well with livers from ECDs. Patients with fulminant hepatic failure often require urgent transplantation before the onset of brain-stem herniation or overwhelming sepsis. Some patients with well-compensated liver disease develop HCC and may require transplantation as a cure of their cancer rather than for criteria dictated by MELD.

Deceased organ donors

The vast majority of livers used in transplantation continue to come from deceased donors who have met brain death criteria. According to the Scientific Registry of Transplant Recipients, at the end of 2008 there were 16 450 patients wait-listed for liver transplant, with 6069 deceased donor transplantations and 249 living donor transplantations performed in 2008. Of the donors, 41.5% had a cerebrovascular accident and 16.4% trauma from a motor vehicle accident; 79.1% of all deceased donors were between the ages of 18 and 64.

In the past decade, the number of livers transplanted from DCDs, also known as non-heart beating donors (NHBDs), has increased dramatically, from 33 DCDs (0.9% of total donors) in 2000 to 277 DCDs (4.7% of total donors) used for 60 different programs in 2006. Graft survival of DCD liver allografts is inferior to survival from deceased donors meeting brain death criteria (Figure 10.5). In addition, biliary complications are more common with

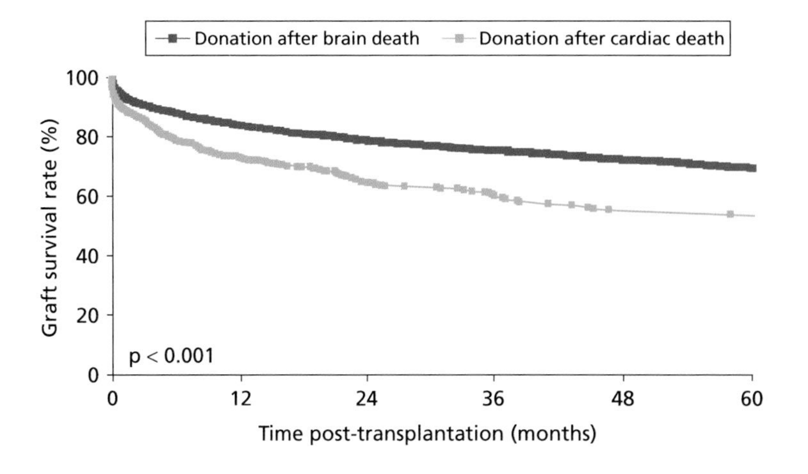

Figure 10.5 Adjusted graft survival for donor after cardiac death and brain dead donor liver transplants, 2001–2006.

DCD livers. Thus, specific criteria may be used in assessing the suitability DCD donors for liver transplantation (see "Donation after cardiac death").

Standard versus extended criteria donors
A "standard" or "reference donor" implies a very low risk of initial poor function or early allograft failure leading to death or requiring retransplantation. Additional factors such as transmissible disease, which do not directly affect the risk of graft failure, must also be considered in the definition of extended criteria. Factors that are not directly related to the donor, such as technical difficulties during the procedure, surgical complications, or disease recurrence, should not be included in the definition. An ideal allograft is different from an ideal donor. The ideal allograft category may be influenced by variables that are introduced after procurement, such as the prolonged cold ischemia time, or technical variants, such as those occurring with allograft reduction (e.g., split-liver allograft). These variables should not be included in the definition of the ECD because the aim is to assess risk before procurement.

In the past, a reference (or ideal) donor was defined according to the following criteria: age <40 years, trauma as the cause of death, donation after brain death, hemodynamic stability at the time of procurement, no steatosis or any other underlying chronic liver lesion, and no transmissible disease. An ECD, on the other hand, implies higher risk in comparison with a reference donor. The risk may be manifested as increased incidence of poor allograft function or allograft failure, or transmission of a donor-derived disease.

Key points 10.2 The characteristics of the ideal deceased donor for liver transplantation

Age <40 years

Trauma as the cause of death

Donation after brain death

Hemodynamic stability at the time of procurement

No steatosis or any other underlying chronic liver lesion

No transmissible disease

At the Paris Consensus Meeting on Extended Criteria Donors in Liver Transplantation (March 2007), broad recommendations were made with regard to donor type, donor history, and donor allograft quality in the evaluation of grafts to be used in liver transplantation. Specific distinction was made between factors that affect initial donor allograft function and factors independent of donor graft function (such as infectious disease or donor-derived malignancy). The conference highlighted the reality that donor allografts represent a continuum of risk that is impossible to separate into fixed categories, but is better viewed as high or low probability of both initial function and long-term allograft survival. This probability index can then be weighed against the risk profiles, comorbidities, and expected mortality rates of potential recipients.

Further attempts at codifying an "extended criteria liver" include various objective criteria: age >55 years, aspartate transaminase (AST) >150 IU/L, serum bilirubin >2 mg/dL, serum sodium >150 mmol/L, high doses of any vasoactive pressor, period of cardiac arrest, intensive care unit (ICU) stay >5 days, and moderate or severe macrosteatosis. Various studies have concluded that the use of such ECD livers, when carefully selected for the appropriate recipient and implanted efficiently, is viable and safely expands the numbers of liver transplantations, thereby diminishing the number of deaths on the waiting list.

Older age donors

Advanced donor age was once considered a contraindication to liver donation because it was feared to increase the risk of poor graft function. In fact, the outcome of transplantation using older donors without any other risk factors has been shown to be similar to that of using younger donors. Accordingly, the UNOS data show that the upper age limit for liver donation has increased over the past decade. In 1996, 25% of all transplanted livers were from deceased donors aged >50 years. Ten years later, that percentage had increased to 34%.

Although advanced donor age is not by itself a contraindication, careful assessment must be made on a case-by-case basis. Older livers tend to be smaller and more fibrotic than younger livers, but these morphologic changes might not impair functional hepatic capacity. Possible explanations for the relatively good results with aged livers include great functional reserve, regenerative capacity, and dual blood supply, which far exceed the metabolic needs of the recipient. However, older donors in general have a higher incidence of severe atherosclerosis and fatty infiltration in the liver. In addition, the combination of older donor age and moderate-to-severe steatosis adversely impacts early allograft survival. Transmission of malignancy is another consideration with aged donors because of the higher incidence of unrecognized malignancies in elderly people. Advanced donor age may also be associated with early severe recurrent liver disease in patients with hepatitis C.

Hepatic steatosis

The prevalence of steatosis in liver donors ranges from 13% to 26%, with two histologic patterns of fatty infiltration typically observed: microvesicular steatosis, in which the cytoplasm contains diffuse small-droplet vacuolization, and macrovesicular steatosis, in which large vacuole deposits displace the nuclei. The outcome of transplantation is not affected by microsteatosis in the donor liver, regardless of the severity. In addition, grafts with mild macrosteatosis (<30%) can be used safely, because the outcomes of such liver allografts are similar to those of non-steatotic grafts. Donor livers with severe macrosteatosis (>60% of hepatocytes having large fat deposits within the cytoplasm) do have a significant risk of graft failure and are generally not used for transplantation. As a result of impaired hepatic microcirculation, steatotic livers have reduced tolerance for ischemia–reperfusion injury.

Key points 10.3 Impact of hepatic steatosis on selection of liver donors

Microvesicular steatosis (cytoplasm containing diffuse small droplet vacuolization):
- no contraindication to donation

Macrosteatosis (large vacuole deposits displacing nuclei):
- <30% of hepatocytes affected– usually acceptable for donation
- >60% of hepatocytes affected – usually not acceptable for donation

Prolonged ischemia

Prolonged ischemia remains one of the major causes of early graft dysfunction, with clear evidence that preservation times affect the incidence of PNF, as well as overall outcomes, in liver transplantation. Prolonged cold ischemic time, defined as the time from cross-clamping and perfusion with preservative solution in the donor operation to the time of reperfusion with blood in the liver recipient, increases the risk of PNF and is an independent risk factor for hepatic ischemia–reperfusion injury. The vulnerability of individual grafts to cold ischemia varies, however. Total ischemic times of <12–16 h are well tolerated by donor livers without any other risk factors, but not by marginal grafts. In the modern era of liver preservation, the incidence of ischemia–reperfusion injury and PNF is low if recipients are transplanted with standard grafts. In extended criteria grafts, however, with such risk factors as steatosis, donor age >50 years, DCD source, or reduced size, it is essential that cold ischemia time be minimized.

Split-liver transplants

Surveys in western populations indicate that split-liver transplantation in adults is associated with significant increases (about 10%) in graft failure and recipient morbidity. Results are notably better in children. Even if split-liver allografts are procured from young donors with normal parenchyma and short cold ischemia times, they should be considered extended criteria grafts for the following reasons: .

- The graft volume is generally lower than the recipient's standard liver volume and may be insufficient to adequately meet the metabolic demand during the early postoperative course.
- There are higher technical requirements, and non-optimal positioning of the partial graft may result in compromised venous outflow.

As a result, biliary leakage, hepatic artery thrombosis, focal or global outflow obstruction, and poor early graft recovery are more frequent in comparison with whole organ transplantation.

Donation after cardiac death

In the past 10 years, a number of transplant programs have begun to use livers from DCDs, or non-heart-beating donors. DCDs can be divided into two categories: uncontrolled and controlled donation. In uncontrolled DCDs, death has occurred without life-support equipment in place. As a result of prolonged warm ischemia before cold perfusion, the organs suffer severe ischemic insult. Liver transplantation using uncontrolled DCDs has resulted in inferior outcomes. In an early study from Pittsburgh in 1995, three of six allografts from uncontrolled DCDs did not function and the 1-year graft survival rate was 17%. Otero et al. reported that the incidence of PNF was 25% in uncontrolled DCDs ($n = 20$), with graft and patient survival rates of 55% and 80%, respectively (see Further reading).

In contrast, in controlled DCDs, life support is carefully withdrawn in the operating room, when donor surgeons are available, resulting in minimal hypotension and warm ischemia. Under these circumstances, the outcomes of liver transplantation are acceptable. In an early report from Pittsburgh, although the 1-year graft and patient survival rate was 50%, there was no incidence of PNF. D'Alessandro et al. reported that the rate of PNF was 10.5% in controlled DCD donors (see Further reading). The 1-year graft survival rate in recipients from DCDs was lower than that from donation after brain death (53.8% vs 80.9%; $p = 0.007$) but there was no difference in patient survival. Abt et al. reported that controlled DCD livers had a higher incidence of intrahepatic ischemic-type biliary strictures compared with DBD livers (33.3% vs 9.5%; $p < 0.01$), but the two types of livers had similar graft and patient survival.

Nationwide data have confirmed inferior outcomes from DCD livers. UNOS data between 1993 and 2001 characterized 117 DCD grafts as controlled, 11 as uncontrolled, and 16 as unknown or not identified. When the controlled DCD and DBD livers were compared, the graft survival rate at 1 year was lower in controlled DCD (72.3% vs 80.4%; $p = 0.056$). DCD recipients had a higher incidence of PNF (11.8 vs 6.4%; $p = 0.008$) and re-transplantation (13.9% vs 8.3%; $p = 0.04$) compared with DBD recipients. However, patient survival was similar in both. Predictors of early graft failure within 60 days of transplantation were prolonged cold ischemia time and use of recipient life support at time of transplantation (e.g., pressors). Merion et al. examined a national cohort of DCD ($n = 472$) and DBD ($n = 23\,598$) liver transplantations between 2000 and 2004 using the Scientific Registry of Transplant Recipients (SRTR) database (see Further reading). There was no categorization of DCD donation such as controlled/uncontrolled status in their analysis. The adjusted relative risk of DCD graft failure was 85% higher than that for DBD grafts.

Mateo et al. reported the importance of risk evaluation to improve graft survival in a DCD setting using the UNOS database between 1996 and 2003. They identified six significant risk factors in recipients for graft loss: a history of a previous liver transplantation, being on life support, being hospitalized or in an ICU, having received dialysis, serum creatinine value >2.0 mg/dL at time of transplantation, and age >60 years. Graft survival rates at 1 year (n = 367) were significantly inferior to those with DBD donors (80% and 72%; $p < 0.001$). However, low-risk recipients with low-risk DCD livers (warm ischemia time <30 min and cold ischemia time <10 h; n = 226) achieved graft survival rates at 1 and 3 years (81% and 67%) not significantly different from those of recipients with DBD livers (n = 33 111). In addition, increasing donor age was more highly predictive of poor outcomes in DCD, especially in recipients in poor preoperative condition.

Although there is, as yet, no consensus on the use of DCD livers, the preponderance of data suggests three things:

- DCD allografts from younger donors (<40 years) fare better over both the short and the long term.
- DCD livers must be used in technically efficient operations with resultant short ischemia times.
- DCD grafts should be used in recipients who tend to be younger and have fewer comorbidities, especially with regard to renal dysfunction.

As these general guidelines are used more frequently, it is possible that, although the use of DCDs may not expand significantly, outcomes will improve.

Living donors

Consideration of a living donor involves both medical and psychosocial evaluation. Donors are evaluated on the basis of suitability of the quality of organ to be donated as well as for the safety and risk to the donor. Evaluation of the donor begins with pre-clinical criteria, followed by extensive medical and psychosocial evaluation. If patients are deemed to be appropriate from both a medical and a psychosocial standpoint, further anatomical evaluation of the organ is performed to determine suitability for the intended recipient. The general format for evaluation of potential donors is outlined in Table 10.6.

The initial evaluation of the living donor begins once recipients have been determined to be suitable candidates for liver transplantation. Often, the public views living donation as a "get out of jail free" card. It is important for recipients and families to understand that, given the magnitude of risk to the potential donor, recipients are required to be deemed appropriate candidates first for transplantation, at which point various donation options can be considered. In general, given the risk of potential coercion, recipient and donor pairs are separated with respect to the hepatologist and transplant surgeon caring for them as well as the coordinator involved with the evaluation. In general, potential donors have to have basic medical suitability to include age ≥18 or ≤50, good medical health, and a blood type compatible with the recipient.

Once a potential donor is identified and the preclinical evaluation found to be suitable, the medical evaluation continues to identify potential health risk to the donor. The general medical evaluation is listed in Table 10.6. In addition to the general evaluation of medical health, potential donors are evaluated by the psychosocial team to determine psychiatric stability, financial and social support, and whether there is any evidence of potential coercion. During this process, patients are educated as to the risks and outcomes of donation. They are required to meet independently with a separate donor advocate who has knowledge of the transplant process but is not part of the transplant team caring for the patient or donor.

Finally, if it appears that there are no medical or psychosocial barriers to donation, the donor undergoes anatomic evaluation of the organ to ensure adequate volume for both the donor and recipient. Donor remnant volumes of at least 35% must be weighed against adequately sized donor grafts. A graft to recipient body weight ratio of ≥0.8% and graft weight as a percentage of standard liver mass of >40% result in improved outcomes for recipients.

Given the need for extensive evaluation of both the donor and the recipient in the setting of LDLT, it is estimated that only 15–28% of potential donors are ultimately found to be suitable for donation. In the adult-to-adult living donor liver transplantation registry, major reasons for disqualification included medical (28%), anatomical (19%), psychosocial (9%), graft (11%), and declining to donate (11%). In addition, 11% of recipients received a deceased donor graft before LDLT and an additional 7% died or were removed from the waiting list before surgery.

Surgical techniques and complications

Liver transplantations are performed in an orthotopic manner and consist of three phases: the hepatectomy

Table 10.6 Evaluation of living donors

Preclinical
Age ≥18 or ≤50 years
Identical or compatible ABO blood type with recipient
Absence of significant medical conditions
Medical
Evaluation by transplant coordinator with consent for evaluation
Evaluation by transplant hepatology
Laboratory evaluation:
Basic biochemistries and blood count
Screening tests for undiagnosed liver disease
Viral serologies: HCV antibody, HBsAg, HBcAb, HBsAb, CMV, EBV
Chest radiograph
EKG
Doppler ultrasonography of the liver
Echocardiogram
Psychosocial
Social work
Psychiatry
Independent donor advocate
Anatomic evaluation of donor organ
Abdominal MRI/CT with volumetric assessment
Liver biopsy (as clinically indicated)
Arteriogram (as clinically indicated)
Final evaluation
Transplant surgery (with consent for donation)
Evaluation by multidisciplinary team for review of information and discussion

CMV, cytomegalovirus; EBV, Epstein–Barr virus; HBcAb, hepatitis B core antibody; HBsAb, hepatitis B surface antibody; HBsAg, hepatitis B surface antigen; HCV, hepatitis C virus.

phase, the anhepatic phase, and the post-perfusion or post-implantation phase. The liver is removed by one of two techniques: conventional (bicaval) (Figure 10.6a) or "piggyback" (caval preserving) (Figure 10.6b). The conventional technique may be done with or without use of venovenous bypass, depending on the recipient's hemodynamic stability and ability to tolerate temporary clamping of the inferior vena cava and the associated decrease in preload due to interruption of venous return to the heart.

Although most studies comparing the two techniques are retrospective, there is evidence that the piggyback method requires one less venous anastomosis and thus lends itself to shorter warm ischemia times. The method also facilitates re-transplantation (particularly important in patients with hepatitis C), and is associated with shorter anhepatic phases, less blood loss and blood product usage, and shorter postoperative ICU stays. On the other hand, it may be associated with higher incidence of venous outflow obstruction which may lead to ascites.

The four main anastomoses involved in liver transplantation are the aforementioned inferior vena cava anastomosis, portal vein anastomosis, hepatic artery anastomosis, and bile duct anastomosis. A brief review of the technical aspects of each of these steps follows, with discussion of the diagnosis and management of potential complications.

Biliary complications are the most common technical complications after liver transplantation, reported in between 6 and 34% of all liver transplant recipients. Their incidence varies with the type of liver allograft (whole vs partial, brain dead vs DCD). The two most common types of biliary reconstruction are choledochocholedochostomy (CC) (Figure 10.7a) and choledochojejunostomy (CJ), usually with a roux-en-Y loop (Figure 10.7b). More than 75% of adult full-size OLTs are performed as a CC. More common reasons for use of a CJ reconstruction are re-transplantation, living donor or split-liver transplantation, pediatric grafts, presence of ductal disease in the recipient, or significant donor-to-recipient duct discordance.

An acute elevation in alkaline phosphatase or bilirubin with relatively little change in transaminases should prompt a diagnostic work-up of a potential biliary stricture or sphincter of Oddi dysfunction (in the case of CC anastomoses), or, less commonly in

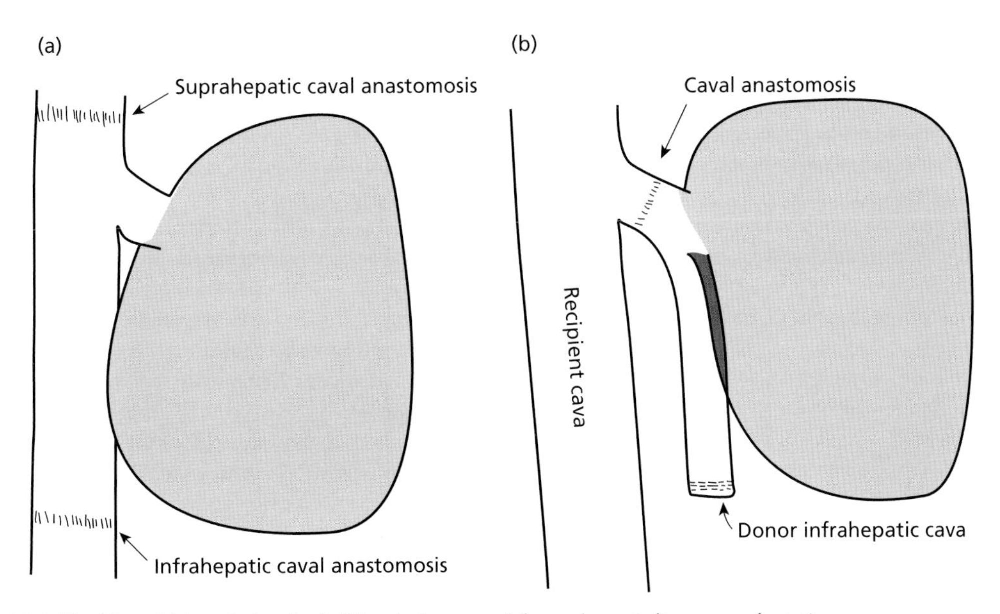

Figure 10.6 The bicaval (a) and piggyback (b) techniques used for orthotopic liver transplantation.

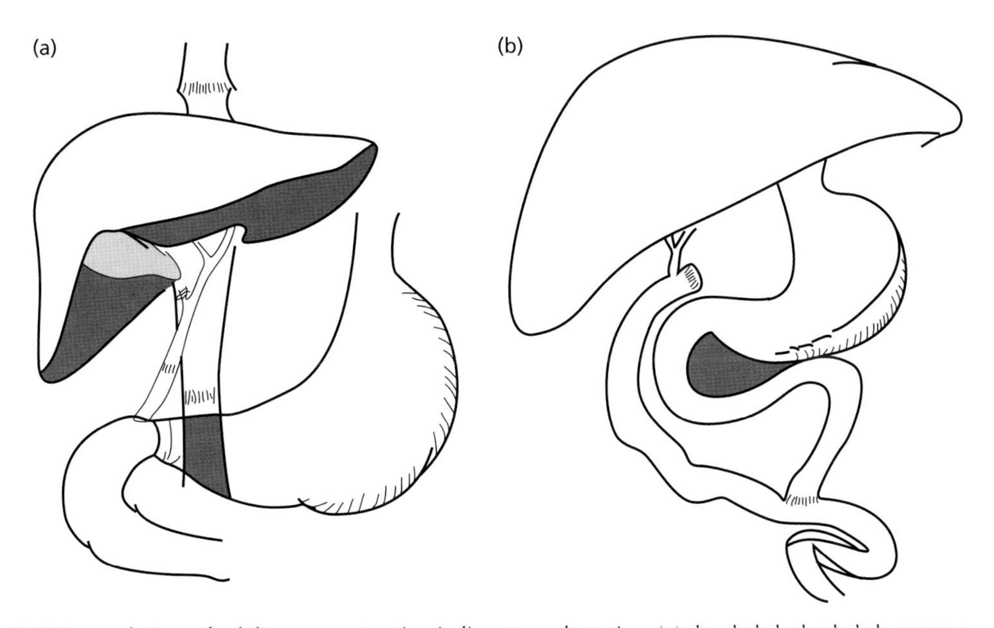

Figure 10.7 Two techniques for biliary reconstruction in liver transplantation: (a) the choledochocholedocostomy or "duct-to-duct" technique; (b) the choledochojejunostomy with roux-en-Y loop technique.

the CJ patient, ascending cholangitis. With no valve to limit reflux of enteric contents, some patients with roux-en-Y CJ post-OLT will have episodes of ascending cholangitis requiring admission for intravenous antibiotics followed by short-term outpatient oral treatment.

Patients with CC-type anastomoses may have T-tube stents, internal stents, or no stents placed. With the advent and experience of endoscopic retrograde cholangiopancreatography (ERCP), the relative risks of T-tubes and internal stents has caused a shift away from surgically placed stents, but with greater use of ERCP post-transplant for diagnosing and treating strictures. Patients with CJ may need evaluation of their biliary–enteric anastomosis with CT, magnetic resonance cholangiopancreatography (MRCP), or percutaneous transhepatic cholangiogram (PTC) post-transplantation, with the last affording the option of placing internal stents for dilation alone or internal–external stents for drainage.

Strictures in the post-transplant period may be anastomotic (usually due to technical issues, vascular insufficiency, or fibrotic healing), or non-anastomotic. Both types may be diagnosed and treated by ERCP or PTC, but non-anastomotic strictures with the presence of biliary casts or stones should prompt careful evaluation of the hepatic arterial supply. In some studies, approximately 50% of patients with non-anastomotic strictures also have hepatic artery stenosis or thrombosis.

Although most biliary complications are related to strictures or bile duct redundancy, leaks also occur in 2–10% of OLTs. Early leaks, defined as those occurring within a month post-transplantation, are usually technical in nature and should be managed with surgical exploration and conversion of a CC to a CJ anastomosis, or a redo of the initial CJ anastomosis. Leaks that occur over 1 month post-transplantation are usually related to ischemia or infection. Careful attention should be paid to the hepatic artery in these patients, while the leak is generally best managed with ERCP or PTC in concert with percutaneous drainage of potential abdominal abscesses or collections.

Hepatic artery thrombosis (HAT) is the most common vascular complication after OLT, and the most common technical complication requiring re-transplantation. Recent reviews document an HAT rate of 1.6–4% in adult recipients and 12–30% in children. Split-liver and living donor liver transplants, in addition to having a higher rate of biliary complications, have an increased incidence of HAT. Mortality rates for HAT range from 11% to 35% depending on the interval after OLT, symptoms on presentation, and mode of therapy.

Patients with HAT will develop acute or chronic symptoms, with the types of symptoms dependent on the time interval between OLT and development of HAT. Signs may range from fulminant hepatic necrosis in the early postoperative period to transaminitis, biliary strictures or abscesses, relapsing bacteremia, or recurrent fevers. Imaging studies, including hepatic duplex ultrasonography, CT angiography and, the gold standard, celiac angiography, have been used to diagnose HAT.

Patients with early HAT who are asymptomatic or mildly symptomatic are candidates for graft salvage with surgical exploration and arterial reconstruction, including the possible use of aortic jump grafting, preferably using an autogenous vein. Acute HAT within the first week post-transplantation is an absolute indication for relisting a patient as status 1 (i.e., the highest priority patient, taking precedence over all other patients listed regardless of MELD score). Patients in whom late HAT develops but who have biliary sepsis are also best served by r-transplantation.

Catheter-directed therapies, with angioplasty, stenting, and long-term use of either warfarin or antiplatelet agents, have also had some success in salvaging allografts when patients are discovered to have HAT by routine ultrasonography or CT. The goal of therapy is to prevent progression to complete occlusion as a result of the diminished blood flow, and consequently to avert associated ischemic biliary strictures and sepsis. The long-term results of such therapies are still under investigation.

Case

One year after an otherwise successful liver transplant performed for alcoholic cirrhosis, a 51-year-old man is admitted for evaluation of fever and abdominal pain. Abdominal CT scan reveals a large hepatic abscess that is drained percutaneously. Further imaging with Doppler ultrasonography reveals thrombosis of the hepatic artery. The patient completes 6 weeks of antibiotic therapy. Follow-up CT shows no residual abscess and the patient continues to be managed as an outpatient.

Other, rarer hepatic artery complications include pseudoaneurysm, which occurs in less than 1% of patients and is usually due to trauma or infectious processes. Treatment almost always requires urgent surgical reconstruction, although occasionally cases can be managed with interventional techniques.

Less common than either biliary or hepatic arterial technical complications are hepatic venous outflow or portal vein stenoses. Hepatic vein outflow obstruction, which occurs more commonly with the piggyback technique (2–10% incidence), may be corrected with catheter-guided venous stent placement with or without subsequent anticoagulation. Portal vein stenosis, reported in 1–2% of patients, may also be corrected with venous stenting, although surgical reconstruction should also be considered in such cases.

Immunosuppression

Immunosuppression after liver transplantation, as with all solid organ transplantation, is guided by the principle that the incidence of rejection is greatest soon after transplantation and declines with time. In contrast, complications associated with immunosuppressive medications accrue the longer a patient is "out" from the transplantation. Chronic rejection is an unusual cause of graft loss or death, but over half of liver transplant recipients will die from complications attributable to antirejection medications including cardiovascular disease, renal failure, infection, and malignancy. As a result, there is a general strategy of using multiple medications at high doses early on and fewer medications at lower doses later.

Traditionally, most liver transplant centers used a regimen of three medications early after transplant. These include the primary long-term immunosuppressant, typically either cyclosporine or tacrolimus, corticosteroids and an antimetabolite usually mycophenolate mofetil (MMF), mycophenolic acid (MPA), or azathioprine. The corticosteroids are administered at high doses intravenously in the days immediately proceeding transplantation and then tapered off typically within a few months to a year. The antimetabolite (MMF or MPA) may be discontinued 3–6 months after the corticosteroid and many patients are maintained on either a dual (with cyclosporine) or single agent (with tacrolimus) regimen depending on the calcineurin agent used.

Immunosuppression after liver transplantation is in evolution as efforts are made to avoid complications and side effects. There are several recent trends of note. There is a tendency to taper corticosteroids more rapidly than in the past to diminish the incidence of steroid side effects. Several new approaches are designed to reduce the burden of renal insufficiency which is associated with the use of cyclosporine or tacrolimus. Antibody-mediated "induction therapy" with antibodies that either deplete T cells or block the interluekin-2 receptor (IL-2RA) is being used with greater frequency to help minimize the use of steroids or to delay the introduction of cyclosporine or tacrolimus to preserve renal function. Typically MMF or MPA is also discontinued within a year of transplantation. However, there is evidence that, if MMF/MPA is continued, lower doses of tacrolimus and cyclosporine can be used with a resulting improvement in renal function. Finally, the newer agent, sirolimus, is being used in some patients in an effort to avoid renal dysfunction. Rapamycin can either be used instead of tacrolimus or cyclosporine or with lower doses of one of these agents.

Cyclosporine and tacrolimus

Both cyclosporine and tacrolimus suppress the immune system through the inhibition of calcineurin, a protein that drives production of cytokines such as IL-2 that drive T-cell activation. Collectively, the two drugs are called calcineurin inhibitors (CNIs) and they are the workhorses of solid organ transplantation. The vast majority of liver transplant recipients are maintained on one or the other indefinitely. Before the advent of cyclosporine, corticosteroids and azathioprine were used with a 1-year survival rate of 25–35%. Cyclosporine, a fungally derived peptide, was approved in 1983, resulting in markedly improved survival. It is lipophilic and requires enterohepatic circulation for absorption. This can be problematic in liver transplant recipients with biliary T-tubes or those with poor graft function. Generic formulations of cyclosporine have been available since 2000. Tacrolimus is a macrolide agent of bacterial origin that was approved for use in liver transplantation in

1994. The primary commercial form of tacrolimus is Prograf but generic forms were released in 2009.

Both tacrolimus and cyclosporine are oral agents taken every 12 hours though a modified formulation of tacrolimus that be given once daily is anticipated. Cyclosporine is available in 25 and 100 mg pills and tacrolimus in 0.5, 1, and 5 mg pills. The dosage is based on trough levels of the drugs and is highly individualized. Higher trough levels are sought initially after transplantation when the risk of rejection is high and lower levels are sought later when concerns about adverse effects start to predominate. Typical trough levels for cyclosporine are 200–300 ng/mL initially and 50–150 ng/mL long term. Typical trough levels for tacrolimus are 5–15 ng/mL with the higher end targeted early after transplantation.

CNIs have significant side effects and nephrotoxicity is their Achilles' heel. Renal insufficiency is a major cause of morbidity and mortality after liver transplantation. Other side effects common to both drugs are hyperkalemia, hypertension, and neurotoxicity, ranging from headaches and tremor to neuropathy and seizures. Cyclosporine is more commonly associated with hyperlipidemia, and gingival hyperplasia, whereas tacrolimus is more frequently associated with diabetes. There is significant debate over the merits of the two drugs. What is clear is that tacrolimus is now used in 89% of OLT patients in the USA at the time of initial discharge. Tacrolimus is associated with less rejection than cyclosporine and this may explain its appeal early on. Both drugs are comparable in their deleterious effects on renal function.

Antibody induction therapy

A strategy that has grown in popularity in the MELD era is the use of potent intravenous antibody preparations that deplete or inhibit T lymphocytes early after transplantation. These agents can be used to delay the introduction of calcineurin inhibitors (CNIs) to facilitate recovery of renal function or to minimize exposure to corticosteroids and lower the incidence of diabetes and osteoporosis. The most commonly used agents include rabbit antithymocyte globulin (Thymoglobulin), daclizumab (Zenapax), and basiliximab (Simulect). However, production of Zenapax has recently been halted. Thymoglobulin is a polyclonal antibody formulation made by immunizing rabbits with human T lymphocytes. Thymoglobulin binds multiple antigens on lymphocytes and leads to T-lymphocyte depletion. It is administered at a fixed dose for 7–14 days and fevers and chills can be seen in up to a third of patients.

Daclizumab and basiliximab are monoclonal antibodies that bind to CD25 or the IL-2R and inhibit T-cell activation. Basiliximab is typically given in two doses, at the time of transplantation and on day 4. Daclizumab has been used in two-, three- and five-dose regimens. Both agents are well tolerated with few specific side effects. OKT3 (Muromonab-CD3) is used less often now because of toxicity and the advent of newer agents, and alemtuzumab (Campath-1H) has not found widespread use in liver transplantation.

Induction therapy can be used to delay the introduction of CNIs for up to a week and it has a beneficial effect on renal function in this setting. In addition, induction therapy is a mainstay in steroid avoidance protocols. In some randomized studies, induction therapy is associated with a lower incidence of acute rejection and it is not clearly associated with an increased incidence of severe recurrent hepatitis C. The use of induction therapy is not as widespread in liver transplantation as it is with other organ transplantations but its use is growing in popularity especially in patients with renal insufficiency at the time of transplantation.

Corticosteroids

Corticosteroids are potent immunosuppressant drugs that inhibit T-lymphocyte, monocyte, and macrophage activity. Corticosteroids are administered at high doses intravenously in the days immediately preceding transplantation. Methylprednisolone may be given at doses of 500–1000 mg/day and then tapered to doses of 10–20 mg/day after 1–2 weeks. There is a tendency to taper corticosteroids more rapidly than in the past. Most centers eliminate corticosteroids within a year but many aim to do so within 3 months or sooner. This has been shown to result in less hypertension, diabetes, hyperlipidemia, and infection. There are several reports of effective induction antibody-based regimens that avoid steroids and these regimens are currently used in up to 20% of liver transplant recipients. Corticosteroids may be continued for longer durations at reduced doses in some patients with autoimmune liver diseases or recurrent rejection.

Antimetabolites

Antimetabolites are a group of drugs that interfere with purine nucleotide synthesis which leads to preferential inhibition of T and B lymphocytes. Azathioprine was a mainstay of immunosuppression early in organ transplantation but, in recent years, mycophenolate mofetil (MMF, CellCept) and enteric-coated mycophenolate sodium (MPA, Myfortic) are used more commonly in liver transplantation. Azathioprine can be associated with cholestatic hepatitis. MMF and MPA do not exhibit this toxicity and are more potent. Antimetabolites are not potent enough to be used as the primary immunosuppressive agent but are important as adjunct agents, especially in the first few months to a year after transplantation. MMF is typically given at 1–2 g daily in two divided doses and MPA is typically given at 720–1440 mg daily in two divided doses. Side effects are frequent and include marrow suppression and gastrointestinal side effects such as gastritis, nausea, diarrhea, and abdominal pain. These agents are typically discontinued by 1 year after liver transplantation. However, several reports suggest that they may be beneficial for longer periods by facilitating lower doses and levels of CNIs.

Sirolimus (mTOR inhibitors)

Sirolimus (Rapamune), similar to tacrolimus, is a macrolide. It is named after the Easter Island of Rapa Nui where it was discovered. Unlike tacrolimus, sirolimus is not a CNI but targets T cells through cell cycle inhibition via the mammalian target of rapamycin (mTOR) pathway. Sirolimus is a newer immunosuppressant agent that is touted as being potent enough to be used as a primary immunosuppressive agent but without the nephrotoxicity of CNIs. Sirolimus can therefore be considered as an alternative to a CNI or, in some instances, in combination with lower doses of one of the CNIs. Sirolimus has been associated with hepatic artery thrombosis and graft loss in new liver transplant recipients in some but not all trials. It has received a "black box warning" from the Food and Drug Administration, which suggests avoiding the drug in the first month after liver transplantation.

The combination of sirolimus and MMF has been compared with a CNI and MMF in a randomized study in patients 4–12 weeks post-liver transplantation. In patients randomized to receive sirolimus, there was a 22.1% increase in glomerular filtration rate from baseline to year 1 compared with a 6.2% increase in patients receiving the CNI, and this difference was significant. There was a higher incidence of rejection in the sirolimus arm. Based on randomized trials, there does not appear to be a clear benefit of converting patients to sirolimus in stable liver transplant recipients. A major drawback to this medication is its side -profile. Side effects include hyperlipidemia, cytopenias, poor wound healing, lymphoceles, and oral ulceration. There is also an association with an unusual but potentially fatal aseptic pneumonitis. Between 25% and 30% of liver transplant recipients who receive the drug are not able to tolerate it.

Drug interactions

Tacrolimus, cyclosporine, and sirolimus all have clear dose-related toxicity and relatively narrow therapeutic windows. As a result the knowledge of drug interactions is critical. Certain medications can affect CNI levels by inducing or inhibiting the cytochrome P450 (CYP) 3A4 pathway, as discussed extensively in Chapters 2 and 7. Allopurinol, by blocking xanthine oxidase, can increase levels of azathioprine to toxic levels. Non-steroidal anti-inflammatory medications can potentiate CNI-induced nephrotoxicity and spironolactone can increase CNI-induced hyperkalemia. Carvedilol has been shown to increase CNI levels by inhibiting the P-glycoprotein pathway. Grapefruit products can dramatically raise CNI levels.

Drugs that are felt to be well tolerated include amlodopine, nifedipine, angiotensin-converting enzyme (ACE) inhibitors, angiotensin II AT_1-receptor blockers (ARBs), and β blockers (excluding carvedilol) for hypertension; oral hypoglycemics, metformin, sulfonylureas, and thiazolidinediones for diabetes mellitus; HMG-CoA reductase inhibitors for hyperlipidemia; and gabapentin and evetiracetam for seizures. Antibiotic agents including penicillins, cephalosporins, quinolones, and sulfonamides should not affect immunosuppressant levels. Narcotics are safe outside their addictive potential and antidepressants are typically well tolerated. Up to 4 g/day of acetaminophen can be given to liver transplant recipients with functioning grafts.

Table 10.7 Snover's criteria for diagnosis of acute cellular rejection

Presence of mixed portal infiltrate
Presence of bile duct injury
Presence of endothelial cell damage

Rejection in liver transplantation

Diagnosis

Acute cellular rejection (ACR) is the most common cause of early allograft dysfunction. The median time to ACR is 8 days with 48% of patients experiencing rejection by 6 weeks and 65% experiencing rejection by 1 year. Early rejection correlates with suboptimal immunosuppression, lower recipient age, prolonged ischemia time, and older donor age. In addition, females and those with autoimmune disorders show a higher frequency of ACR in some studies.

Patients may present with elevated transaminases or cholestasis. They may have fever, right upper quadrant pain, or leukocytosis. More commonly, with mild ACR, patients are asymptomatic. The use of biochemistries to distinguish ACR from other etiologies has not proven to be helpful. Currently, the only reliable way to diagnose either ACR or chronic rejection (CR) is with liver biopsy.

The histologic diagnosis of ACR is based on Snover's criteria (Table 10.7) which include: (1) mixed portal infiltrate, (2) bile duct inflammation and damage, and (3) endothelialitis of either the portal or terminal hepatic vein branches. The minimum criteria for a diagnosis of ACR are at least two of the above in addition to biochemical evidence of liver injury. Of these three findings, the most specific for a diagnosis of ACR is the presence of endothelialitis (see Figure 10.8).

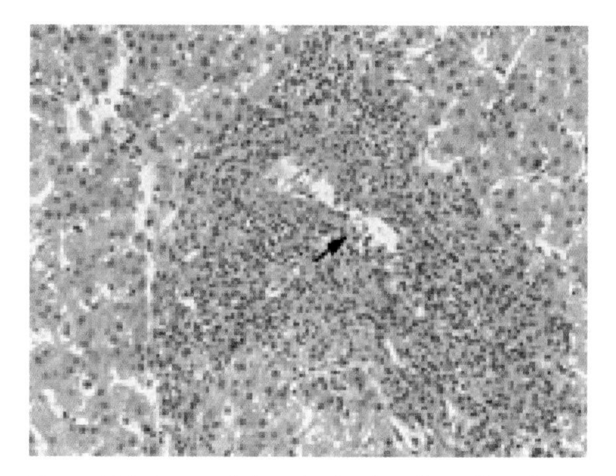

Figure 10.8 Acute cellular rejection in a liver allograft characterized by mixed portal infiltrate, bile duct damage, and endothelialitis, here consisting of a perivenular lymphocytic infiltrate.

Atypical presentations of ACR can include central perivenulitis and plasma cell rejection. Central perivenulitis can be a component of early ACR in association with characteristic portal tract changes. However, isolated perivenulitis has been described and may represent a more severe form of ACR that is less likely to respond to conventional immunosuppression. Differential diagnosis in these isolated cases includes ischemia–reperfusion injury, vascular ischemia, viral or autoimmune hepatitis, or drug toxicity (tacrolimus or azathioprine). Plasma cell ACR may also occur in the setting of recurrent hepatitis C and is a poor prognostic factor for patient and graft survival. Whether this represents a form of ACR or, alternatively, a new form of autoimmune hepatitis is unclear.

For both adults and children, rejection is uncommon more than 12 months post-transplantation. Late rejection more often correlates with reduction in immunosuppression, or poor compliance, which may be more common in adolescents. Late rejection may have histological features different from those seen in acute rejection, and include a predominantly mononuclear portal inflammatory infiltrate and less inflammation of the bile ducts or vascular endothelium. Both interface and lobular hepatitis may be present and, in these cases, it is important to rule out viral hepatitis as a potential cause. Increased immunosuppression and reinforcement of adherence to medications is paramount to prevent progression to chronic rejection.

CR occurs in 3–5% of patients undergoing liver transplantation. It is almost always preceded by one or more episodes of ACR. Additional risk factors for the development of CR include younger recipient age, primary diagnosis of immune disease, relatively lower baseline level of immunosuppression, and non-white recipient race. Features may include progressive duct injury with cholestasis, loss of hepatic synthetic function, or pruning of the intrahepatic arteries on angiography. A less common form of CR targeting hepatocytes has also been described. Bile duct injury is not prominent and patients present with elevated transaminases as opposed to a more cholestatic picture. Diagnostic criteria developed by the Banff group include: (1) senescent changes with cytoplasmic eosinophilia, cell enlargement and multinucleation, uneven nuclear spacing, and loss of polarity affecting a majority of the bile ducts with or without bile duct loss; (2) convincing foam cell obliterative arteriopathy; or (3) bile duct loss affecting more than 50% of the portal tracts. A significant proportion of these patients will progress to cirrhosis and up to half will require re-transplantation. If diagnosed at an early stage and treated with additional immunosuppression, CR has been shown to be reversible in some patients.

Differentiating ACR from recurrent hepatitis C can be difficult. This is an important distinction because treatment of ACR with bolus steroids has been associated with more aggressive recurrence of hepatitis C virus (HCV). ACR and recurrent HCV often share common features and both may be present simultaneously. Bile duct injury may be seen in both ACR and recurrent HCV. Although ACR often occurs in the first month after, with HCV recurring later, significant overlap may exist, making diagnosis and treatment decisions difficult. Marked elevations of HCV RNA may be present with recurrence; however, viral loads cannot be used to distinguish the two. Other features that may suggest recurrent HCV over rejection include the presence of steatosis, predominance of lymphocytes within portal tracts, acidophilic bodies, and lack of endothelial cell damage.

Case

Two months after a liver transplantation performed for cirrhosis resulting from hepatitis C, a 39-year-old man has a liver biopsy for evaluation of a recent rise in serum alanine transaminase (ALT), AST, and alkaline phosphatase levels. The biopsy shows mixed portal inflammation with a predominance of lymphocytes. There is mild endothelialitis involving branches of portal venules. Mild steatosis is noted as well. The pathologic diagnosis is recurrent hepatitis C and possible mild acute rejection. As a result of concerns that additional immunosuppression might increase the replication of hepatitis C, no additional therapy is administered for rejection. The patient's liver function tests gradually stabilized.

Treatment

High-dose corticosteroids are usually the first-line therapy for ACR after liver transplantation. Treatment regimens vary between centers but generally include intravenous methylprednisolone from 500 mg to 1000 mg daily for up to 3 days. Tapering regimens of 1000 mg followed by a 6-day taper from 200 mg/day down to 20 mg/day is effective and may result in fewer complications than high-dose steroids for 3 consecutive days. Using one of these regimens, ACR is controlled in approximately 80% of cases.

Ten to twenty percent of patients will experience steroid-resistant ACR. Rescue therapies including rabbit ATG and OKT3 have been used to treat these episodes. Resolution of rejection is generally seen in 60–80% of patients treated. After treatment, further adjustments in baseline immunosuppression are required to prevent early recurrence. Consideration of increased baseline immunosuppression must be weighed against potential side effects and often varies from center to center.

Treatment of rejection in the setting of HCV requires careful consideration. The use of corticosteroid boluses and OKT3 clearly has a negative impact in HCV-infected individuals. Therefore, it is critical to clearly define significant rejection and minimize over-treatment in equivocal cases or in cases with overlap. Many centers do not aggressively treat mild rejection in the setting of HCV. Consideration of increasing baseline immunosuppression and avoiding bolus corticosteroids should be made. What is clear is that immunosuppression in patients with HCV needs to be individualized and careful consideration of biopsy findings with an experienced pathologist should be considered before any changes in medical therapy.

Recurrent disease

Hepatitis C

Hepatitis C currently accounts for most liver transplants performed at many large centers. It is the most common diagnosis for transplantation in the USA. Current estimates suggest that the overall prevalence of HCV antibodies in the USA is 1.8%. Statistics from the Centers for Disease Control (CDC) indicate that approximately 4 million Americans are infected with

HCV and, of these, an estimated 2.7 million have chronic HCV infection. Chronic liver disease from hepatitis C is the tenth leading cause of death among American adults and accounts for approximately 25 000 deaths each year, or 1% of all deaths in the USA. Once exposed, approximately 75% of patients remain chronically infected.

The NHANES III database shows that this cohort of patients chronically infected with HCV is aging. In the 1990s the 30- to 39-year-old group had the highest prevalence of HCV antibody, 3.9%, for an estimated 1.6 million HCV-infected individuals in this age group. Currently, people aged 40–59 years have the highest prevalence of HCV infection and, in this age group, the prevalence is highest in African–American individuals (6.1%). These aging individuals are at increasing risk of fibrosis and consequences of long-term infection such as HCC, decompensation, and liver transplantation. Computer projections have corroborated CDC predictions that mortality from HCV-related liver disease may increase two- to three-fold over the next 10–20 years.

In addition, HCV accounts for an estimated third of HCC cases in the USA and is currently the most common risk factor for HCC. HCC rarely occurs in the absence of cirrhosis or advanced fibrosis. The incidence of HCV-related HCC continues to rise in the USA and worldwide, in part because of the increasing numbers of people who have been chronically infected for decades, the presence of comorbid factors, and the longer survival of people with advanced liver disease due to improved management of complications. The increased risk of HCC places further burden on transplant centers as patients present for consideration.

Key points 10.4 Facts about hepatitis C in the USA

Most common cause of end-stage liver disease requiring liver transplantation

1.8% prevalence of antibodies to hepatitis C in the US population

Tenth leading cause of death among adult Americans with approximately 25 000 deaths annually

Currently the prevalence of hepatitis C is highest in patients between the ages of 40 and 59 years

The earliest studies of the outcome of OLT for HCV reported post-transplant patient and graft survival similar to those achieved after OLT for other chronic liver diseases. These were usually single-center reports limited by small numbers and relatively short periods of follow-up. Several large registry analyses have recently reported reduced graft and patient survivals in recipients with HCV. An analysis of the UNOS database shows that 3-year patient survival rate was 78% in HCV-positive liver transplant recipients versus 82% in HCV-negative patients. Likewise, 3- and 5-year graft survivals are significantly reduced in patients undergoing OLT with HCV compared with non-HCV-infected patients.

Later studies have shown that up to 40% of patients with recurrent HCV develop cirrhosis within 5 years, suggesting that HCV is becoming more aggressive in transplant recipients in recent years. Stronger immunosuppressive agents, rapid steroid withdrawal, and increasing donor age are possible explanations, although increased diagnosis due to more liberal use of diagnostic biopsies may also be important. Unlike non-HCV-infected patients in whom graft survival has consistently improved over time, patients with HCV have shown a worsening of graft survival rates over time, again suggesting that some change in practice may have negatively influenced HCV recurrence and/or progression.

The natural history of HCV progression is accelerated after transplantation. As noted above, up to 40% of patients develop cirrhosis within 5 years, compared with 30% after 20–30 years in the non-transplant setting. Once patients have cirrhosis, clinical decompensation is also accelerated: 60% exhibit decompensation 3 years after the diagnosis of cirrhosis in HCV transplant recipients compared with only 10% at 10 years in immunocompetent patients. Finally, once patients have evidence of decompensation, death is accelerated with less than 10% survival at 3 years versus 60% in immunocompetent patients.

HCV RNA levels decrease significantly after hepatectomy during the anhepatic phase. During the first 12–24 h after OLT, HCV RNA levels may fall further or plateau but then start to rise progressively, reaching levels 12 times pretransplant levels by months 1–4. The clinical spectrum of recurrence is highly variable. In 20–30% of patients, progression is not quickly apparent and liver injury remains mild or absent for the first few months. These patients may eventually progress to chronic hepatitis or may remain with minimal injury over several years. A small percentage of patients will develop early, severe recurrence, termed "fibrosing cholestatic hepatitis." This is a severe form of liver injury with progression to cirrhosis and death within a few months of liver transplantation. Most patients will develop what appears to be an acute hepatitis early post-transplantation which develops into chronic hepatitis and progressive fibrosis over time. Currently 10% of patients will require re-transplantation for cirrhosis and HCV after OLT.

Several factors have been shown to be associated with accelerated fibrosis in patients with HCV undergoing OLT. In addition to factors related to immunosuppression, including steroid boluses as well as rapid *withdrawal* of steroids, other host, viral, and donor factors likely influence disease progression. The age of the donor has been found to be independently associated with disease severity, progression, and graft and patient survival. The increasing age of the donor population over time may be one of the most significant contributors to the increased severity of recurrent HCV disease in recent years. Several studies have shown that pretransplant HCV levels in the serum or in the explanted liver correlates with the severity of HCV recurrence, with a high pretransplant viral load being associated with increased mortality and graft loss. The number and severity of rejection episodes and treatment with steroid boluses are associated with increased severity of HCV recurrence and the development of cirrhosis. Interestingly, early and rapid steroid withdrawal has also been shown to be associated with increased development of fibrosis. By contrast, there is really no convincing evidence to date that choice of CNI influences outcome.

There are several strategies employed to decrease morbidity and mortality of recurrent HCV before and after OLT. Before transplantation, HCV is treated primarily to prevent fibrosis progression to cirrhosis. This would be the ideal time to treat most patients because treatment is reasonably tolerated and safe with sustained virologic response (SVR) rates in excess of 50%. Once a patient has developed cirrhosis, one might consider treatment either to prevent decompensation or to reduce HCV RNA levels in the liver before transplantation. Unfortunately, treatment in patients with advanced liver disease is poorly tolerated and associated with high rates of infection and low rates of response.

After transplantation, treatment can be either pre-emptive or delayed once disease is established. The advantage of pre-emptive therapy may be that HCV RNA levels are lower during the first 1–3 months after OLT; however, immunosuppression levels are the highest. In addition, numerous medications during this time period contribute to bone marrow suppression, making effective treatment challenging. Certainly the main goal in treating HCV after OLT is prevention of graft loss and improved graft and patient survival. Given that recurrence of HCV is almost 100% after OLT, treatment before transplantation should be considered in appropriate individuals.

It is well known that higher pretransplant HCV RNA correlates with increased mortality and graft loss. However, tolerability in patients with more advanced liver disease is poor, with a significant rate of serious adverse events and systemic infections. Several authors have reported on treatment of HCV in patients with advanced liver disease. Everson from the University of Colorado reported results on 124 patients with cirrhosis treated with interferon and ribavirin, with a mean Child's score of 7.4 and a MELD score of 11 (see Further reading). On treatment virologic response was 46% with SVR of 24%. Recurrent HCV infection was prevented in all patients achieving SVR. Overall, the data suggest that on treatment responses and SVR rates are generally lower than in patients with less advanced disease. In addition, dose reduction occurs in the majority of patients with very high rates of discontinuation as compared with patients with less advanced disease.

Many patients present for transplantation with decompensation and have limited or no opportunity for antiviral therapy before transplant. After OLT, viral eradication becomes the primary goal of therapy. Interferon-based therapies have been shown to eradicate virus both pre- and post-transplantation. Recently, Veldt from Mayo Clinic performed a cohort study evaluating the impact of treatment of HCV after OLT on graft survival. The incidence of graft failure was lower for patients treated within 6 months of recurrence compared with patients not treated within this time period (log rank $p = 0.002$). Time-dependent multivariate Cox's regression analysis showed that treatment of recurrent HCV infection was associated with a decreased risk of overall graft failure (hazard ratio [HR] 0.34; confidence interval [CI] 0.15–0.77; p = 0.009) and a decreased risk of graft failure due to recurrent HCV (HR 0.24; CI 0.08–0.69; p = 0.008). In conclusion, although a cause and effect relationship cannot be established, treatment of recurrent HCV infection after liver transplantation is associated with a reduced risk of graft failure.

Several challenges with the use of interferon are seen after OLT, including poor tolerance, limited eligibility, and lower efficacy. After transplantation there is an initial decline in HCV RNA levels with a variable rate of increase over the first 2 weeks to peak values 3–4 months after OLT. A pre-emptive strategy initiates treatment within the first few weeks after OLT when HCV RNA values are lowest and histologic injury is minimal. Treatment in the early phase of infection may be easier than with established chronic disease. These benefits have only partially been seen with pre-emptive clinical studies. Rates of SVR have been variable ranging from 8% to 35%. Most studies used combination ischemia–reperfusion with studies using monotherapy having the lowest SVR. Dose reductions were required in a significant portion of patients. Although several early studies reported a trend toward reduced severity of recurrent HCV at the end of treatment in patents receiving pre-emptive therapy, compared with untreated controls, this strategy is applicable only to patients without significant post-transplant complications and whose clinical status is sufficiently stable to allow initiation of antiviral treatment within a few weeks of OLT. Other studies have evaluated the efficacy of treatment within the first 6 months after OLT. Tolerability appeared to be somewhat better than that seen in studies with earlier treatment with fewer patients requiring discontinuation.

Finally, there have been numerous studies evaluating treatment of established recurrent HCV infection after OLT. Most of these studies have been uncontrolled and retrospective with relatively small sample sizes. Two systematic reviews of the efficacy of interferon/pegylated interferon and ribavirin for 6–12 months have also been published. Wang included studies of both non-pegylated and pegylated interferon with ribavirin (P/R). A total of 38 studies published between 1980 and 2005 were included. The pooled estimate of SVR was 20% for interferon and ribavirin and 24% for P/R. End-of-treatment virologic response (EOTR) rates were 34% and 42% respectively, indicating close to a 50% relapse rate for most studies. A second systematic review from Berenguer focused on studies of P/R between 2003 and 2007: 611 patients were included with overall EOTR and SVR rates of 42.2% and 30.2%. The mean SVR was 28.7% in G1 patients. Baseline factors associated with SVR included non-1 genotype, low pretreatment HCV, absence of prior antiviral therapy, and endovascular repair (EVR). Failure to achieve a decline in HCVRNA during the first 3 months of treatment was highly predictive of non-SVR. Relapse occurred in a substantial number of patients 43% and 21% in the Wang and Berenguer reviews respectively (see Further reading).

Liver transplantation for viral hepatitis continues to increase. Recurrence of virus post-transplantation leads to increased morbidity and mortality. Management of liver recipients with HCV is post-transplant treatment of recurrent disease. New strategies are needed to improve outcomes based on patient selection and use of current antiviral treatment. Improved therapies are needed both pre and post transplantation to reduce the need for transplantation and improve outcomes following transplant.

Hepatitis B

Early in the history of liver transplantation, hepatitis B was considered a relative contraindication to transplantation. Patients frequently experienced reinfection of the graft with significantly decreased patient and graft survival rates. In the early 1990s, trials using hepatitis B immunoglobulin (HBIg) showed that recurrence of the disease could be prevented in a significant number of patients. Trials using HBIg showed that recurrence of disease could be prevented in up to 90% of patients with long-term intravenous administration. As a result, 5-year graft survival rates for patients transplanted with hepatitis B have improved from 53% to 76%, equivalent to survival rates of patients transplanted for other diseases.

Further studies, combining a nucleos(t)ide analogs with HBIg showed additional opportunities for the prevention of recurrent disease. The first agents used included lamivudine and adefovir, both of which showed added efficacy when combined with HBIg. In these studies, recurrent HBV occurred in only 4–8% of patients.

Concerns about cost and viral resistance led to further investigations with different regimens of HBIg administration and use of newer nucleos(t)ide analogues. With traditional intravenous administration of HBIg, yearly costs could approach US$100 000. Studies using intravenous HBIg in a modified regimen, including lower doses of HBIg administered intramuscularly, have proven to be both efficacious and cost-effective, reducing costs by approximately 50%.

Currently, there are five oral agents approved for the treatment of HBV. Several studies evaluating the efficacy of these agents in patients with end-stage liver disease have shown both improvement in Child–Pugh scores and resolution of clinical sequelae of liver failure, such as ascites. However, the emergence of viral resistance to some drugs such as lamivudine and adefovir poses a challenge in these patients. Once resistance occurs, decompensation can return and treatment after transplantation becomes more challenging. As a result, current practice suggests that oral agents associated with a very low risk of inducing viral resistance, such as entecavir or tenofovir, be considered in patients with cirrhosis or decompensated liver disease.

After transplantation, most centers continue patients on HBIg and a nucleos(t)ide agent indefinitely. Although the original trials used lamivudine in combination with HBIg, current practice is to combine an oral agent such as entecavir or tenofovir with less risk of inducing viral resistance. The surface antigen of HBV (HBsAg) should be measured regularly to monitor for recurrence of HBV. A positive HBsAg on two or more occasions documents recurrence. Once recurrence occurs, HBIg is no longer useful and should be discontinued. Patients should be managed with oral nucleos(t)ides, the choice depending on prior therapies and the possibility of viral resistance from prior treatment.

Primary biliary cirrhosis

Primary biliary cirrhosis (PBC) has been shown to recur in up to 50% of patients undergoing liver transplantation for that diagnosis. PBC usually recurs 3 years or more after OLT but has been reported to recur earlier in some patients and has not been identified as having significant impact on either quality of life or the need for re-transplantation.

Diagnosis of recurrent PBC is dependent on histologic features. Antimitochondrial antibody titers persist after transplantation and cannot be used as an indicator of disease recurrence. The gold standard for defining recurrent PBC are histologic features, including florid duct lesions with granulomatous cholangitis or destructive lymphocytic cholangitis within a dense portal infiltrate. Early or mild recurrence may limit the identification of these features. The diagnosis of recurrent PBC can be established in a patient with a history of PBC before transplantation, a persistent positive antimitochondrial antibody level, and three of the following five histologic features: (1) mononuclear inflammatory infiltrate, (2) lymphoid aggregate formation, (3) epithelioid granulomas, (4) lymphocytic cholangitis with biliary epithelial eosinophilia, and (5) the presence of ductular proliferation with portal and periportal fibrosis small bile duct loss, foamy hepatocytes, and lysosomal pigments with copper deposition in periportal hepatocytes.

Risk factors for recurrent PBC probably include a genetic predisposition. Associations between PBC and common genetic variants in HLA class II, IL12A, and IL-12 receptor β_2 loci have been demonstrated. Some authors have suggested that a smaller number of HLA-A, HLA-B, and HLA-DR mismatches between donor and recipient may be an independent risk factor for disease recurrence after OLT. Others have suggested that tacrolimus may be an independent risk factor for recurrence and that cyclosporine may be protective. A recently discovered association of betaretrovirus with PBC suggests that this virus may also play a role in recurrence; however, this has not been further elucidated.

Most studies have concluded that recurrent PBC is unlikely to affect long-term patient or graft survival. Few patients have been identified with organ dysfunction resulting from recurrence, and re-transplantation for recurrent PBC is rare.

Primary sclerosing cholangitis

The diagnosis of recurrent primary sclerosing cholangitis (PSC) includes a confirmed diagnosis of PSC before OLT, cholangiographic evidence of non-anastomotic biliary strictures with beading, or a liver biopsy revealing fibrous cholangitis and /or biliary–obliterative lesions of large bile ducts in the absence of other potential causes. Several entities can mimic

PSC in the post-transplant setting when there is injury of biliary epithelium resulting from a variety of insults. Biliary strictures may occur with severe recurrent acute rejection, chronic ductopenic rejection, ABO incompatibility, hepatic arterial thrombosis or stricture, and after use of a DCD donor.

Histologically, early stages of recurrent PSC are characterized by mild, non-specific pericholangitis or cholangitis. Portal inflammation may be present and small bile duct loss may be observed. Later features include cholestasis, intralobular foam cell clusters, and copper deposition. Fibro-obliterative lesions may be observed involving the medium and small bile ducts. Radiographically, a cholangiogram revealing non-anastomotic biliary strictures of the intra-/extra-hepatic biliary tree with beading and irregularity, occurring more than 90 days post-transplantation is essential for the diagnosis.

Predictive factors for recurrent PSC may include the presence of specific HLA haplotypes; however, this has not been confirmed. Certain factors such as recipient age, male gender, donor–recipient gender mismatch, coexistence of inflammatory bowel disease, CMV infection, recurrent ACR, or steroid-resistant ACR all have been implicated in recurrence of PSC after OLT.

Recurrent PSC can affect graft survival; however, there are limited data with regard to specific treatment. Currently, use of corticosteroids or altered immunosuppression has not been shown to be beneficial in these patients. Ursodeoxycholic acid is often utilized; however, neither pre- nor post-transplant studies have demonstrated definite benefit. Re-transplantation for recurrent disease and graft loss has been described and should be considered in select patients.

Autoimmmune liver disease

Recurrence of autoimmune hepatitis (AIH) occurs in up to 27–42% of patients after OLT. Histologic features include lobular and interface necroinflammatiory activity with a predominance of plasma cells. Serologic features may include positive autoantibodies in titers ≥1:40, but patients may have evidence of histologic recurrence in the absence of positive autoantibodies. The criteria for diagnosis should include a combination of biochemical changes, histological features, and corticosteroid dependency.

Studies have suggested that patients with HLA-DR3 may have increased risk of recurrence. In addition, patients with type I AIH (antinuclear antibody [ANA]/anti-SMA [smooth muscle antibody] positive) vs type II (anti-LKM positive) may have increased risk of recurrence as well. In most patients with suspected recurrence, biochemical and histological response occurs with increased immunosuppression. Severe recurrence has been documented and graft loss and need for re-transplantation reported. In addition, typical features of AIH have been reported in recipients transplanted for both PBC and PSC. This raises the issue of whether these cases represent new AIH or a recurrence of an overlap syndrome.

Transplantation for HCC

The incidence of HCC is 1–3 per 100 000 in the USA and Europe, nearly doubling in the past two decades. An estimated 8500–11 000 new cases of HCC occur each year in the USA. HCV-associated HCC is expected to further double in the next 20 years, and outcomes for patients with HCC and cirrhosis remain poor without liver transplantation, with expected 1-year survival often less than 1 year.

During the NIH consensus development conference in Washington DC in 1982, liver transplantation was accepted as a treatment modality for patients with end-stage liver disease (ESLD) and unresectable tumors of the liver. A quarter century later, OLT has become the standard of care for all forms of ESLD, including HCC. In providing complete oncologic resection and correcting the hepatic dysfunction in patients with cirrhosis and HCC, OLT is well suited to such patients. Although early experience with OLT for cancer resulted in poor patient survival and high recurrence rates, methods of patient selection have been refined, and results have improved dramatically.

The so-called Milan criteria were born as a result of a 1996 study by Mazzaferro and colleagues, which reviewed radiologic and histologic results of patients with ESLD and HCC who received liver transplants. They reported that, in patients with a solitary tumor ≤5 cm or no more than three tumors, each no larger than 3 cm, overall and recurrence-free survival rates after transplantation were 85% and 92%, respectively. Overall HCC recurrence was 8% at the 4-year follow-up. Patients who exceeded the criteria showed an actuarial survival rate of 50%, only 59% of whom were recurrence free. The Milan criteria are currently the standard by which the UNOS and Medicare to guide selection of patients for cadaveric OLT in the USA, with some variation established by regional review boards.

Over the past decade, several studies have challenged the Milan criteria, reporting comparable outcomes after transplantation for more advanced stages of HCC. Yao and colleagues showed a 5-year survival rate of 70.2% in patients with HCC fulfilling so-called University of California, San Francisco (UCSF) criteria. These criteria, based on explant pathology, allowed inclusion of single tumors ≤6.5 cm, or a maximum of three tumors ≤4.5 cm, and a cumulative tumor size ≤8 cm.

The Barcelona Clinic Liver Center has developed a system for treatment of HCC with OLT, based on tumor stage, liver function, physical status, and cancer-related symptoms. Their emphasis is on drop-out rates and intention-to-treat analyses, and their expanded criteria include one tumor <7 cm, three tumors <5 cm each, or five tumors <3 cm each, or downstaging to conventional Milan criteria with pretransplant adjuvant therapies. Using this expanded approach, the Barcelona group has achieved 5-year post-transplant survival rate in excess of 50%, versus 20% for palliative treatment alone.

Studies that followed UCSF and the Barcelona group seemed to support their criteria, and such observations led to the description of the so-called "Metro Ticket Paradigm," formulated by Mazzaferro using a decision analysis model. The larger the tumor diameter and/or the higher the number of nodules, the higher the "price of the ticket" in terms of potentially higher HCC recurrence rates.

Pretransplant adjuvant therapy

Within the framework of persistent organ shortage and high wait-list drop-out rates due to HCC growth, pretransplant patient selection has become the determining factor in treating HCC in patients with ESLD, and pretransplant adjuvant therapies a routine component of this process. Controlling tumor growth during the wait-list time may have several advantages, including preventing drop-out, influencing HCC recurrence rates post-transplantation, and overall survival for this subgroup of patients.

Current strategies to control tumor growth focus mainly on surgical and radiologic interventions, as systemic chemotherapy has had little success thus far in treating HCC. Transarterial chemoembolization (TACE) and transarterial embolization (TAE) are frequently used in HCC patients who are not candidates for surgical resection, either because they are beyond Child's class A, they have bilobar tumors, or they have significant medical comorbidities. TACE in particular has been shown in some centers to allow for significantly longer disease-free survival post-OLT, but the effectiveness of TACE seems to depend in large part on tumor stage and the degree of tumor necrosis. Moreover, a French multicenter study by Decaens and colleagues demonstrated no overall effect from TACE on overall and disease-free survival. No controlled randomized trials comparing patients with HCC with or without TACE before liver transplantation are available to date. Further qualifying the use of TACE is the theory that incomplete TACE can invoke a neoangiogenic reaction and promote tumor growth through increased levels of vascular endothelial growth factor (VEGF) and β-fibroblast growth factor (β-FGF).

The other main modality for pretransplant adjuvant therapy is radiofrequency ablation (RFA), a relatively easy method of inducing coagulation necrosis in a tumor by heat generated by electrical current. It is a viable option for tumors up to 4 cm in size, and is sometimes used in combination with percutaneous ethanol injection (PEI) in larger tumors, under ultrasound or CT guidance. Recurrence rates after RFA differ depending on whether the success is assessed by radiologic methods or explant pathology, though tumor necrosis induced by RFA is uniformly higher than necrosis induced by TACE or TAE. Recurrence rates after transplantation in patients where RFA achieved complete or nearly complete tumor necrosis is very low, ranging from 0% to 6% in retrospective studies.

Although single treatment modalities are effective in slowing tumor progression in many patients with HCC, multimodality treatment may allow for increased rates of complete tumor necrosis, and thus better post-transplant recurrence-free survival. Several centers, most notably Yao and colleagues from UCSF, have shown in uncontrolled studies that multimodality approaches can offer a low drop-out rate during the waiting time, favorable survival figures, and a low recurrence rate after transplantation. Also, Freeman showed similar results in a retrospective review of the Scientific Registry of Transplant Recipient (SRTR) data on liver transplantation in the USA from 1997 to 2006. He observed a significant survival advantage at 3 years post-transplantation of patients with HCC exemptions and local ablative therapies during the waiting time.

Case

A 48-year-old man with chronic liver disease due to hepatitis C is referred for possible liver transplantation. Imaging studies reveal three solid lesions in the liver parenchyma and biopsy confirms hepatocellular carcinoma. One of the tumors is 3 cm in diameter and the other two are each 4 cm in diameter. Radiofrequency ablation is performed on each tumor, successfully shrinking each tumor to <2 cm in diameter. Now satisfying the Milan criteria, the patient is subsequently wait-listed for liver transplantation.

Selection of patients with HCC for liver transplantation

Overall, series reporting use of expanded criteria for OLT in patients with HCC, with or without preoperative locoregional therapy of some sort, have uniformly achieved a 50% 5-year survival rate when the tumor burden is categorized based on explant pathology. Furthermore, series comparing pretransplant imaging and pathologic data generally show higher overall survival using the latter, particularly for tumors beyond the Milan criteria. Possible explanations include understaging of HCC by preoperative imaging, a lag period between last imaging and OLT during which tumor size and extent may progress, or variability in radiologists' interpretations of tumor size and number among regenerative nodules in cirrhotic livers.

In the largest, prospectively collected, single-institution study of HCC in OLT to date, from the University of California at Los Angeles (UCLA), factors that predicted poor survival included increased tumor number, presence of lymphovascular invasion, and poor tumor differentiation. These findings echo the results of prior series, and underscore the key principle that tumor biology, more than size or number, determines outcome after OLT for HCC. This has led several researchers to surmise that tumors that respond favorably by radiologic images to pretransplant therapy, be it TACE or RFA, possess a more favorable biologic profile. More study needs to be done to elucidate this theory, especially with regard to the best means of assessing tumor biology pretransplant, be it by serologic or radiologic testing.

Based on these findings, Duffy and colleagues from UCLA propose that preoperative tumor staging is best accomplished with CT or MRI within 6 months of the time of OLT, as well as liver biopsies to assess histologic grade and the absence or presence of lymphovascular invasion. As there are real concerns about liver biopsies in patients with cirrhosis and the risks of sampling error, bleeding, or risk of tumor dissemination, others have recommended using tumor biopsies only in cases of large tumors that approach ≥3 cm, or tumors that do not respond well to locoregional therapy.

Long-term complications of liver transplantation

The major sources of long-term morbidity and mortality after OLT, not related to graft loss, include malignancy, infections, and metabolic complications leading to renal insufficiency and cardiovascular events. Although there remains an appreciation that renal insufficiency and many of the metabolic complications associated with transplantation are associated with immunosuppressive medications, there is a growing awareness that many of these complications are related and are a manifestation of a liver transplantation-associated metabolic syndrome. Post-transplant metabolic syndrome (PTMS) includes the constellation of obesity, hypertension, diabetes, and hyperlipidemia mediated by underlying insulin resistance. PTMS can affect over half of liver transplant recipients compared with 27% of the adult US population overall. It is associated with increased morbidity from cardiovascular events after liver transplantation and potentially graft loss.

The influence of PTMS on outcomes after liver transplantation is further complicated by a complex interplay between metabolic complications, renal insufficiency and recurrent HCV after transplantation. A preponderance of evidence suggests that infection with HCV is a significant risk factor for the development of type 2 diabetes in both liver transplant and non-transplant recipients infected with HCV. HCV has also been identified as an independent risk factor for renal insufficiency after liver transplantation. Conversely, type 2 diabetes and insulin resistance are associated with accelerated damage to the post-transplant liver from recurrent HCV.

As patients liver longer after liver transplantation and as so many transplantations are done in individuals with HCV or non-alcoholic fatty liver disease (NAFLD), PTMS will become an increasingly important target in efforts to improve liver transplantation outcomes.

Renal insufficiency

Renal insufficiency is a major source of morbidity and mortality after liver transplantation. In 2003, Ojo et al. published a seminal paper marrying the SRTR database with the Centers for Medicare and Medicaid Services (CMS) database to establish that liver transplant recipients had an 18.1% chance of chronic renal failure (GFR ≤29 mL/min per m^2) by 5 years after OLT. Traditionally, renal insufficiency after organ transplantation is felt to be largely mediated by nephrotoxicity from CNIs. However, the incidence of renal failure after liver transplantation exceeded rates for all other non-renal solid organ transplants with the exception of the intestine, despite the perception that the allogeneic liver is more tolerizing than other organs and requires less immunosuppression. This may result partially from the fact that HCV infection was a risk factor for post-transplant renal failure in the analysis and HCV is prevalent only in liver transplant recipients. Moreover, several reports clearly show that liver transplant recipients who require renal replacement therapy have markedly diminished survival. Finally, as pretransplant renal function is an important predictor of post-transplant renal function and as the MELD allocation system gives priority to patients with an elevated serum creatinine, there is concern that the burden of renal insufficiency after liver transplantation will only increase.

To date, there does not appear to be diminished outcomes in the MELD era, in part because survival for any given level of pretransplant renal insufficiency has improved. Although there has been a greater use of combined kidney–liver transplants in the MELD era, much of the improvement is likely due to newer immunosuppressive strategies. One intervention that has had a substantial effect on renal function and survival in patients with diminished renal function before liver transplantation is the use of antibody-based induction therapy with agents such as rabbit antithymoglobulin and IL-2R antagonists. These agents allow a delay in the initiation of CNIs and, as a result, may protect the kidneys in the delicate immediate post-transplant period before nephrotoxic CNIs are introduced. The use of induction therapy has grown significantly in liver transplant recipients when comparing the pre-MELD and MELD eras.

Another agent that has been used to preserve renal function after OLT is sirolimus. Sirolimus is one of a few agents potent enough to be used as a primary immunosuppressant that is not a CNI. Although sirolimus has a variety of adverse reaction and is not tolerated by up to a third of patients, it is not clearly nephrotoxic. In patients randomized to receive sirolimus, as opposed to a CNI, within 4–12 weeks of a liver transplantation, there was a 22.1% increase in GFR from baseline to year 1 compared with a 6.2% increase in patients receiving the CNI, and this difference was significant. There was a higher incidence of rejection in the sirolimus arm. There does not appear to be a clear benefit in randomized trials to sirolimus conversion in stable liver transplant recipients who are further out from liver transplantation.

In patients who develop renal insufficiency after liver transplantation aggressive efforts should be make to control factors associated with diminished renal function including hypertension and diabetes. In addition, nephrotoxic drugs should be avoided and an effort made to decrease CNI exposure. Multiple studies have also shown that OLT patients can experience benefit in renal function from succinct efforts to lower CNI levels often together with an antimetabolite such as MPA. As with sirolimus, these efforts have the most efficacy when initiated early.

Diabetes mellitus

Diabetes is frequent after liver transplantation and can occur in about a third of patients with insulin resistance in up to 45% of patients. Risk factors for post-transplant diabetes mellitus (PTDM) include corticosteroid and tacrolimus use, multiple courses of steroid-resistant rejection, infection with HCV, diabetes before transplantation, and obesity. The increase in NAFLD as an indication for transplantation has the potential to increase the incidence of PTDM. The association between HCV and PTDM is especially compelling. In many HCV patients with PTDM, the onset of diabetes coincides with recurrence of allograft hepatitis and effective antiviral therapy can improve glycemic control. It should be noted that chronic liver disease and cirrhosis are diabetogenic and liver transplantation has the potential to cure diabetes. In one report of 618 OLT patients, 37 of 66 patients who had diabetes pretransplantation did not have diabetes afterwards. However, patients with type 1 diabetes pretransplantation typically maintain their need for insulin.

PTDM is associated with diminished outcomes and appropriate control of hyperglycemia is desirable. Patients may benefit from adjustments in immunosuppressive medications when possible. The use of more rapid steroid tapers and steroid-sparing protocols in recent years is associated with a decline in the incidence of PTDM. In addition, tacrolimus at higher levels is associated with diabetes and lowering or eliminating the medication can be helpful in some patients. Azathioprine and MPA derivatives are not associated with hyperglycemia. Management of PTDM is similar to management of diabetes in non-transplant patients in most other ways. All patients should be counseled on diet and lifestyle modifications with an emphasis on weight loss. Oral hypoglycemic drugs are typically well tolerated although patients receiving metformin and thiazolidinediones should be monitored for lactic acidosis and hepatotoxicity, respectively.

Hypertension

Hypertension is frequent after liver transplantation and can occur in between 40% and 70% of patients, with the incidence increasing over time. Patients with ESLD typically have low systemic vascular resistance and blood pressure as a manifestation of their cirrhosis but this reverses almost immediately after transplantation with the functioning of a non-cirrhotic allograft and the use of CNIs and corticosteroids. CNIs elicit a potent vasoconstriction of renal afferent arterioles with subsequent sodium reabsorption through activation of the renin–angiotensin system. As with diabetes and metabolic syndrome in general, the use of steroid minimization or elimination protocols has the potential to decrease the incidence of hypertension. Aggressive control of hypertension has the potential to diminish the impact of both renal insufficiency and cardiovascular complications after OLT.

The Ad Hoc Group on "Prevention of Post-Transplant Cardiovascular Disease" recommends maintaining the systolic blood pressure <140 mmHg and the diastolic <80 mmHg. Efforts can start with minimization of both corticosteroids and CNIs. As with non-transplant patients, OLT patients should pursue lifestyle modifications including weight loss, salt restriction, and avoidance of nicotine and caffeine. The ideal pharmacologic management of hypertension post-transplantation has not been defined but, in practice, calcium channel blockers (CCBs) have proven to be effective and well tolerated. They are potent vasodilators and have the ability to reverse the vasoconstriction induced by CNIs. Diltiazem, verapamil, and nicardipine all have the potential to raise CNI levels and amlodipine, nifidepine, and felodipine have emerged as popular choices because they do not. β Blockers are less effective than CCBs, but can be used, especially as adjunct agents. With the exception of carvedilol, they do not affect CNI levels; labetolol is an effective agent. Diuretics can be used especially in patients with fluid retention but have the potential to exacerbate hyperuricemia and azotemia. ACE inhibitors and ARBs have the potential to be very effective agents and to reduce the progression of diabetic nephropathy. In practice, they can exacerbate hyperkalemia, especially soon after transplantation, and they are often abandoned if the serum creatinine starts to rise.

Hyperlipidemia

Hyperlipidemia, defined as hypercholesterolemia and/or hypertriglyceridemia, is common after OLT and affects approximately 40% of transplant recipients. Potential risk factors include female sex, cholestatic liver disease, a pre-OLT cholesterol level >141 mg/dL, diabetes, and obesity. Immunosuppressant medications associated with hyperlipidemia include cyclosporine, corticosteroids, and sirolimus. Sirolimus is associated with unusually high levels of both cholesterol and triglycerides, and its use can be limited in some individuals on this basis. Treatment begins with minimization of exacerbating medications, and lifestyle and dietary modifications including weight loss, exercise, and a diet less rich in refined sugars and low saturated fats. Patients may benefit from conversion of cyclosporine to tacrolimus. Oral contraceptives, β blockers and thiazide diuretics also have the potential to exacerbate hyperlipidemia. The HMG-CoA reductase or "statin" drugs are effective and typically well tolerated in OLT patients and do not interfere with CNI levels. Patients should be monitored for myositis and elevated transaminases but these complications are unusual. Fibric acids can be used but the incidence of myotoxicity rises significantly when a fibric acid is used with a statin. Bile acid sequestrants, orlistat, and ezitimibe can affect CNI levels. When necessary, all other medications should be given 1 hour before or 2 hours after these agents and CNI levels, especially cyclosporine, should be monitored.

Obesity

Few problems in the long-term management of liver transplant recipients are as challenging as obesity because there are few successful options. There has been a dramatic increase in obesity in patients undergoing liver transplantation. Before 1996, 17% of transplant recipients had a BMI >30 but, between 2001 and 2004, 32% of patients did so. In addition, 22% of non-obese patients will become obese within 2 years post-transplantation. Risk factors for obesity after OLT include greater recipient BMI, greater donor BMI, being married, and higher cumulative doses of prednisone.

It should be noted that it has been difficult to demonstrate that an elevated BMI is associated with worse survival after outcome. Numerous single center studies and an analysis of the 704 patients in the National Institutes of Diabetes and Digestive and Kidney Diseases (NIDDK) did not show an association between BMI and patient and graft survival. An analysis of the UNOS database showed diminished survival only in the "very severely obese" population with a BMI >40. Even here, most of the difference in survival occurred early and much of the difference was due to infectious complications. This may be a result, in part, to the fact that obese patients are screened for cardiac disease pretransplantation and no doubt exposed to the selection bias. The impact of obesity on survival did increase if patients had coexisting diabetes or coronary artery disease.

Few interventions have had success in treating obesity. Dietary interventions are no more successful in OLT patients than in the population at large, which is minimal. Few medical options are available. Orlistat has been shown to be safe in transplant recipients on tacrolimus although tacrolimus levels frequently had to be adjusted. The medication did not result in weight loss. Bariatic surgery with gastric banding either at the time of transplantation or subsequently has been described at the case report level.

Bone disease

Metabolic bone disease is common after liver transplantation. Cirrhosis itself is a risk factor for bone loss. Up to 25% of patients with cirrhosis will have bone density at the less than thee fractures threshold and the number is higher in patients with cholestatic liver disease. Other risk factors include a history of smoking or heavy alcohol use, low BMI, postmenopausal state, physical inactivity, and advanced age. Bone loss accelerates in the period right after transplantation as a result of immobilization and corticosteroid use and nadirs between 3 and 6 months post-transplantation. The risk of fracture is greatest during this period. Bone density increases after this period although no further improvement occurs after the end of the second year. Although a third of OLT patients have traditionally been left with bone density below the fracture threshold, this number has been clearly declining in recent years, in part because of steroid minimization and medical intervention.

There are few uniform recommendations for management of bone loss in transplant recipients. A dual energy X-ray absorptiometry (DXA) scan is the preferred modality to monitor bone loss and a baseline study at the time of transplant evaluation is useful followed by yearly studies initially. Patients should be mobilized and should avoid alcohol and nicotine. Corticosteroid use should be minimized and patients with renal insufficiency should be evaluated for renal osteodystrophy. All patients should receive 1500 mg calcium and 800 IU vitamin D daily, which is typically adequate to provide normal levels. Estrogen therapy can be considered in postmenopausal women and testosterone replacement in men with low testosterone. Prospective randomized studies with bisphosphonates, oral alendronate, and intravenous pamidronate have shown significant improvements in bone density after OLT. Their effect on the incidence of fractures is still unclear.

Malignancy

In all series of late term mortality after liver transplantation, new malignancies are a major source of mortality. The immunosuppression associated with solid organ transplantation places patients at an increased risk of both lymphoproliferative and solid tumor malignancies. In addition, many OLT patients have engaged or continue to engage in the high-risk behaviors of nicotine and excess alcohol use. Finally viral infections including the Epstein–Barr virus (EBV), human papillomavirus (HPV) and herpesvirus are associated with malignancy post-transplantation. The incidence of new malignancy increases with the age of the patient and the time from transplantation with an incidence of up to 50% in patients many years from transplantation. Surveillance for malignancy is an integral aspect of the long-term care of these patients.

PTLD is a specific entity observed in all solid organ transplant recipients. It is most common in the first year after transplant but can occur at any time. It is classically a B-cell lymphoproliferative disorder associated with infection with the EBV which has the potential to immortalize B-cell clones. It occurs in 1–2% of adult liver transplant recipients but is more common in pediatric liver transplant recipients who may naive to EBV post-transplantation and who frequently require intense immunosuppression. There are more unusual forms of PTLD that are not B-cell derived, including a T-cell malignancy. PTLD can present in the liver, lymph nodes, and other solid organs such as the gut and bone. It is always a consideration in patients with unexplained fevers, night sweats, or weight loss. It can respond to significant reductions in immunosuppression and antiviral agents such as ganciclovir. Patients should be considered for surgical resection when applicable. In recent years, an anti-CD20 monoclonal antibody or rituximab has been used commonly in patients with B-cell PTLD and has shown considerable activity.

Liver transplant recipients are at increased risk for solid cancers with an incidence of 2.5 times that seen in age- and sex-matched non-transplant individuals. Malignancies are more common after the first year and the risk increases over time. The most common malignancy in OLT patients is cutaneous cancer of the skin and lip, with an incidence 31 times that seen in non-transplant patients. Squamous cell carcinoma predominates although basal cell carcinoma and melanoma can be seen. Risk factors for cutaneous cancer are similar to those for the population at large including age, sun exposure, and a history of skin cancer or actinic keratosis. Additional risk factors include the duration of immunosuppression and a history of HPV infection. Other solid malignancies with an increased risk in liver transplant recipients include kidney cancer (relative risk [RR] 3.1), pancreatic cancer (RR 3.9), oral cancer (RR 2.5), colon cancer (RR 2.6), and lung cancer (RR 1.4). The incidence of colon cancer may be related to an increased incidence of rectal cancer and to the transplantation of patients with colitis. There is no clear increased risk of breast, cervical, and genitourinary cancer.

Recommendations for OLT patients should generally follow the recommendations of the American Cancer Society. Patients with a history of colitis should undergo yearly colonoscopic examination with biopsies. All patients should avoid nicotine use, limit exposure to sun and ultraviolet light, and undergo yearly dermatologic screening. It should also be noted that patients with a history of colon, breast, bladder, or symptomatic renal cell cancer even 5 years pretransplantation have a >20% chance of recurrence after liver transplantation.

Immunizations

The hepatitis A and B vaccines and the pneumococcal vaccine should be given preferentially pretransplantation but may be administered safely post-transplantation. Patients should receive the yearly influenza immunization typically in the fall. Inactivated vaccines are considered safe whereas live attenuated vaccines are generally avoided. The inactivated and injected influenza vaccine is administered instead of the inhaled, live, attenuated form. Other live attenuated vaccines that are avoided include Bacille Calmette–Guérin (BCG), measles, mumps, oral polio, rubella, vaccinia, and varicella.

Further reading

Abbasoglu O, Levy MF, Brkic F, et al. Ten years after liver transplantation: an evolving understanding of late graft loss. *Transplantation* 1997;**64**:1801–7.

Abbasoglu O, Levy MF, Vodapayy MS, et al. Hepatic artery stenosis after liver transplantation: incidence, presentation, treatment, and long- term outcome. *Transplantation* 1997;**63**:250–5.

Abt P, Crawford M, Desai N, Markmann J, Olthoff K, Shaked A. Liver transplantation from controlled non-heart-beating donors: an increased incidence of biliary complications. *Transplantation* 2003;**75**:1659–63.

Balan V, Batts KP, Porayko MK, Drom RA, Ludwig J, Wiesner RH. Histological evidence for recurrence of primary biliary cirrhosis after liver transplantation. *Hepatology* 1993;**18**:1292–398.

Bambha K, Kim WR, Kremers WK, et al. Predicting survival among patients listed for liver transplantation: an assessment of serial MELD measurements. *Am J Transplant* 2004;**4**:1798–804.

Berenguer M. Management of hepatitis C virus in the transplant patient. *Clin Liver Dis* 2007;**11**:355–76.

Berenguer M. Systematic review of the treatment of established recurrent hepatitis C with pegylated interferon in combination with ribavirin. *J Hepatol* 2008;**49**:274–87.

Bostom AD, Brown RS, Chavers BM, et al. Prevention of Post-transplant cardiovascular disease – report and recommendations of an Ad Hoc Group. *Am J Transplant* 2002;**2**;491–500.

Burton JR, Rosen HR. Acute rejection in HCV-infected liver transplant recipients: the great conundrum. *Liver Transplant* 2006;**12**(suppl):S38–47.

Busuttil RW, Klintmalm GB, eds. *Transplantation of the Liver*. Philadelphia, PA: Elsevier, 2005.

Busuttil RW, Farmer DG, Yersiz H, et al. Analysis of long-term outcomes of 3200 liver transplantations over two decades: a single center experience. *Ann Surg* 2005;**241**: 905–16.

Campsen J, Zimmerman MA, Trotter JFD, et al. Clinically recurrent primary sclerosing cholangitis following liver transplantation: a time course. *Liver Transplant* 2008;**14**: 181–5.

Charatcharoenwitthaya P, Pimentel S, Talwalker JA, et al. Long-term survival and impact of ursodeoxycholic acid treatment for recurrent primary biliary cirrhosis after liver transplantation. *Liver Transplant* 2007;**13**:1236–45.

Charlton M, Seaberg E, Wiesner R, et al. Predictors of patient and graft survival following liver transplantation for hepatitis C. *Hepatology* 1998;**28**:823–30.

Darcy MD. Management of venous outflow complications after liver transplantation. *Tech Vasc Interv Radiol* 2007; **10**:240–5.

Demetrius AJ, Batts KP, Dhillon AP et al. for an international panel. Banff Schema for Grading Acute Liver Allograft Rejection: an international consensus document. *Hepatology* 1997;**25**:658–63.

Demetris A, Adams D, Bellamy C, et al. Update of the international Banff schema for liver allograft rejection: working recommendations for the histopathologic staging and reporting of chronic rejection. An international panel. *Hepatology* 2000;**31**:1300–6.

Demetris AJ, Sebagh M. Plasma cell hepatitis in liver allografts: variant of rejection or autoimmune hepatitis? *Liver Transplant* 2008;**14**:750–5.

Duffy JP, Hong JC, Farmer DG, et al. Vascular complications of orthotopic liver transplantation: experience in more than 4200 patients. *J Am Coll Surg* 2009;**208**:896–905.

Duffy JP, Vardanian A, Benjamin E, et al. Liver transplantation criteria for hepatocellular carcinoma should be expanded. *Ann Surg* 2007;**246**:502–11.

Everson GT. Treatment of advanced hepatitis C with a low accelerating dosage regimen of antiviral therapy. *Hepatology* 2005;**42**:255–62.

Flechner SM, Kobashigawa J, Klintmalm G. Calcineurin inhibitor-sparing regimens in solid organ transplantation: focus on improving renal function and nephrotoxicity. *Clin Transplant* 2008;**22**:1–15.

Foley DP, Fernandez LA, Leverson G, et al. Donation after cardiac death: the University of Wisconsin experience with liver transplantation. *Ann Surg* 2005;**242**:724–31.

Garcia-Tsao G, Sanyal AJ, Grace ND, Carey W. Prevention and Management of gastroesophageal varices and variceal hemorrhage in cirrhosis. AASLD Practice Guidelines. *Hepatology* 2007;**46**:922–38.

Gautam M, Cheruvattath R, Balan V. Recurrent autoimmune liver disease after liver transplantation: a systematic review. *Liver Transplant* 2006;**12**:1813–24.

Ghany MG, Strader DB, Thomas DL, Seeff LB. Diagnosis, management, and treatment of hepatitis C: An update. *Hepatology* 2009;**49**:1335–74.

Ghobrial RM, Gornbein J, Steadman R, et al. Pretransplant model to predict post transplant survival in liver transplant patients. *Ann Surg* 2002;**236**:315–23.

Gonzalez-Koch A, Czaja AJ, Carpenter HA, et al. Recurrent autoimmune hepatitis after orthotopic liver transplantation. *Liver Transplant* 2001;**7**:302–10.

Graziadei JW. Recurrence of primary sclerosing cholangitis after liver transplantation. *Liver Transplant* 2002;**8**: 575–81.

Haddad E, McAlister V, Renouf E, Malthaner R, Kjaer MS, Gluud LL. Cyclosporine versus tacrolimus for liver transplanted patients (review). *Cochrane Database Syst Rev* 2009;(4): CD005161.

Holt AP, Thorburn D, Mirza D, Gunson B, Wong T, Haydon G. A prospective study of standardized nonsurgical therapy in the management of biliary anastomotic strictures complicating liver transplantation. *Transplantation* 2007;**84**:857–63.

Hubscher SG. Transplantation pathology. *Semin Liver Dis* 2009;**29**:74–90.

Jiang Y, Villeneuve PJ, Fenton SS, et al. Liver transplantation and subsequent risk of cancer: findings from a Canadian cohort study. *Liver Transplant* 2008;**14**: 1588–97.

Kamath PS, Weisner RH, Malinchoc M, et al. A model to predict survival in patients with end-stage liver disease. *Hepatology* 2001;**33**:464–70.

Klintmalm GBG, Washburn WK, Rudich SM, et al. Corticosteroid-free immunosuppression with daclizumab in HCV+ liver transplant recipients: 1-year interim results of the HCV-3 study group. *Liver Transplant* 2007;**13**: 1521–31.

Lesurtel M, Mullhaupt B, Pestalozzi BC, et al. Transarterial chemoembolization as a bridge to liver transplantation for hepatocellular carcinoma: an evidence based analysis. *Am J Transplant* 2006;**6**:2644–50.

Llovet JM, Schwartz M, Mazzaferro V. Resection and liver transplantation for hepatocellular carcinoma. *Semin Liver Dis* 2005;**25**:181–200.

Lok AS, McMahon BJ. Chronic hepatitis B: Update 2009. *Hepatology* 2009;**50**(3):1–36.

McCashland TM. Management of liver transplant recipients with recurrent hepatitis C. *Curr Opin Organ Transplant* 2009;**14**:221–4.

McGuire BM, Rosenthal P, Brown CC, et al. Long-term management of the liver transplant patient: recommendations for the primary care doctor. *Am J Transplant* 2009;**9**:1–16.

Markmann JF, Markmann JW, Desai NM, et al. Operative parameters that predict the outcomes of hepatic transplantation. *J Am Coll Surg* 2003;**196**:556–72.

Mateo R, Cho Y, Singh G, et al. Risk factors for graft survival after liver transplantation from donation after cardiac death donors: an analysis of OPTN/UNOS data. *Am J Transplant* 2006;**6**:791–6.

Mazzaferro V, Regalia E, Doci R, et al. Liver Transplantation for the treatment of small hepatocellular carcinomas in patients with cirrhosis. *N Engl J Med* 1996;**334**:693–9.

Meier-Kriesche H-U, Lib S, Gruessner RWG, et al. Immunosuppression: Evolution in practice and trends 1994–2004. *Am J Transplant* 2006;**6**:1111–31.

Merion RM, Pelletier SJ, Goodrich N, Englesbe MJ, Delmonico FL. Donation after cardiac death as a strategy to increase deceased donor liver availability. *Ann Surg* 2006;**244**:555–62.

Merion RM, Schaubel DE, Dykstra DM, et al. The survival benefit of liver transplantation. *Am J Transplant* 2005;**5**: 307–13.

Moonka D, Teperman L, Sher L, et al. Spare-the-nephron (STN) trial in liver transplant recipients: interim efficacy and safety of mycophenolate mofetil (MMF)/sirolimus (SRL) maintenance therapy after CNI withdrawal. *Transplantation* 2008;**86**(suppl 2):97.

Ojo AO, Held PJ, Port FK, et al. Chronic renal failure after transplantation of a nonrenal organ. *N Engl J Med* 2003; **349**:931–40.

Patterson SJ, Angus PW. Post-liver transplant hepatitis B prophylaxis: the role of oral nucleos(t)ide analogues. *Curr Opin Organ Transplant* 2009;**14**:225–30.

Pfau PR, Kochman ML, Lewis JD, et al. Endoscopic management of postoperative biliary complications in orthotopic liver transplantation. *Gastrointest Endosc* 2000;**52**: 55–63.

Reuben A. Long-term management of the liver transplant patient: diabetes, hyperlipidemia, and obesity. *Liver Transplant* 2001;**7**:S13–21.

Rosen HR, Martin P. A model to predict survival following liver retransplantation. *Hepatology* 1999;**29**:365–70.

Saab S, Wang V, Ibrahim AB, et al. MELD score predicts 1-year patient survival post-transplantation. *Liver Transplant* 2003;**9**:473–6.

Samuel D. The option of liver transplantation for hepatitis B: where are we? *Dig Liver Dis* 2009;**41**(suppl 2):S185–9.

Snover DC, Freese DK, Sharp HL, et al. liver allograft rejection: an analysis of the use of biopsy in determining outcome of rejection. *Am J Surg Pathol* 1987;**111**:1–10.

Steinman T, Becker B, Frost A, et al. Guidelines for the referral and management of patients eligible for solid organ transplantation. *Transplantation* 2001;**71**:1189.

Strasberg SM, Howard TK, Molmenti EP, Hertl M. Selecting donor livers: Risk factors for poor function after orthotopic liver transplantation. *Hepatology* 1994;**20**:829–38.

Sylvestre PB, Batts KP, Burgart LJ, et al. Recurrence of primary biliary cirrhosis after liver transplantation: histologic estimate of incidence and natural history. *Liver Transplant* 2003;**9**:1086–93.

Veldt BJ. Impact of pegylated interferon and ribavirin treatment on graft survival in liver transplant. *Am J Transplant* 2008;**8**:2426–33.

Vera A, Molendina S, Gunson B, et al. Risk factors for recurrence of primary sclerosing cholangitis of liver allograft. *Lancet* 2002;**360**:1943–4.

Verdonk RC, Buois CI, Porte RJ, Haagsma EB. Biliary complications after liver transplantation: a review. *Scand J Gastroenterol* 2006;**41**:89–101.

Wang CS. Interferon based combination antiviral treatment for hepatitis C after liver transplantation: a review and quantitative analysis. *Am J Transplant* 2006; Jul **6**(7): 1586–99.

Wiesner R, Edwards E, Freeman R, et al. UNOS liver disease severity score committee. Model for end-stage liver disease

(MELD) and allocation of donor livers. *Gastroenterology* 2003;**124**:91–6.

Wiesner R, Lake JR, Freeman RB, Gish RG. Model for end-stage liver disease (MELD) exception guidelines. *Liver Transplant* 2006;**12**:S85–7.

Wiesner RH, Demetris AJ, Belle SH, et al. Acute hepatic allograft rejection: incidence, risk factors and impact on outcome. *Hepatology* 1998;**28**:638–45 .

Wiesner RH, Shorr JS, Steffen BJ, et al. Mycophenolate mofetil combination therapy improves long-term outcomes after liver transplantation in patients with and without hepatitis C. *Liver Transplant* 2005;**11**:750–9.

Yao FY, Kinkhabwala M, LaBerge JM, et al. The impact of pre-operative locoregional therapy on outcome after liver transplantation for hepatocellular carcinoma. *Am J Transplant* 2005;**5**(4 Pt 1):795–804.

Zu-hua Gao. Seeking beyond rejection: An update on the differential diagnosis and a practical approach to liver allograft biopsy interpretation. *Adv Anat Pathol* 2009; **16**:97–117.

Multiple choice questions

Chapter 1

1. Which of the choices shown below correctly completes the following statement? The frequency of T cells in a normal individual capable of directly recognizing allogeneic MHC molecules is:
   A. Almost undetectable before transplantation
   B. About the same as that of T cells directed to a given nominal antigen (e.g., measles virus)
   C. Many times higher than that of T cells directed to a given nominal antigen
   D. Zero because T cells recognize antigen only in association with self-MHC molecules
   E. Unrelated to acute rejection of organ allografts

Many times higher than that of T cells directed to a given nominal antigen

2. Which of the choices shown below correctly completes the following statement? Minor histocompatibility antigens are:
   A. The major rejection problem in MHC-mismatched renal transplantation
   B. Of no consequence in allograft rejection
   C. Critical targets during hyperacute rejection of organ allografts
   D. Recognized as polymorphic donor peptides associated with self-MHC antigens
   E. Encoded by genes located within the MHC

The correct answer is: "Recognized as polymorphic donor peptides associated with self-MHC antigens."

3. Which of the choices shown below correctly completes the following statement? Allografts are grafts transplanted:
   A. Between genetically different individuals of the same species
   B. Between genetically identical individuals of the same species
   C. In the same individual, i.e., the donor is the recipient
   D. Between individuals of different species

4. Which is the following statements is NOT correct?
   A. Second set rejection of allografts exhibits memory and specificity
   B. Allograft rejection can be mediated by lymphocytes
   C. Second set rejection of allografts occurs in recipients who receive a second transplant from the same donor
   D. Allograft rejection does not occur if donor and recipient are matched for MHC alleles

Allograft rejection can occur even when donor and recipient are matched for MHC alleles due to the response to minor histocompatibility antigens.

5. Antibodies of which of the following specificities can trigger antibody-mediated rejection?
   A. Antibodies to HLA antigens
   B. Antibodies to non-MHC molecules
   C. Antibodies to ABO blood group antibodies
   D. All of the above

Antibody-mediated rejection can be caused by antibodies directed to HLA antigens, non-MHC molecules, and ABO blood group antigens.

6. Which of the following statement about antibody-mediated rejection is NOT correct?
   A. Antibody-mediated acute rejection occurs only at early time points after organ transplantation
   B. Risk factors for antibody-mediated rejection include multiple transplantation, previous pregnancies, and a history of blood transfusions
   C. hyperacute rejection is mediated by high levels of pre-existing anti-donor antibodies
   D. The cross-match assay is performed to prevent hyperacute rejection

Antibody-mediated acute rejection can occur at any time after transplantation.

Primer on Transplantation, 3rd edition.
Edited by Donald Hricik.

7. Which of the following statements regarding C4d deposition is NOT correct?
   A. C4d is a fragment of C4 produced during the classic complement activation pathway
   B. C4d deposition is known to cause severe graft injury in renal transplantation
   C. C4d deposition in the peritubular capillaries correlates with the presence of circulating anti-donor antibodies
   D. C4d is highly stable and persists at the cell surface for a long time periods

C4d deposition in the PTC is a marker of antibody-mediated rejection, but there is no evidence that it is causally related to graft injury.

8. T-cell maturation (positive and negative selection) occurs in what organ?
   A. Bone marrow
   B. Thymus
   C. Thyroid
   D. Pancreas

9. Is the following statement true or false? Foreign peptides not expressed in association with MHC molecules do not induce a T-cell response.
   A. True
   B. False

10. Typically, which of the following stimuli do T cells require to become fully activated by an antigen presenting cell?
   I. TCR stimulation by a specific peptide/MHC complex
   II. Activation of co-stimulatory molecules
   III. IL-2-induced proliferation
   A. I, II
   B. I, III
   C. II, III
   D. I, II, III

11. Fill in the blank. The direct allogeneic antigen presentation involves the recognition of peptides through intact MHC molecules displayed on ______ APCs while indirect allogeneic antigen presentation involves the recognition of ______ through self-MHC displayed on ______ APCs.
   A. Donor; host MHC; host
   B. Host; host MHC; donor
   C. Donor; donor MHC; host
   D. Host; donor MHC; donor

12. Immunosuppressive drugs that inhibit T cell responses to transplanted organs utilize various mechanisms. These may include which of the following?
   A. Inhibiting cytokine production
   B. Inhibiting cellular division
   C. Inducing cellular death
   D. Blocking cellular processes
   E. All of the above

13. Immunological tolerance is defined as what?
   A. Accelerated response to an antigen that is induced by a previous exposure to the antigen
   B. Unresponsiveness to an antigen that is induced by a previous exposure to an unrelated antigen
   C. Unresponsiveness to an antigen that is induced by a previous exposure to the same antigen
   D. Spontaneous unresponsiveness to an antigen

14. Which of the following statements about xenotransplantation is NOT true?
   A. Xenotransplantation is a potential solution to the current shortage of donor organs for clinical transplantation
   B. Antibodies to the α-Gal carbohydrate moiety dominate the humoral response to xenografts
   C. Innate immune responses may contribute to immune destruction of xenografts
   D. Anti-α-Gal antibody is the only kind of antibody that can trigger humoral rejection after xenotransplantation

In addition to anti-α-Gal antibody, other kind of antibodies also can trigger humoral rejection of xenografts.

Chapter 2

1. Which of the following statements about type I drug toxicity is correct?
   A. It can result from exposure to small quantities of the drug
   B. It results from idiosyncrasies in drug metabolism
   C. It is predictable and dose-related
   D. It is sometimes caused by immune reactions to the drug

2. According to US FDA pregnancy categories, which of the following best describes a drug in category D?
   A. There is evidence for fetal risk based on human studies
   B. There is evidence for fetal risk in animals but not in humans
   C. Controlled studies have failed to demonstrate fetal risk in humans

3. Which of the following agents is associated with decreased blood levels of calcineurin inhibitors?
   A. Clarithromycin
   B. Diltiazem
   C. Ketoconazole
   D. St John's wort

4. Which of the following monoclonal antibodies binds to the CD3 complex adjacent to the T-cell receptor?
   A. Rabbit anti-thymocyte globulin
   B. OKT3
   C. Daclizumab
   D. Alemtuzumab

5. Compared with cyclosporine, tacrolimus is less often associated with which of the following?
   A. New onset of diabetes mellitus
   B. Gingival hyperplasia
   C. Impaired wound healing
   D. Nephrotoxicity

6. All of the following drugs are metabolized by hepatic cytochrome CYP3A4, EXCEPT:
   A. Sirolimus
   B. Cyclosporine
   C. Tacrolimus
   D. Mycophenolate mofetil

7. The terminal half-life of basiliximab is approximately:
   A. 6 hours
   B. 24 hours
   C. 7 days
   D. 14 days

8. Decreased expression of NF-κB is a major mechanism of action of which class of immunosuppressant drugs?
   A. Corticosteroids
   B. Calcineurin inhibitors
   C. Antimetabolites
   D. Target of rapamycin inhibitors

9. Which of the following drugs impairs metabolism of azathioprine?
   A. Tacrolimus
   B. St John's wort
   C. Allopurinol
   D. Clarithromycin

10. Which of the following drugs is LEAST likely associated with anemia?
   A. Azathioprine
   B. Tacrolimus
   C. Mycophenolate mofetil
   D. Sirolimus

11. Which of the following drugs is most commonly associated with impaired wound healing?
   A. Azathioprine
   B. Cyclosporine
   C. Tacrolimus
   D. Sirolimus

Chapter 3

1. Which of the following conditions would NOT fulfill the criteria for brain death?
   A. Absence of brain-stem reflexes
   B. No response to painful stimuli in all four extremities
   C. Absence of electroencephalographic activity in a sedated patient
   D. Absence of blood flow on brain scan

2. Which of the following electrolyte abnormalities results from the effects of brain death on the posterior pituitary gland?
A. Hyponatremia
B. Hypernatremia
C. Hyperkalemia
D. Hypokalemia
E. Hypocalcemia

3. Hormonal replacement therapy for brain dead donors includes administration of all of the following, EXCEPT:
A. Growth hormone
B. Vasopressin
C. Thyroxine
D. Corticosteroids

4. Which of the following characterizes the decreased left ventricular ejection fraction observed early after brain death?
A. It usually occurs because of myocardial infarction
B. It represents an absolute contraindication to procurement of the heart
C. It is often reversible
D. It may contribute to hemodynamic instability

5. Which of the following cytokines has been associated with pulmonary inflammation associated with brain death?
A. IL-2
B. IL-6
C. IL-5
D. IL-8

6. All of the following characterize pulmonary inflammation associated with brain death, EXCEPT:
A. It is correlated with poor outcomes in the recipient of the procured lung
B. It can be associated with endothelial injury and accumulation of alveolar fluid
C. It is not present in ideal lung donors

7. Which of the following conditions is an absolute contraindication to organ donation?
A. Bacteremia
B. Squamous cell cancer of the skin
C. HIV infection
D. Hospital-acquired pneumonia

8. After declaration of brain death, a potential donor becomes hypernatremic (serum sodium 160 mmol/L) and central venous pressure is 2 cmH_2O. Initial fluid replacement should consist of:
A. Isotonic saline
B. Hyptonic saline
C. Ringer's lactate
D. Albumin

9. Which of the following characterizes the use of vasopressors in management of a potential organ donor?
A. Their use precludes procurement of the kidneys
B. Only agents devoid of inotropic activity should be used
C. Norepinephrine is the agent of choice
D. The choice of agents must be individualized based on physiologic parameters

10. Which of the following elements of an apnea test would determine that a potential donor is NOT brain dead after removal from the respirator for 10 min?
A. $PaO_2 > 13.3$ kPa (100 mmHg)
B. Absence of chest movements
C. $PaCO_2 < 5.3$ kPa (40 mmHg)
D. $PaO_2 < 6.7$ kPa (50 mmHg)

11. Consent for organ donation is best obtained by:
A. A transplant surgeon
B. An intern
C. A professional trained in dealing with organ donation issues

12. In potential lung donors, the PaO_2:FiO_2 ratio ideally should be:
A. >300
B. <300

13. How many potential solid organ transplant recipients can receive organs from a single deceased donor?
A. 2
B. 4
C. 6
D. 8
E. 12

Chapter 4

1. Which of the following infections is LEAST likely in the first 4 weeks after an otherwise successful liver transplantation?
   A. Pulmonary aspergillosis
   B. *E. coli* urinary tract infection
   C. Staphylococcal bacteremia
   D. West Nile virus meningitis

2. Which of the following antimicrobial agents is most likely to increase calcineurin inhibitor blood levels?
   A. Azithromycin
   B. Cefazolin
   C. Rifampin
   D. Clarithromycin

3. Which of the following fungi is most commonly found in catheter-related infection?
   A. Cryptococci
   B. *Candida* spp.
   C. *Aspergillus* spp.
   D. *Coccidioides* spp.

4. In the early period after solid organ transplantation, pneumonia is most often:
   A. Community acquired
   B. Nosocomial
   C. Opportunistic

5. Nocardiosis is most common in patients transplanted with which of the following organs?
   A. Kidney
   B. Pancreas
   C. Lung
   D. Liver

6. Which of the following pathogens is most commonly associated with acute meningitis in kidney transplant recipients?
   A. *Listeria monocytogenes*
   B. *Strongyloides stercoralis*
   C. JC polyoma virus
   D. BK polyoma virus

7. All of the following are features of cytomegalovirus syndrome, EXCEPT:
   A. Fatigue
   B. Fever
   C. Leukocytosis
   D. Thrombocytopenia
   E. Myalgias

8. Epstein–Barr virus-induced lymphoma is most often characterized by uncontrolled proliferation of which of the following cell lines?
   A. T cells
   B. B cells
   C. Natural killer cells
   D. Macrophages

9. Which of the following viruses is the causative agent in Kaposi's sarcoma?
   A. Herpes zoster virus
   B. HHV-8
   C. Herpes simplex virus
   D. HHV-6
   E. Epstein–Barr virus

10. Which of the following viruses is the causative agent in progressive multifocal leukoencephalopathy?
   A. Epstein–Barr virus
   B. Cytomegalovirus
   C. JC polyoma virus
   D. BK polyoma virus
   E. Herpes simplex virus

11. Which transplanted organ is mostly frequently affected by BK polyoma virus?
   A. Kidney
   B. Heart
   C. Lung
   D. Liver

12. Which of the following viruses has been identified as a causative agent in some post-transplant squamous cell skin carcinomas?
   A. BK polyoma virus
   B. HHV-8
   C. Human papillomavirus
   D. Human immunodeficiency virus
   E. Cytomegalovirus

13. Coccidioidomycosis is an endemic cause of post-transplant central nervous system infections in which part of the USA?
   A. Midwest
   B. South-west
   C. North-west
   D. North-east

14. For sulfa-allergic patients, which of the following antimicrobial agents can be used for prophylaxis against *Pneumocystis jiroveci*?
   A. Linezolid
   B. Dapsone
   C. Ciprofloxacin
   D. Ganciclovir

15. The risk of infection in solid organ transplant recipients is related most closely to which of the following variables?
   A. The net state of immunosuppression
   B. The white blood cell count
   C. CD4 lymphocyte counts
   D. Epidemiologic exposures
   E. B and C
   F. A and D

Chapter 5

1. Which viral infection has been associated with aplastic anemia in transplant recipients?
   A. Cytomegalovirus
   B. Parvovirus
   C. Hepatitis C
   D. Epstein–Barr virus

2. Which of the following immunosuppressants is associated with hirsutism?
   A. Cyclosporine
   B. Tacrolimus
   C. Sirolimus
   D. Mycophenolate mofetil

3. Which of the following drugs can be effective in treating post-transplant erythrocytosis?
   A. Metoprolol
   B. Doxazosin
   C. Verapamil
   D. Minoxidil
   E. Lisinopril

4. Which of the following infections is most commonly associated with leukopenia?
   A. Aspergillosis
   B. Cytomegalovirus infection
   C. BK polyoma nephropathy
   D. Candida pyelonephritis

5. Which of the following immunosuppressants is most commonly associated with gout?
   A. Tacrolimus
   B. Sirolimus
   C. Cyclosporine
   D. Azathioprine

6. Which of the following characterizes the use of HMG-CoA reductase inhibitors in heart transplant recipients?
   A. Their use is associated with a reduced incidence of cardiac allograft vasculopathy
   B. They effectively lower LDL-cholesterol levels
   C. They can cause rhabdomyolysis
   D. All of the above

7. Risk factors for new onset of diabetes mellitus after transplantation include all of the following, EXCEPT:
   A. Hepatitis C infection
   B. African–American ethnicity
   C. Cytomegalovirus infection
   D. Older age
   E. Obesity

8. The incidence of end-stage renal disease is highest after which of the following non-renal organ transplants?
   A. Liver
   B. Heart
   C. Pancreas
   D. Lung

9. Which of the following is the most common cutaneous malignancy in transplant recipients?
   A. Melanoma
   B. Kaposi's sarcoma
   C. Squamous cell carcinoma
   D. Basal cell carcinoma

10. Post-transplant lymphoproliferative disease is most often associated with infection with which of the following viruses?
   A. Epstein–Barr virus
   B. Hepatitis C
   C. Parvovirus
   D. West Nile virus
   E. Hepatitis B virus

11. Which of the following classes of antihypertensive drugs are effective in treating post-transplant hypertension?
   A. β Blockers
   B. α Blockers
   C. Calcium channel blockers
   D. Angiotensin-converting enzyme inhibitors
   E. All of the above

12. Which of the following classes of antihypertensive drugs has been associated with the development of anemia?
   A. β Blockers
   B. α Blockers
   C. Calcium channel blockers
   D. Angiotensin-converting enzyme inhibitors
   E. All of the above

13. In diabetic transplant recipients, bone fractures most commonly occur in which part of the skeleton?
   A. Lumbar spine
   B. Feet
   C. Hands
   D. Hips

14. Which of the following immunosuppressants most commonly affects spermatogenesis?
   A. Sirolimus
   B. Tacrolimus
   C. Cyclosporine
   D. Azathioprine

15. Which of the following is associated with increased metabolism of cyclosporine?
   A. Ginseng
   B. St John's wort
   C. Garlic
   D. All of the above

16. Which of the following antihypertensive agents is associated with gingival hyperplasia?
   A. Irbesartan
   B. Nifedipine
   C. Metoprolol
   D. Diltiazem

17. Which of the following fetal/maternal complications are common in kidney transplant recipients compared to age matched controls?
   A. Higher incidence of pre-eclampsia
   B. Higher incidence of prematurity
   C. Lower birth weights
   D. All of the above

18. Which of the following is the most common psychiatric disorder in transplant recipients?
   A. Schizophrenia
   B. Borderline personality
   C. Depression
   D. Mania

19. All of the following drugs affect metabolism of calcineurin inhibitors, EXCEPT:
   A. Diazepam
   B. Phenytoin
   C. Verapamil
   D. Erythromycin
   E. Ketoconazole

20. Which of the following immunosuppressants is most commonly associated with hyperlipidemia?
   A. Tacrolimus
   B. Azathioprine
   C. Sirolimus
   D. Mycophenolate mofetil

Chapter 6

1. Which of the following is the most common cause of end-stage renal disease in children?
   A. Diabetes mellitus
   B. Congenital renal/urologic anomalies
   C. Hypertension
   D. Glomerulonephritis

2. True or false. The incidence of post-transplant lymphoproliferative disease is greater in children than in adults
   A. True
   B. False

3. Compared with adults, the annual mortality rate for children maintained on chronic dialysis is:
   A. Higher
   B. Similar
   C. Lower

4. Of the following, which is the most common disorder leading to liver transplantation in children?
   A. Wilson's disease
   B. Alcoholic cirrhosis
   C. Biliary atresia
   D. Autoimmune hepatitis

5. Which of the following can be indications for native nephrectomy as an adjunct to kidney transplantation?
   A. Renal concentrating defects with polyuria
   B. Heavy proteinuria
   C. Severe hypertension
   D. All of the above

6. After kidney transplantation, graft survival rates are lowest in:
   A. Infants
   B. Children aged 6–10 years
   C. Adolescents

7. In children, the highest rates of acute rejection have been reported in recipients of which of the following organs?
   A. Liver
   B. Intestine
   C. Kidney
   D. Pancreas

8. Side effects of corticosteroids include all of the following, EXCEPT:
   A. Gingival hyperplasia
   B. Weight gain
   C. Acne
   D. Growth retardation

9. Since the institution of PELD and MELD scores used for allocating liver allografts, the number of children wait-listed for liver transplantation has:
   A. Decreased
   B. Remained unchanged
   C. Increased

10. The most common indication for lung transplantation in adolescents is:
   A. Surfactant deficiency
   B. Chronic obstructive pulmonary disease
   C. Cystic fibrosis
   D. Idiopathic pulmonary fibrosis
   E. Pulmonary hypertension

11. Adult-to-child kidney transplantation can be performed in infants weighing as little as:
   A. 2 kg
   B. 4 kg
   C. 6 kg

12. The minimum allowable age for live kidney donors is:
   A. 14 years
   B. 16 years
   C. 18 years
   D. 21 years

13. Compared with adults, conversion rates among potential pediatric organ donors tend to be:
   A. About the same
   B. Higher
   C. Lower

14. In a randomized trial of pediatric kidney transplant recipients, the major benefit of using OKT3 for induction therapy was:
   A. Increased patient survival
   B. Increased graft survival
   C. Delayed onset of acute rejection
   D. Decreased severity of acute rejection episodes

15. The most common cause of death after pediatric liver transplantation is:
   A. Malignancy
   B. Infection
   C. Cardiovascular disease

16. The most common cause of graft failure beyond the first post-transplant year in pediatric lung transplantation is:
- **A.** Bronchiolitis obliterans
- **B.** Pneumonia
- **C.** Recurrent disease
- **D.** Acute rejection

17. Which of the following viral infections increases the risk of Epstein–Barr virus-mediated post-transplant lymphoproliferative disease?
- **A.** Hepatitis C virus
- **B.** Parvovirus
- **C.** Cytomegalovirus
- **D.** HIV

Chapter 7

1. All of the following are characteristic of recipients of kidney transplants from non-heart-beating deceased donors (DCDs), EXCEPT:
- **A.** Delayed graft function rate is higher than in standard criteria donor recipients
- **B.** 1-year graft survival is comparable to standard criteria donor recipients
- **C.** 1-year graft survival is inferior to expanded criteria donor recipients

2. Most pancreas transplantations are performed as:
- **A.** Pancreas after kidney transplantation
- **B.** Simultaneous pancreas and kidney transplantation
- **C.** Pancreas transplantation alone

3. Which of the following is an absolute contraindication to kidney transplantation?
- **A.** Human immunodeficiency virus infection
- **B.** History of renal cell cancer requiring nephrectomy 10 years earlier
- **C.** Ongoing chemotherapy for metastatic breast cancer
- **D.** Recent coronary artery stent placement

4. How much higher are rates of graft loss expected to be in recipients of expanded criteria donors compared with standard criteria donors?
- **A.** 70%
- **B.** 50%
- **C.** 30%
- **D.** 10%

5. The incidence of post-transplant lymphoproliferative disease in adult kidney transplant recipients is:
- **A.** >20%
- **B.** 15%
- **C.** 10%
- **D.** <5%

6. Compared with cyclosporine, tacrolimus is associated with a higher incidence of:
- **A.** Hyperlipidemia
- **B.** Hypertension
- **C.** Diabetes mellitus
- **D.** All of the above

7. Which of the following antibodies is approved by the Food and Drug Administration for use as induction therapy to prevent acute rejection after kidney transplantation?
- **A.** Basiliximab
- **B.** Alemtuzumab
- **C.** Rabbit anti-thymocyte globulin
- **D.** All of the above

8. Which of the following immunosuppressants is associated with the highest incidence of lymphocele?
- **A.** Cyclosporine
- **B.** Tacrolimus
- **C.** Sirolimus
- **D.** Mycophenolate mofetil

9. Which of the following is the histologic hallmark of antibody-mediated renal allograft rejection?
- **A.** C4d deposition in glomeruli
- **B.** IgG deposition in arterioles
- **C.** C4d deposition in peritubular capillaries
- **D.** IgA depositions in glomeruli

10. Which of the following drugs interacts adversely with azathioprine?
   A. St John's wort
   B. Diltiazem
   C. Erythromycin
   D. Allopurinol

11. Which of the following diseases recurs least commonly after kidney transplantation?
   A. Primary oxalosis
   B. Lupus nephritis
   C. Focal and segmental glomerulosclerosis
   D. Membranoproliferative glomerulonephritis

12. Which of the following pathologic lesions results as a consequence of anti-donor antibodies?
   A. Transplant glomerulopathy
   B. Hyperacute rejection
   C. Antibody-mediated acute rejection
   D. All of the above

13. The drug most commonly used to treat steroid-resistant acute cellular rejection is:
   A. Basiliximab
   B. Rabbit anti-thymocyte globulin
   C. Dalizumab
   D. Rituximab

14. The National Organ Transplant Act of 1984 prohibited which of the following activities in the field of transplantation?
   A. Sale of organs
   B. Use of living unrelated donors
   C. Use of donors after cardiac death
   D. All of the above

15. Compared with dialysis, a survival advantage of kidney transplantation is characteristic of which of the following patient groups?
   A. Patients with diabetes aged 20–39 years
   B. Patients without diabetes aged 40–59
   C. Patients with diabetes aged 40–59
   D. All of the above

16. Which of the following conditions would preclude living kidney donation?
   A. Only one of six HLA antigen matches
   B. Creatinine clearance of 90 mL/min
   C. 24-hour urine total protein excretion of 450 mg
   D. Recent basal cell carcinoma

17. All of the following are risk factors for new onset diabetes mellitus after kidney transplantation, EXCEPT:
   A. Smoking
   B. Hepatitis C infection
   C. African–American ethnicity
   D. Older age

18. Which of the following are causes of sensitization to HLA antigens?
   A. Previous pregnancies
   B. Previous organ transplantation
   C. Blood transfusions
   D. All of the above

19. Which of the following characteristics is NOT a component of the current definition of an expanded criteria donor?
   A. History of hypertension
   B. History of diabetes mellitus
   C. Cerebrovascular accident as the cause of death
   D. Age >60 years

20. Which of the following abnormalities are independently associated with a risk for cardiovascular disease after kidney transplantation?
   A. Proteinuria
   B. Low glomerular filtration rate
   C. Hypertension
   D. All of the above

21. True or false? For laparoscopic donor nephrectomies, the right kidney is harvested more often than the left kidney.

22. The actions of sirolimus are initiated by binding to which of the following intracellular molecules?
A. Calcineurin
B. Target of rapamycin (TOR)
C. FK-binding protein (FKBP)

23. Calcineurin is best described as a:
A. Phosphatase
B. Kinase
C. Dehydrogenase

24. Everolimus belongs to which of the following classes of immunosuppressants?
A. Calcineurin inhibitor
B. TOR inhibitor
C. Lymphocyte-depleting antibody
D. Non-lymphocyte-depleting antibody

25. Which of the following is the most common cause of pancreas allograft failure in the first week after transplantation?
A. Acute rejection
B. Infection
C. Thrombosis
D. Recurrent autoimmune disease

26. All of the following immunosuppressants cause bone marrow suppression, EXCEPT:
A. Prednisone
B. Sirolimus
C. Mycophenolate mofetil
D. Azathioprine

Chapter 8

1. The most common reason for referral for heart transplantation is:
A. Life-threatening arrhythmias
B. Hypertrophic cardiomyopathy
C. Left ventricular systolic dysfunction
D. Angina pectoris refractory to medical therapy

2. Contraindications to heart donation include all of the following, EXCEPT:
A. Prolonged cardiac arrest with multiple intracardiac injections
B. Cardiopulmonary resuscitation (CPR) before declaration of brain death
C. Penetrating cardiac trauma
D. Known coronary artery disease

3. Which of the following characteristics identify an ideal heart donor?
A. Age <30 years
B. No history of substance abuse
C. Ischemia times <2 h
D. Absence of infection
E. All of the above

4. The most common surgical technique used for implantation of a cardiac allograft is:
A. Heterotopic implantation
B. Total excision of recipient atria with pulmonary vein implantation
C. Bicaval technique
D. Biatrial technique

5. Which of the following arrhythmias is most common in the early postoperative period after heart transplantation?
A. Bradycardia
B. Atrial fibrillation
C. Atrial flutter
D. Ventricular fibrillation

6. Which of the following drugs is most useful in treating pulmonary hypertension early after heart transplantation?
A. Nitric oxide
B. Digoxin
C. Milrinone
D. Vasopressin

7. Denervation of the donor heart results in all of the following phenomena, EXCEPT:
   A. Decreased utility of digoxin for rate control in patients with atrial fibrillation
   B. Decreased efficacy of atropine in controlling bradycardia
   C. Decreased sensitivity to adenosine
   D. Absence of typical angina pectoris as a symptom of ischemia

8. Predictors of successful steroid withdrawal after heart transplantation include all of the following, EXCEPT:
   A. Absence of previous acute rejection
   B. Older age
   C. Female gender
   D. Higher degrees of HLA matching

9. The most accurate test for diagnosing acute rejection in heart transplant recipients is:
   A. Magnetic resonance imaging
   B. Endomyocardial biopsy
   C. Echocardiography
   D. Radionuclide imaging

10. True or false. Antibody-mediated rejection after heart transplantation is more common in patients who required the use of ventricular assist devices (VADs).
   A. True
   B. False

11. Which of the following echocardiographic findings are characteristic early signs of acute cardiac allograft rejection?
   A. Increased end-diastolic pressure
   B. Mitral valve regurgitation
   C. Rapid diastolic filling
   D. All of the above

12. All of the following are true of acute cardiac allograft rejection associated with hemodynamic compromise, EXCEPT:
   A. It occurs in <10% of cases
   B. It is more common in patients with diabetes mellitus
   C. It is more common in males

13. Which of the following characteristics distinguish cardiac allograft vasculopathy from atherosclerotic coronary artery disease?
   A. Angiographically determined narrowings tend to be distal and diffuse, rather than proximal and focal
   B. Cholesterol is intracellular, not extracellular
   C. Calcification is less common
   D. It develops more quickly
   E. All of the above

14. Donor factors associated with the development of cardiac allograft vasculopathy include all of the following EXCEPT:
   A. Female gender
   B. Obesity
   C. Older age
   D. Hypertension

15. Which of the following recipient factors is associated with an increased risk for development of cardiac allograft vasculopathy?
   A. Female gender
   B. African–American ethnicity
   C. Younger age

16. Which of the following are contraindications to heart re-transplantation?
   A. Graft failure within 2 weeks of transplantation
   B. Age >55 years
   C. Non-compliance
   D. All of the above

17. All of the following are true of heart transplantation in the past decade, EXCEPT:
   A. Patient survival has gradually improved
   B. The number of transplantations has increased
   C. Most recipients are male

Chapter 9

1. The most common indication for lung transplantation in children is:
   A. Chronic obstructive lung disease
   B. Cystic fibrosis
   C. α_1-Antitrypsin deficiency
   D. Idiopathic pulmonary fibrosis

2. Bilateral (as apposed to single) lung transplantation is preferred in patients with which of the following types of lung disease?
   A. Suppurative
   B. Obstructive
   C. Interstitial

3. Which of the following pathogens represents the LEAST likely contraindication for lung transplantation in a patient with cystic fibrosis?
   A. *Pseudomonas aeruginosa*
   B. *Burkholderia cepacia*
   C. *Aspergillus fumigatus*

4. Efforts to expand the pool of donor lungs available for lung transplantation have included:
   A. Use of donors after cardiac death
   B. Expansion of traditional criteria for acceptability of brain dead donors
   C. Living lobar transplantation
   D. All of the above

5. Which of the following statements correctly characterizes the new UNOS lung allocation system?
   A. It applies only to patients aged >12 years
   B. Size matching no longer plays a role
   C. Time on the waiting list is no longer a consideration
   D. The new system eliminates the need for ABO blood group compatibility

6. Which form of "matching" is essential for successful lung transplantation?
   A. HLA match
   B. ABO blood group compatibility
   C. Gender match
   D. Matching of CMV antibody status

7. Which of the following factors influences mortality in lung transplant recipients with primary graft dysfunction?
   A. Age
   B. Graft ischemic time
   C. Impaired gas exchange
   D. All of the above

8. The 2007 report of the International Society for Heart and Lung Transplantation indicated which of the following regarding immunosuppression for lung transplantation?
   A. Increasing use of cyclosporine as the calcineurin inhibitor of choice
   B. Increasing use of azathioprine as the purine inhibitor of choice
   C. A trend toward better graft survival with use of induction antibodies
   D. Lower rates of acute rejection with inhaled cyclosporine

9. Which of the following statement regarding histologic grade A1 acute rejection of a lung allograft is INCORRECT?
   A. It is most often detected by surveillance transbronchial lung biopsy
   B. Its discovery mandates an increase in immunosuppression
   C. It may be a risk factor for bronchiolitis obliterans
   D. It is rarely accompanied by symptoms or changes in lung function

10. Detection and grading for bronchiolitis obliterans is most often accomplished by noting changes in:
   A. FEV_1
   B. Oxygen saturation
   C. Bronchoalveolar lavage
   D. Chest radiograph

11. Risk factors for bronchiolitis obliterans include which of the following?
   A. Gastroesophageal reflux
   B. HLA mismatches
   C. Prior episode(s) of acute rejection
   D. Cytomegalovirus infection
   E. All of the above

12. Five-year graft survival rate after lung transplantation in adults is approximately:
   A. 20%
   B. 35%
   C. 50%
   D. 80%

13. Five-year graft survival rate after detection of bronchiolitis obliterans is approximately:
   A. 10–20%
   B. 30–40%
   C. 50–60%
   D. 70–80%

14. Which of the following diseases can recur after lung transplantation?
   A. Sarcoidosis
   B. Cystic fibrosis
   C. Pulmonary fibrosis

Chapter 10

1. Which of the following changes occurred after the implementation of the MELD system of organ allocation for liver transplantation?
   A. Increased national median waiting time.
   B. Reduction of wait-list mortality
   C. Increased allocation of organs to less ill patients.
   D. Identification of a threshold for patients too ill to transplant

2. Which of the following would be an absolute contraindication to liver transplantation?
   A. Coronary heart disease status post-coronary artery bypass grafting.
   B. Documented hepatocellular cancer with three lesions, the largest lesion being 2.9 cm.
   C. Human immunodeficiency virus infection
   D. Mechanical ventilation in a patient with ongoing requirement for blood pressure support in the setting of infection

3. With regard to living donor liver transplantation, which of the following statements is true?
   A. 1- and 3-year patient survivals are equivalent to cadaveric liver transplantation
   B. 1- and 3-year graft survivals are improved when compared with cadaveric liver transplantation
   C. The percentage of living donor liver transplants/total liver transplantations in the USA continues to increase

4. Which of the following factors is used to calculate the Child–Pugh score?
   A. Uncontrolled variceal bleeding
   B. Nutritional status
   C. Encephalopathy
   D. Renal Insufficiency

5. In the adult-to-adult living donor liver transplant registry, which of the following is the most common indication for rejection of a donor?
   A. Anatomic anomalies of the donor organ
   B. Donor declines to donate
   C. Associated medical conditions of the donor
   D. Psychologic or social issues of the donor

6. Which of the following is the most common technical complication after liver transplantation?
   A. Portal vein thrombosis
   B. Hepatic arterial stenosis
   C. Bile duct leak or stricture
   D. Inferior vena caval stenosis

7. Which of the following donor/recipient ratios results in the best outcomes for living donor liver transplant?
   A. Donor remnant size of at least 20%
   B. Graft to recipient body weight ratio of ≥70%
   C. Graft weight as a percentage of standard liver mass >40%

8. Which of the following liver grafts would be expected to function least well?
   A. A 40-year-old graft with 50% macrosteatosis
   B. A 40-year-old graft with 100% microsteatosis
   C. A 70-year-old graft with no steatosis

9. Which of the following statements about split-liver adult liver transplantation is true?
   A. Biliary complications are lower compared with whole organ transplantation
   B. Graft survivals are higher compared with whole organ transplantation
   C. Outflow obstruction is higher compared with whole organ transplantation
   D. Hepatic arterial thrombosis is lower compared with whole organ transplantation

10. Which of the following most closely reflects the increased risk of graft loss when using a deceased donor liver graft compared with a standard graft?
   A. 85%
   B. 50%
   C. 35%

11. Routine consideration of performing a choledochojejunostomy compared with a duct-to-duct biliary anastomosis include all of the following except:
   A. History of prior cholecystectomy
   B. History of primary sclerosing cholangitis
   C. Re-transplantation
   D. Living donor liver transplantation

12. A 35-year-old patient undergoes liver transplantation for autoimmune hepatitis. Six months after transplantation, the patient presents with acute abdominal pain. ALT is elevated to 109/L (baseline 36), alkaline phosphatase is elevated to 173/L (baseline 85) and bilirubin is elevated to 2.2 mg/dL (baseline 0.9). A CT of the abdomen shows a solitary area of lucency in the right lobe. Which of the following is the next best study to investigate this finding?
   A. ERCP
   B. Doppler ultrasonography
   C. Percutaneous aspiration of the lesion
   D. MRI

13. Which of the following drugs may be associated with cholestatic hepatitis and fibrosis?
   A. Cyclosporine
   B. Azathioprine
   C. Mycophenylate
   D. Tacrolimus
   E. Prednisone

14. Which of the following features is most commonly seen in liver grafts with acute cellular rejection?
   A. Endothelial cell damage
   B. Perivenular fibrosis
   C. Central zone cholestasis and ballooning
   D. Steatosis
   E. Acidophilic bodies

15. Risk factors for chronic rejection in a liver recipient include all of the following except:
   A. White recipients
   B. Younger recipient age
   C. Recipient diagnosis of immune liver disorder
   D. Previous episodes of acute cellular rejection

16. Which of the following is true with regard to liver transplantation in patients with hepatitis C?
   A. 3-year patient survival is equivalent to recipients without hepatitis C
   B. 3-year graft survival is lower compared with recipients without hepatitis C
   C. Graft survivals in patients with hepatitis C have improved over time
   D. 20% of patients undergoing liver transplantation for hepatitis C with have negative viral levels after liver transplantation

17. Which of the following patients would be considered to fall outside the Milan criteria for hepatocellular cancer?
   A. A 50-year-old man with four lesions, 2.7 cm, 1 cm, 1 cm and 1.5 cm
   B. A 70-year-old man with a solitary lesion 4.7 cm in the right lobe
   C. A 50-year-old woman with two lesions, 3 cm and 2 cm
   D. A 50-year-old woman with three lesions, 2.9 cm, 2.2 cm and 1.7 cm involving both left and right lobes
   E. A 70-year-old man with a 7.2 cm lesion now measuring 4.3 cm after chemoembolization

18. Which of the following has been associated with hepatitis C after liver transplantation?
   A. Increased risk of hypertension
   B. Increased risk of diabetes
   C. Increased risk of hyperlipidemia
   D. Increased risk of skin malignancy

19. Which of the following best estimates the risk of renal failure 5 years after liver transplantation?
   A. 5%
   B. 20%
   C. 40%

20. Risk factors for the development of post-transplant diabetes in liver recipients includes all of the following except:
   A. Hepatitis C
   B. Hepatitis B
   C. Steroid-resistant rejection
   D. Obesity

21. Risk factors for obesity after liver transplantation include which of the following?
   A. Increased donor BMI
   B. Married status
   C. Higher cumulative doses of prednisone
   D. All of the above

22. A 20-year-old patient undergoes liver transplantation for autoimmune hepatitis. The patient has not been previously immunized for any childhood illnesses. Which of the following immunizations would be contraindicated in this patient?
   A. Hepatitis B
   B. Hepatitis A
   C. MMR (measles, mumps, rubella)
   D. H1N1 immunization
   E. Polio

Answers to multiple choice questions

Chapter 1

1. C
2. D
3. A
4. D
5. D
6. A
7. B
8. B
9. A
10. D
11. C
12. E
13. C
14. D

Chapter 2

1. C
2. A
3. D
4. B
5. B
6. D
7. C
8. A
9. C
10. B
11. D

Chapter 3

1. C
2. B
3. A
4. C
5. D
6. C
7. C
8. A
9. D
10. C
11. C
12. A
13. D

Chapter 4

1. A
2. D
3. B
4. B
5. C
6. A
7. C
8. B
9. B
10. C
11. A
12. C
13. B
14. B
15. F

Chapter 5

1. B
2. A
3. E
4. B
5. C
6. D
7. C
8. A
9. C
10. A
11. E
12. E
13. B
14. A
15. B
16. B
17. D
18. C

Primer on Transplantation, 3rd edition.
Edited by Donald Hricik.

19. A
20. C

Chapter 6

1. B
2. A
3. C
4. C
5. D
6. C
7. B
8. A
9. A
10. C
11. C
12. C
13. B
14. C
15. B
16. A
17. C

Chapter 7

1. C
2. B
3. C
4. A
5. D
6. C
7. A
8. C
9. C
10. D
11. B
12. D
13. B
14. A
15. D
16. C
17. A
18. D
19. B
20. D
21. False
22. C
23. A
24. B
25. C
26. A

Chapter 8

1. C
2. B
3. E
4. C
5. A
6. A
7. C
8. C
9. B
10. A
11. A
12. C
13. E
14. A
15. B
16. D
17. B

Chapter 9

1. B
2. A
3. C
4. D
5. A
6. B
7. D
8. C
9. B
10. A
11. E
12. C
13. B
14. A

Chapter 10

1. B
2. D
3. B
4. C
5. C
6. C
7. C
8. A
9. C
10. A
11. A
12. B
13. B

14. A
15. A
16. B
17. A
18. B
19. B
20. B
21. D
22. C

Index

Primer on Transplantation, 3rd edition.
Edited by Donald Hricik.